Heaven and Earth

Heaven and Earth

Arturo Riojas

To order additional copies of this book, contact:
Xlibris
1-888-795-4274
www.Xlibris.com
Orders@Xlibris.com
744940

Contents

About the Book

From the heavens they came to our Mother Earth; through a different dimension, they moved freely to examine the fruits of the seeds they had planted several millennia ago. Their race was characterized by a highly developed intellect, evolving only after the conquest of the poisoned environment of their world and the maladies that had nearly driven their race to extinction. They traveled the galaxy on a search. This tale of intrigue involves national secrets that NASA, DHS, the Air Force, the CDC, and the FDA cannot disclose. From a web of misinformation and concealment that spans the nation from coast to coast, the truth must be extracted and revealed. Why are we being "protected" from the truth—the existence of a race of alien beings and the known environmental causes of problems ailing our society—and what is the price we pay for this protection?

The story unfolds drawing parallels between their world and our own—conspiracies to exploit the masses, events and conditions that are not as they appear, the universal need to know, the conflict between self-interests and the universal good, and the ultimate triumph of valor over fear.

This is a story involving different kinds of races. For the space travelers, it is a race against time and a message traversing the vast emptiness of space at the speed of light. For Earthlings, it is a race to reverse an environmental tailspin leaving death in its wake. A tale of mass deceit and denial, conquest without overt violence, insidious enemies, and turbulent battles fought within, *Heaven and Earth* explores the very sources of pain and suffering and offers a surprise ending to free two races from oppression and exploitation. But the battles . . . are just beginning.

About the Author

Arturo Riojas holds four engineering degrees (two chemical engineering and two civil engineering with specialization in environmental engineering) and is a licensed professional engineer in the State of Texas. Dr. Riojas has over thirty-five years of professional experience in industrial, consulting, and academic settings. It is his concern regarding the carcinogenic heavy metal, cadmium, in our water and food supplies and his interest in science fiction that have prompted him to write this book.

Dr. Riojas possesses hands-on experience gained in the petroleum refining and chemical industries and experience with the environmental regulatory processes associated with CERCLA and RCRA. His industrial experience includes water and wastewater engineering, soil and groundwater remediation/restoration, process engineering and optimization, preparation and review of remediation- and water-related assessments and work plans, and review of solid waste handling and landfill design projects. He has extensive experience working at U.S. military facilities and has worked on water/wastewater-related projects in Venezuela, Honduras, Mexico, Central Europe, and the Republic of Korea.

Dr. Riojas has also taught graduate- and undergraduate-level classes at The University of Texas at San Antonio.

To comfort and reassure my mother that she would survive her illness, my then wife told her that when we returned home, I would move *Heaven and Earth* to find the cure for her cancer.

This book is dedicated to my mother, Giovanna, and all the members of my family, those who are alive and those who have passed on after having endured the pain and suffering associated with what I am convinced should be our nation's foremost health concern— cadmium poisoning. It continues to go virtually unnoticed, and the problems that it causes fail to be properly diagnosed. The time has come to address the cause rather than treat the symptom.

If only I had known then what I know now . . . about cadmium.

Purpose

The purpose of this book is twofold. First and foremost, this book was written to disseminate information regarding a serious health issue that is plaguing our society. The issue is cadmium poisoning. Second, the book will hopefully be a stimulating and thought-provoking source of entertainment for the reader, touching on a wide variety of themes—some based on reality, others on conjecture, and still others on pure fantasy.

The storyline of the book, a science-fiction "aliens from another planet" theme, is laid out in chapters, with information related to cadmium appended at the end of each chapter. Readers who have no interest in the cadmium issue can skip over these "Cadmium Poisoning Facts" appendices, focus on the sci-fi plot of the book, and still benefit from new insights into the problem. Hopefully, most readers will find the appendices informative, gaining a new perspective on our common malady . . . one that has multiple, seemingly unrelated symptoms.

To all my readers—I wish you an entertaining journey on a cross-country adventure. Enjoy the read, and enjoy the ride!

Disclaimer

All characters and the story portrayed in this book are fictional. Any semblance of the characters to actual people is coincidental. Some locations, organizations, and facilities mentioned herein are real; others are not and were fabricated to enhance the plot. Documents, plans, and events described herein are either fabricated or based on accounts found on the Internet.

Many of the health issues addressed and suggestions for consideration contained in this book are based on studies and reports available on the Internet and personal experience. Nothing in this book is intended to diagnose, treat, cure, or prevent any disease, and individuals with health issues should seek the advice of a medical doctor. The author is not a medical doctor and accepts no legal liability or responsibility for individuals initiating self-treatment, with or without the advice and/or supervision of a medical doctor.

Neither the author nor the author's agent(s) makes any warranty, expressed or implied, or assumes any legal liability or responsibility for the accuracy, completeness, safety, or usefulness of any information, apparatus, product, or process disclosed or described. References herein to any specific commercial product, process, or service by trade name, trademark, manufacturer, or otherwise, does not necessarily constitute or imply its endorsement, recommendation, or favoring by the author or the author's agent(s). The views and opinions expressed herein do not necessarily state or reflect those of the author or his agent(s).

Prologue

Many thousands of years ago, visiting spacecraft came to our beloved Mother Earth, like an interstellar Johnny Appleseed—planting seeds everywhere they found life-forms that "showed promise." They found a planet fragmented by vast seas of separation and mountains that divided more than regions of continents. They encountered many diverse species that adapted themselves to their environment, but one appeared to be able to adapt to all environments it encountered. It was that species, with minor variations in appearance, that had spread across the face of the planet. One curious feature of the species was that many of the subgroups were unaware and oblivious to the existence of most of the others. Perhaps it was the distances between them that impeded communication. Perhaps it was their primitive technologies, coupled with the natural barriers of the planet's surface that isolated them so. Or perhaps it was that they too often fell victim to other species or members of their own species, fighting among themselves rather than uniting to conquer the elements of their environment. Their life expectancies were presently too short to expect very much, but with a few "seeds" they might prove themselves worthy of future interaction.

Chapter One

Earth Revisited

The spacecraft hovered weightlessly over Atlanta as the information continued to stream up from the surface, undetected by the primitive sensors of the naive subjects of their survey. "They keep looking in the wrong dimension." The beady-eyed young officer chortled as he gazed out from one of the expansive curved windows on the observation deck. This was the first of several stops scheduled to canvass progress made by the inhabitants of the planet. Egroeg, the son of a powerful lord of the ruling Drutsab Clan and Head Officer of Total Security and High Intelligence of Treretum, was on this milquetoast assignment because it was a means of keeping him out of trouble and harm's way while meeting his civil service duty. But Egroeg missed home, his beloved Treretum. He felt that he was too far from it, even though it was a mere 8.6 light-years from the site of their assignment. He resented the fact that he had to spend any time from his prime years with the Unenlightened on a trek that would likely prove fruitless due to the contaminated surroundings of the survey subjects.

I suppose that the heavy metal contaminants must be limiting their mental capacity, he thought to himself disdainfully. Having been programmed at a very early age, Egroeg was aware that he had been designated as one of the future leaders of Treretum, and he anxiously awaited his chance to race along the path on which his forefathers had been plodding for eons.

Back on the third planet from the center of their binary star system, Sirius, the Treretumians required every able-bodied male, female, and neutered drone to serve in the Drutsab Corps. This served the interests of the Drutsab Egral, an elite group that, over the millennia, had amassed the combined wealth of all their neighboring planets. Because their planet's orbit circumscribed two stars having different volumes and masses, the conditions on their planet could be severe, but the severity of the climate changed with each orbit of the stars around their center of mass. And because the Drutsab offered food, shelter, and social status to the members of the corps, Treretumians served, asking no questions about their assignments, simply performing their duty to what all were convinced was protecting their loved ones and the Treretumian way of life.

Egroeg gazed out of the expansive window, almost in a trance, mumbling stories from his childhood that Hsubdab and his grandfather, the one they called the *Ancient One*—a nickname used for most grandfathers on the planet, had told of planet Earth. It was Egroeg's father, Hsubdab, who after being part of the "Second Stage of Sharing" had authorized this third stage of sharing information with the subjects in this star system, thinking that the information would continue to stimulate and accelerate the development of the hearty Earthlings. He felt strongly that in spite of the fact that reconnaissance visits indicated that the primitive beings lived in a highly contaminated environment, this planet would be of great importance to Treretum in the future. At Hsubdab's insistence, plans for the third mission were launched, and the responsibility of commanding the lead ship befell upon his son, Egroeg. He offered convincing arguments before the ruling body of the Drutsab Egral, assuring that his son's mission would be different from his own which, more than anything, had served to demonstrate how technologically primitive the subjects were.

Egroeg remembered his father saying that although the advancements made by the time of his mission were evident at the initial survey, the tragic ending of that mission had left him with the desire to do more.

Perhaps it was that they had been given too much too soon in the relationship, as was rumored on Treretum, that had contributed to the tragic end of the second mission. Or perhaps it was the presence of a third party that enticed some of the indigenous inhabitants to partake of certain *gifts* that had been placed on the planet prematurely, forbidden from introduction to the Earthlings due to their lack of maturity and the associated potential for mass destruction. But no one could have known . . . .

Egroeg also remembered many stories that the Ancient One, a member of the original Treretumian mission to Earth, had shared about their first encounters with Earth cave dwellers and the great promise that the indigenous inhabitants had shown. The Ancient One often recounted tales of the first mission: about how *the teachers* had trained Earthlings to construct bridges from the primitive raw materials available in their environment that would span vast gorges, how his Treretumian construction team had built a few large pyramids on Earth along with duplicates on the fourth planet of the star system to designate suitable landing sites for future missions, and how they showed their newfound friends where they came from by pointing at what had been the tri-star system of Sirius, explaining that the third tiny star had been extinguished many thousands of years ago and now constituted the nearest planet in the system, still mostly molten as it slowly cooled, forming a thin crust, and still seething with volcanic activity.

Again, thinking back upon the adventures described by his father during the second mission, Egroeg recalled his father saying that Treretumians encountered a great deal of interest in stories about the stars, confirmed by observatories in various parts of the planet. They also found that those same groups had mimicked their building of pyramids, and because of the apparent interest, they assisted with numerous additional construction projects. Stones were cut to fit so that a blade of grass could not grow in the gap, and some stones weighing more than twenty tons were transported long distances, and even to mountaintops.

But it was apparent that at that time, there was still a lack of fundamental understanding. He remembered stories about how the

Earthlings were given the formula for an early version of the tough, lightweight, heat-stable skin of the Treretumian's spacecraft, using elements found on the planet; but the recipients did well to record the formula, not knowing about the existence of things such as elements. He recalled accounts of how Earthlings were shown how to perform delicate brain surgery using utensils made of stone and copper. Copper was prescribed to maintain as sterile an environment as possible in a world where the surgeons had no concept of what problems unicellular beings on their planet could cause or, for that matter, that they even existed.

All these stories of previous missions seemed to stew in Egroeg's mind, and now, he was reluctantly in charge of the third mission.

"Egral Egroeg," uttered the tall corps officer as he tapped Egroeg on his narrow, sloping right shoulder. "What will be our destination once we have acquired the data from the primitive information storage units on the surface?"

Egroeg turned his head slowly as he emerged from his trancelike state. He spoke slowly in a low tone, "Sucram Suturb . . . uh . . . yes." Egroeg paused as he returned to the here and now.

Stark contrasts in the physical characteristics of the two Treretumians were evident.

Both had broad foreheads and narrow chins, with their eyes being the dominant feature of their faces. However, the broad-shouldered Suturb had eyes that were very large—twice the size of Egroeg's— almond-shaped, and slanted, while Egroeg's were round and beady. Both had a greenish tint to the skin of their faces, with Egroeg being very pale, compared to the darker skin of his subordinate. Their hands were similar in structure, but Egroeg's hands were smaller and more delicate. Each had hands of five digits—three at the end of the hand, and two farther back, below a flexible joint in the middle of the hand. Two fingers were paired on either side of the hand like the legs of a lizard, with the fifth digit pointing forward. The structure of their five-digit hands was part of their evolution. They were well suited for holding onto branches that could be broken off the parent plants and used as clubs that looked like natural extensions of the Treretumians' arms. The flexible joint between the front three fingers and the back two fingers gave their hands enormous lateral reach. A distinguishing characteristic of several of the clans on the planet was the scaly skin on the backside of their hands, their arms, and their backs, unlike the skin on their faces. Although Egroeg and members of the Drutsab Clan considered themselves more refined because of the smooth skin all over their bodies, the tougher skin of Suturb's clan, along with their size and strength, made members of his clan better suited for hard labor under the harsh Treretumian sun.

Egroeg continued, muttering slowly, "We will adjust the current latitude by 4 degrees to the south, and go up-rotation from our current setting by 10 degrees and 58 minutes to collect data from another set of data banks in a place called Houston. Some vague references from the current data being collected mentioned an alien spacecraft under quarantine." Egroeg paused and stared out the broad, gently curved window of the spacecraft as he raised his right hand in a pensive fashion with one of the three long, slender fingers at the end of his hand to his small mouth. "We shall see. First the data at hand, next Houston, and then perhaps we shall stop to view the activities at a place called Area 51, just 3 degrees and 20 seconds to the north and an additional 9 degrees and 11 minutes up-rotation from Houston. Walk with me."

The two seemed to float as they walked along the perimeter observation deck of their spacecraft, the *Regnellach*. This was one of the many dozens of spacecraft that were launched from their mother station of Treretum over the span of several years, each embarking on exploration of nearby solar systems within a fifty-light-year radius of the mother station. The coastline of the United States to the north was clearly in view.

The green of fresh growth of spring on the surface vegetation, contrasted against the Atlantic blue, was fading into the haze, and tiny specks of civilization's light were beginning to appear as the light of the Earth's sun began to dim. It all seemed to fade behind them as their walk turned the view out to the open sea.

"More than a bak'tun ago, my father told me of the seeds, but he did not tell me of the bizarre behavior," commented Egroeg. "Tell me, how many bak'tuns of data have we obtained in the current probe?"

Suturb replied, "Only about one fourth of one bak'tun—what the Earthlings would call a century. This society is relatively young among the many that have evolved on the planet."

"Since we are but in the middle of our mission," said Egroeg authoritatively, "you should have plenty of time to prepare a separate report dealing specifically with that—the characteristically bizarre behavior of their society."

Surprised to hear what appeared to be a new assignment, the young officer responded, "With what, Egral Egroeg? I am not sure what kind of a report you seek. Their behavior is indeed bizarre, but it is of little consequence. The mission was to—"

Egroeg raised his hand abruptly to stop Suturb in midsentence. "I am well aware of the objectives of this mission, Suturb," rebuffed Egroeg, indignantly. "Shall I remind you that your duty is to do as you are directed? Your assignment is to document the behavior of the masses. This may prove useful to future expeditions. If nothing else, I think that it should make interesting and entertaining reading for the heads of the corps back on Treretum . . . and for my father, Hsubdab."

"I beg your pardon, sir. It is just that Nivla and I were hoping to help investigate the disappearance of the Treretumian spacecraft more than half a century ago. Of course, you know, sir, that Nivla has a special interest in this topic because along with the lost spacecraft disappeared one of his brothers. Because we are both of the Kcalb Clan, I was hoping—"

"Enough!" shouted the physically diminutive commanding officer. "Your assignment stands. And for the remainder of this mission, you are confined to this spacecraft. I was not aware of Nivla's personal connection to this mission. Had I known, I would have disqualified him and his two drones during crew selection. I had some reservations . . ." Egroeg paused. "I should have followed my instincts. Well, it appears that your friend Nivla has earned himself a reprimand to go on his service record . . . and perhaps additional disciplinary actions."

Disturbed by his superior's comments, Suturb interjected, "Sir, I'll take the information to the Navigation Center so that they can prepare our course settings."

"Yes." Egroeg squinted converting his beady eyes into tiny brown slivers against his pale skin. He raised his right hand and squeezed Suturb's arm. "And when you finish, find Nivla and send him to my quarters."

Suturb tilted his head, looking directly at Egroeg's hand as he felt the grip tighten on his arm. "Yes, sir." Suturb was a whole head taller than Egroeg, and his first impulse was difficult to control, but he knew his place. The two disengaged. The message of disdain for the Kcalb Clan was clear. Suturb turned and began to gracefully float down the curved hallway.

They are magnificent but potentially very dangerous, Egroeg thought to himself. *If it weren't for their size and strength . . . . It is better to keep him close so that I can keep my fingers on the pulse of the Kcalb Clan members on board.*

"Stop!" Egroeg roared down the hallway. Suturb turned suddenly looking at Egroeg in alarm. Egroeg continued in a gentle voice, "Come back. We must first discuss your progress reports."

Suturb approached Egroeg, who slowly turned and began to move in the same direction as the tall corps officer was about to reach him.

"I'm sorry if I seemed a bit harsh, but I have much on my mind," Egroeg uttered in a low tone as he reached around Suturb's back to pat him on the far shoulder with one hand and gently took hold of his forearm with the other. Suturb's head jerked first to the right to inspect where he felt Egroeg's hand patting him and then to his left to see Egroeg's hand on his arm. They continued up the hallway slowly. "I understand your first name is Sucram. May I call you Sucram?"

The Kcalb Clansman responded, "Yes, sir, of course."

The Atlantic waters appeared cold and dark in the expansive window of the observation deck. Egroeg continued, "With the completion of your reports and the end of this mission, if all goes well, you can expect a promotion in the corps—a major advancement in your career. A strong Kcalb like you has a bright future ahead of you when we return to Treretum . . . when you know the right individuals in the Drutsab. Who knows, you could have a pair of drones assigned to you . . . like your fellow Kcalb Clansman, Nivla."

"Yes, sir," said Suturb as the two reached an ascension portal. Suturb raised his right hand and a bony finger emerged from the loose sleeve of the robelike uniform he wore to touch the door panel. After about two seconds, the panel seemed to evaporate, Suturb entered, and the two Treretumians parted company.

ᘔᘔᘔᘔᘔᘔᘔᘔᘔᘔᘔᘔᘔᘔᘔᘔᘔᘔᘔᘔᘔᘔᘔᘔᘔᘔᘔᘔᘔᘔ

Egroeg returned to his quarters to rest, but again he began to think about all the tales he had heard about Earth, its inhabitants, and the *gifts* that Treretum had provided previously. These were the seeds they had planted thousands of years ago on this place that their survey subjects called Earth, a relatively tame environment in comparison to the environments of Treretum or of the neighboring planets. An atmosphere that contained primarily one condensable, water, was much more amenable to habitation that one of sulfuric acid or an atmosphere so rarefied that it cannot support life on the surface.

Egroeg knew their task at the Center for Disease Control and Prevention (CDC) was nearing completion, but there was still much to be done before returning home. It was time to check the pulse of the natives at every location where Treretum had assisted with pyramids, observatories, medical procedures, agricultural advances, and more. It was time to assess the environment and the progress that had been made over the millennia in achieving control over it. It was late, and Egroeg was tired. It was time.

CADMIUM POISONING

FACTS

- The cadmium story in this country began around the end of World War II, with the widespread use of phosphate and other commercial fertilizers. Cadmium (chemical symbol Cd) is a carcinogenic heavy metal and a contaminant in phosphate fertilizers that are spread on the fields where crops that we eat are grown—it is in the food chain.

- Cadmium is a sister element of zinc (chemical symbol Zn), an essential nutrient for humans. The chemical properties are similar since the two metals are of the same family in the periodic table (cadmium is found directly beneath zinc and above mercury [chemical symbol Hg]).

- In humans and mammals, in general, Cd bioaccumulates primarily in *the pancreas, the kidneys, the liver, the lungs, and the bones*; however, it is also known to be able to pass through and sometimes accumulate in the *skin* and accumulate to a lesser degree in the *prostate*, the *thyroid*, and elsewhere, causing problems everywhere it accumulates.

- Cadmium is not directly involved in any of the biochemical reactions in the life process, although trace amounts in the tissues tend to stimulate growth. Cadmium is a *carcinogen* and is one of three naturally occurring heavy metals that are not used in the human body. The other two are lead and mercury.

- The great increase in mining of cadmium-laden phosphate deposits for use as fertilizers since around World War II has resulted in the widespread distribution of Cd in the environment and its introduction into the food chain. Phosphorous, contained in phosphates, is an essential ingredient in many fertilizers (the P in NPK fertilizers [nitrogen and potassium are the N and K, respectively]).

- Cadmium is in the *food we eat*. Cadmium accumulates in the center of grains such as wheat and rice, while zinc concentrates on the outside husks. Thus, when we polish grain and remove everything that is not pure and white, we remove the element that is essential for our existence and consume the poison that remains in our bodies with an average biological half-life of thirty years or more.

- Cadmium is present in *water we drink*. Old plumbing systems contain galvanized steel pipe. The zinc coating contains Cd that leaches out of the coating and into the water that flows through the pipe. New plumbing systems contain polyvinyl chloride (PVC) piping that also contains Cd, added as a plasticizer and stabilizer, to improve PVC's durability.

- Cadmium is in the *air we breathe*. Cigarettes and other tobacco products are sources of cadmium for the smoker and the unsuspecting individuals breathing secondhand smoke. Phosphate fertilizers are used on the fields where tobacco is grown, and the cadmium is taken up into the leaves that are harvested to make tobacco products.

Chapter Two

Cause and Effect

"Good night, Mr. Hutchinson," she said as she walked briskly from the elevator doors.

"Another late one!" The custodian knew that this was not an unusual occurrence. "Olga, when are you going to get serious about one of those beaus and start leaving this place at a decent hour? Sometimes I worry about you, sweetie. You need to get a life."

"I love you too, Pops," she responded affectionately as she raised her left hand in a less-than-enthusiastic wave while walking across the lobby to the door leading to the garage. Her hair, pulled back in a ponytail, bounced from side to side as she walked out the door and into the garage. He was probably right, but right now, she had to concentrate on her research project; it was critical that she remain focused for the meeting in Houston, and

. . . "Who am I kidding," she mumbled as she reached the door of her old, but still dependable, boxy, white, '84 Volvo. "He's right."

The young woman was brilliant, having earned her doctorate from the Aeronautical Engineering Department at Stanford University at the ripe old age of twenty-five. She was now one of the principal researchers at NASA's Jet Propulsion Lab in Pasadena, California, focusing on some peculiar events detected in the general direction of Sirius, a neighboring star to our sun but still many light-years away.

She turned the key and smiled as her old reliable cranked itself to life with that characteristic Volvo-starter sound. "I promise, Viejito [Old One (affectionately)], I'll give you the tuneup you deserve after the trip. Hang in there." She again smiled and patted the dashboard gently as she approached the garage exit.

She pulled out of the garage, waved at the guard as she drove past the guard gate, and emerged onto a deceptively serene road with horses and a stable to her right. Although it was late, the silhouettes of the stable and a colt next to an attentive mare in the moonlight was soothing. She continued past the adjacent high school toward the interstate.

She reached the 210, looked to the left, and was nearly blinded by all the approaching headlights. *Dios mío [My God], doesn't this city ever sleep?* she thought to herself. After straightening Viejito out in his lane of traffic and taking a deep breath, she answered aloud, "No, I guess it doesn't."

She had hardly gone a mile or two when Tchaikovsky's "Love Theme" from *Romeo and Juliet* began flowing out of her purse. Except for an initial glance, Olga kept her eyes fixed on the road as she fumbled for her purse with one hand. When she finally got her purse open, she reached in, pulled out her dated cell phone, and flipped it open like a switchblade. "Hello." [Pause.] "Oh, hi, Eagle Man. You beat me to the punch. I was going to call you over the weekend . . . but—" Olga's speech stalled because of the interruption by the party on the other end of the conversation. She continued, "Sorry, but you know my flip phone doesn't slow me down, and besides, if it's good enough for Jerry Jones, it's good enough for me." [Pause.] "I know that it's coming up, and I'm looking forward to the Powwow, as always." Olga started to giggle like a giddy teen. "I said *Powwow*, not *bow wow*! What's wrong with you, you crazy Mexican?" Her giggle turned into a full-fledged laugh. It was Cuauhtémoc Gavilán.

൜൜൜൜൜൜൜൜൜൜൜൜൜൜൜൜൜൜൜൜൜൜൜൜൜൜൜൜൜

She had met Cuauhtémoc Gavilán at the Stanford Powwow during her junior year as an undergraduate. The activities that were open for public observation were compelling for Olga, but she wished she could communicate with the Native American participants in something other than English, the language used to betray their trust so many times in the past. She had tried before to speak Spanish with several individuals but was always disappointed.

They met at a demonstration of a fertility dance with a chieftain dancing in full headdress. The footwork was impressive. "¡Chihuahua, que talento!" [Gosh, what talent!] she heard someone say. She turned quickly and saw a man with Indian features gazing at the dancer, enthralled with the performance. He was only a few steps away. Olga inched her way sideways toward him through the crowd. "¿Es usted mexicano?" [Are you Mexican?]

He seemed startled at first, but when he saw Olga, his startled appearance melted away. "Pues, nacido en México pero educado aquí en los Estados Unidos. ¿Y usted?" [Well, born in Mexico but educated here in the United States. And you?]

There was instant chemistry between them, though he seemed a bit older and worldlier. The dance continued, but he was now finding it difficult to concentrate on the performance with this amazing distraction standing next to him.

"Nacida en San Antonio . . . sí, soy Tejana, y no me falta mucho para recibirme de aquí, Estanford," [Born in San Antonio . . . yes, I'm a Texan, and I'm about to graduate from here, Stanford] she said proudly. She had often caught herself thinking, *Am I an elitist academic snob?* She was convinced that she wasn't, but she just needed to be able to communicate with people, connect on the same level.

Undaunted, the Mexican shouts enthusiastically, "Way to go! My alma mater."

"No way!" she quipped.

"Yes way!" he quickly rebounded.

They looked at each other and slowly turned their heads to watch the dancer. His dance was winding down, and in a minute or so, the chieftain knelt on one knee, leaned forward, and lowered his head in a stance that resulted in his being almost completely covered by his colorful headdress and the many, long feathers attached to his spear. The crowd applauded enthusiastically.

The man turned to Olga and asked, "So what's your major?"

"Aeronautical engineering," she responded.

"¡Fantástico! [Fantastic!] A stargazer. My Mayan ancestors were stargazers. I'm a slightly more vintage product of the Earth Sciences program."

Wow, a knockout with brains! he thought to himself.

Wow, someone I can communicate with, she thought to herself.

"So what caused you to go into engineering?" he inquired.

"Caused? Right on!" she responded. "My curiosity caused me to study engineering. And the person you see before you—this engineer in the making—is the result . . . the effect. Cause and effect have been part of me as far back as I can remember. I remember when I was just four years old, with the moral support of my older brother, I took apart my mother's Baby Ben alarm clock to see what made it tick—literally. My curiosity made me investigate the cause of what I observed, the apparent effect." She moved her head from side to side and continued, "Tick, tock, tick, tock."

Cautiously, Gavilán uttered, "I have to ask—did you get the clock back together?"

Without hesitation, she responded, "And . . . I have to answer—that was my first lesson about approaching the unknown *with caution.* I guess the short answer is no. And what about you? Is there life after Snodfart?"

"That name is still around, I see." With a big grin on his face, Gavilán continued, "Yes, there is life after Stanford, but don't think that graduating means you've learned all you need to know. That degree just represents the basics and the training that you'll need to keep learning . . . to keep investigating."

"That's cool. I intend to be that way 'til the day I die," Olga said resolutely. This was completely consistent with her way of thinking. "There are too many things that we really don't understand, and you know me—cause and effect. I want to know what makes things tick, not just appreciate the fact that there is a tock and another tick coming right behind."

He was taken aback and more impressed with the young lady than he wanted to let on. "Oh, I'm sorry. My name is Cuauhtémoc." He began to extend his hand for a handshake.

In disbelief, Olga blurts out, "No way!"

He was a little startled, and he pulled his hand back. "Yes way. And if you're having trouble believing that, you probably won't believe that my last name is Gavilán either, but that's me. Cuauhtémoc Gavilán—good as gold, like the double eagle in my name."

"You're kidding, right?" she blurted out without thinking.

"No, really!" responded Gavilán with raised eyebrows and wrinkles on his forehead.

She took control of her disbelief and impulsive responses and said, "Well, I'm Olga Ramos." She extended her hand with great deliberation. "Nice to meet you."

"The pleasure is mine," he responded as he took her hand and felt a firm grip develop, followed by three gentle ups and downs. *Gorgeous creature!* he thought.

Olga looked at his face, focused on his eyes, and thought, *Interesting man.*

◧◪◧◪◧◪◧◪◧◪◧◪◧◪◧◪◧◪◧◪◧◪◧◪◧◪◧◪◧◪◧◪

"Are we on for this year's Powwow?" Gavilán asked with anticipation.

"I wouldn't miss it for the world. You know that!" replied Olga. "But this year, I have a conference that I have to attend in Houston the week before the Powwow."

"Ah! I have it! And here is my indecent proposal," he said jokingly with a touch of a giggle in his tone. "I'll meet you in Houston, and we'll take a relaxing drive to the Powwow. That'll give us a chance to catch up."

"Sounds like a deal," responded Olga. "I'll give you more details tomorrow. I don't have the conference agenda in front of me."

"So what's the conference about?" inquired Gavilán.

"Well, it's almost like a command performance. The Department of Defense has requested some hotshot scientists and engineers to attend in the name of national security," answered Olga. She continued, "The DoD's agenda includes a session on my computer-enhanced, high-resolution digital photography. I guess my report on the sightings must have raised some eyebrows at the Pentagon. You know old 'cause and effect' me. I am not satisfied in observing the effect. I need to know what caused it."

In his complementary fashion, Gavilán responded, "It's always so refreshing to talk with you. Unlike my doctor who wants to give me a shot or a pill to treat my every symptoms each time I go to see him, you want to get down to the bottom of things. I guess *he* figures he doesn't see me often enough . . . I don't know. Anyway, while he is happy to treat the symptom rather than the cause, you see the symptom as the effect resulting from something more fundamental, the root cause of the problem. I really like that in you. And now the DoD needs your help. I'm impressed, as usual."

"Oh please!" exclaimed Olga. "You're going to make my newfound fame go to my head. I'm just doing my job. I'm not one of the movers and shakers."

Olga's modesty wasn't too convincing. They both knew the importance of Olga's sightings. Gavilán's tone suddenly turned very firm as he said, "Tú ya sabes que en esta vida, cada quien puede ser causa o effecto. Nosotros escojemos entre los dos. Te conozco, y ya se acual escojiste tú. Yo también, ya escojí, y en ese respeto somos iguales, como te lo he dicho muchas vezes. Y también te he dicho que por mi parte . . . [*he paused with great deliberation*] pues, tú eres mi inspiración." ["You know that in this life, every individual can be a cause or an effect. We choose between the two. I know you, and I know which you chose. I too have chosen, and in that regard we are the same, as I have told you many times. And I have also told you that as for me . . . well, you are my inspiration."]

CADMIUM POISONING

FACTS

- The distribution of cadmium in our environment is widespread and has become more so as a result of man's mining, refining, and extensive use of materials with which Cd is closely related (e.g., phosphates, zinc, copper) and minerals in which it is found in nature. For example, Cd and Zn are typically in the same mineral deposits, and normal refining of zinc leaves small quantities of Cd in the zinc. The exhaust gases from zinc smelters are rich in cadmium. Similarly, phosphate deposits that are mined are laden with cadmium, and wastewater from the processing of phosphates in the manufacture of phosphate fertilizers are typically rich in cadmium.

- The cadmium concentration of the skeleton of a modern human is approximately fifty times that of the skeletal remains of Plains Indians of centuries past. In other words, our current cadmium exposure and assimilation rates are tremendously higher compared to those of centuries past.

- Cadmium is present in the phosphate deposits that are mined (e.g., in Florida, South Carolina, Idaho) and spread on the fields where we grow our crops. Florida phosphate deposits generally have the lowest Cd concentrations, while phosphates from Rocky Mountain deposits contain the highest Cd concentrations.

- Cadmium bioaccumulates in shellfish, crustaceans including shrimp, crab, oysters, and clams, with concentration factors exceeding one thousand times those of fish or meats like chicken, beef, and pork. This means the cadmium intake in a single meal containing a quarter-pound of shrimp and/or oysters is roughly equivalent to the quantity ingested in three years' worth of meals (i.e., one thousand meals), each containing a quarter pound of beef, chicken, or pork (assuming no organ meats). You may have heard that shellfish are rich in zinc, and they are, but the adverse impacts of cadmium in shellfish far outweigh any potential benefit that could be realized by eating shellfish.

- Epidemiological studies on pancreatic cancer show southern Louisiana, especially around New Orleans, to be a hot spot for pancreatic cancer. This part of the country is noted for its shrimp, oyster, crab, and crawfish dishes. However, being at the mouth of the Mississippi River—which is highly polluted by runoff from fields that see heavy annual applications of phosphate fertilizers—coupled with the high cadmium bioaccumulation efficiency of shellfish account for Cd poisoning of our Louisiana friends, and alcohol enhances Cd uptake. However, the prevalence of the disease is formally identified as a "pancreatic cancer" problem rather than a "cadmium poisoning" problem. Why do we choose to ignore the obvious connection?

Chapter Three

For the Good of the Whole

On an unseasonably cool Saturday morning, a young man in a sweater walks into the entrance at the base of the middle leg of the roughly E-shaped building that houses the Centers for Disease Control and Prevention just northeast of downtown Atlanta. He pushes open the large glass doors with his right shoulder. In his right hand, he carries a bag, conspicuously marked with golden arches against a red background and bulging with covered Styrofoam breakfast deluxe plates to appease the masses. Tucked away under his left arm like a football, he carries his Dachshund in a small doggie sweater. He makes his way down the hallway to a large room containing a cubicle maze and his desk where he sets down the bag with the food. He shifts the little dog to both hands and quickly slips his tiny sweater off his long body.

Another young man is working on the computer in his cubicle. "Sam, I don't know where the database is, but I hope you had it backed up."

Sam responds in a mixture of disgust and sarcasm, "I knew that the Hercules System you guys were switching us over to was a mistake. Why can't you just leave well enough alone? You know, Ernie . . . if it ain't broke, don't fix it!"

Ernie straightens up and raises his head from the screen. "Sam, we've been over this ten times, and you know that the old system wasn't going to keep up with all the data that's been coming in and the exponential rate at which it's increasing. Hercules may be a minor inconvenience for a small fraction of the users, but it is for the good of the whole."

"Yeah, yeah, yeah. Well, we all just need to tighten our belts a little. Your progress may have just cost me two months' worth of work to try to reconstruct the missing database from the fragmented pieces that we have in the backup files. The only saving grace about this mess is that I get to call you and your crew out on a Saturday."

The growl of the small Dachshund draws the two men's attention away from the gripe session for a moment. "All right, Agent Cooper!" exclaimed Sam. "You'll have your chance to get your two cents' worth in on the way home to Marietta."

Cooper was a fearless little mutt with a slick reddish-brown coat, willing to take on all comers, including dogs ten times his size, oblivious to the fact that if the big dog didn't back off, he could be snapped in two by the powerful jaws of his "victim." Cooper periodically growled at Ernie, lunging forward two or three steps and quickly retreating behind Sam's pant's leg. Sam assured Ernie, "Don't worry, he's all bark and no bite."

"I'm not. I just want you to know that I haven't had my rabies shots," Ernie said as he pretended to snarl, showing his teeth and shaking his head at Cooper, "so if I bite him back, he may have something to worry about."

Sam snickered. "Well, I hope that Dr. Welch's bite isn't as bad as his bark, because I think that he's going to be barking quite a bit when he hears what's going on."

Ernie raised his head and peeked over the large computer screen. "Uh . . . come on, Sam. You're not bringing in the big guns, are you?"

"I don't have a choice on this one. This is his pet project, and I've been collecting all this data for the statistical analysis that I have a feeling is going to radically change the environmental focus of this country for the foreseeable future." Sam reached for his cell phone and began dialing. "Several industries will suffer as a result, but the truth has to come out. It's for the good of the whole. That's why I came to work for the CDC. This is—by its very name—the Center for Disease Control and Prevention, an organization that works for the good of the whole."

"I see . . . you're going to be a whistleblower," Ernie said in a slight decrescendo, realizing that Sam was on the phone.

Sam raised his hand, indicating that someone was on the other end of the telephone connection. Sam tried to calm Cooper to keep him from barking as he focused on the telephone conversation. "Hello, Dr. Welch? I'm at the office, and I'm afraid I have some bad news about the cadmium database." [Pause.] "Yes, sir. I'll keep on trying, and sir . . . Ernie from Information Services is here doing his best. Yes, sir. I'll be awaiting your arrival."

Ernie stood and patted Sam on the side of his arm as he said, "Thanks for the plug, but he doesn't know me from Adam." The perky dog continued to bark as though his master's life were in danger. "What's that crazy dog of yours barking at? He acts like he's seen a ghost."

The barking was fierce, and the stubby front legs of the brave defender came off the ground with each bark. In a concerned voice and hunched over in the early stages of one of his monster hugs, Sam struggled to catch his defender's attention. "Come on, Coop, what's the matter?" Sam caught a glimpse of something out of the corner of his eye and jumped to his feet. "Did you see that?" he asked Ernie in a startled tone.

"See what?" Ernie exclaimed. Sam looked around the room and regained his composure as his reconnaissance yielded no startling discoveries. But Cooper continued to bark aggressively.

Suddenly, the lights went off, and the barking stopped. Sam exclaimed disgustedly, "Oh great! Now what has one of your ace troubleshooters done? Leaned against the light switch?" In an instant, the lights came back on.

Ernie responded, "Well, I don't know what one of my ace troubleshooters leaned against, but I wish he had done it a couple of hours ago. Look, Sam, the database is there—just like it's supposed to be."

Sam lunged at the monitor in disbelief, but when he saw the same thing Ernie had described, he slowly mumbled, "What the—?"

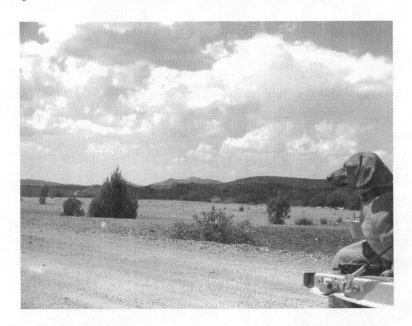

CADMIUM POISONING

FACTS

- Zinc is necessary for the natural maintenance of a healthy immune system (actually four immune systems with the largest one being located in the gut) for fighting infections and maintaining a healthy body. It is also essential for healing. It is involved in over 300 enzymatic reactions in the body. It is directly involved in the firing of the synapses and transferring of signals between adjacent nerve cells and is essential for proper brain function. Two of the largest reservoirs of zinc are the skeleton and the brain; however, zinc is found in every cell of the body, for example, intertwined in the DNA in what are called zinc fingers.

- Cadmium competes with zinc for reaction sites and accumulates in the body. Our bodies exhibit no sign of cadmium poisoning until an organ-specific threshold concentration is reached, at which time the organ begins to malfunction. Unlike cadmium with a 30-year biological half-life, zinc has a half-life of approximately 78 days. Continued presence and accumulation of cadmium typically leads to both zinc deficiency and cancer.

- Cadmium concentrations as low as 200 micrograms/kilogram in the renal cortex is enough to cause kidney disjunction and passing of protein in urine.

- Cadmium accumulation in the pancreas' islets of Langerhans beta cells inhibits the infusion of insulin into the bloodstream in response to fluctuations in blood glucose concentration. This condition is commonly known as Type 2 diabetes.

- Cadmium does not accumulate particularly in the brain. However, because cadmium competes with zinc, the bodies of individuals suffering from cadmium poisoning are typically deficient in zinc.

And since the brain is one of the largest reservoirs of zinc in the body, the brain is often robbed of zinc so that other bodily requirements are satisfied, as is commonly found in Alzheimer's patients.

- Humans are not the only ones being impacted by the drastic shift between zinc and cadmium concentrations in our external and internal environments. The zinc concentration in meat and bone meal is approximately 150 milligrams/kilogram (mg/kg). With the domestication of dogs, we ask man's best friend to adjust his diet from one that is rich in zinc to one containing substantial quantities of corn meal and other grains. The zinc concentration in corn is approximately 10 mg/kg. Comparing 10 with 150, it is not difficult to understand why many dogs may be suffering from a zinc deficiency. Many of the same cadmium poisoning symptoms that humans experience are also experienced by our canine friends especially since many of the dog foods and treats we offer them are wheat based (high-cadmium) or contain organ meats (high-cadmium) of other animals that also accumulate high concentrations of cadmium in the same organs as do humans.

Chapter Four

Moffett Field

Cuauhtémoc Gavilán stood in the shadow of Hangar One, the huge dirigible hangar on the site of his company's latest environmental remediation project at Moffett Federal Airfield, better known by its old name, Moffett Field. The expansive plumes of chlorinated solvents had served as a proving ground for many emerging technologies, beginning with research projects like the one he remembered from years before when he was an undergraduate, just northwest of the site, on the west side of San Francisco Bay. Gavilán was proud to do a small part to repair the damage that man has caused his Mother Earth. But this place was more than just a job. He felt that something special had happened in this place, something that transcended his world. He sensed that spirits were active at this site.

His long black hair seemed to flow in unison with the persistent bay breeze. His large forehead and the pronounced downward inflection in the profile of his nose were characteristic of his ancestry. He was very proud of what he called his natural tan. "Come on, Mike, Danny. Get that rig set up. The probes have to be set up approximately twenty feet apart, and make sure we're splitting soil and groundwater samples. No screwups."

Gavilán had installed his share of remediation systems in his day, and Mike and Danny had worked with Gavilán on many of them. Mike asked, "Why are we switching gears, Gavilán?"

Danny added in, "Yeah, man . . . que pasó?" [What happened?]

"Until the price of iron pellets went through the roof, we focused on my favorite remediation technique—permeable reactive barriers. You know, PRBs." Gavilán paused briefly, thinking back to his years of study at The Farm, not far from there. The application of principles he had learned in classes taken as electives from the chemical and environmental engineering departments had paid off in spades. He had selected well. Gavilán continued, "But now, we have to adjust, and I think that we need to reexamine the whole issue of how to dechlorinate a chlorinated hydrocarbon." His department, the Department of Earth Sciences, had provided the perfect platform for him to learn about his Mother Earth and ways to help her heal.

The economics of PRB remediation projects had changed. Gavilán's new approach required minimal initial capital investment, using probes in the ground that would destabilize the carbon-chlorine bonds in the contaminant molecules. The resonant pulse frequencies were key. This system was different. This was his baby.

Located on flat ground on the south end of San Francisco Bay, Hangar One is visible from many miles away in all directions. Gavilán remembered when he was an undergraduate and the many times he had returned to the Bay Area, the hangar had served as a landmark when he was traveling on Highway 101, the Bayshore Freeway. He always had his bearings as long as he could see where he was with respect to the hangar at Moffett Field. Seeing the hangar meant that his Stanford home was not too far away. It would always be Moffett Field for Gavilán and everyone he knew.

Gavilán's cell phone rang, and he was pleased to see *Olga* appear on the screen. "Hi, sweetie, are you ready to talk now?" [Pause.] "Well, now I'm on a job site, and I'll be tied up here through midafternoon, but are you up for some Chinese tonight at Chef Chu's? I know that I am, but I'm a good guy. I'll call you when they bring those delicately battered prawns to my table." [Pause.] "Okay, okay, Dr. Ramos. We'll save Chef Chu's for the Powwow." [Pause.] "I know that we have a lot to talk about before the Powwow, but it'll have to keep 'til this evening. I'll share my Foster Freeze gourmet meal with you over the phone."

[Pause.] "Chile and bean burrito and pineapple milk shake—the Bay Area's very best!" Gavilán chuckled. Once the humor subsided, Gavilán apologetically said, "I'm sorry, Olga, but I really do have to go now. I have a rig and a crew out here, and we need to make hay while the sun shines. I'll call you this evening from the Foster Freeze. Take care." As he put his cell phone in his pocket, Gavilán thought to himself, *Damn, she makes me feel good.*

Gavilán returned to the push-rig that was about fifty yards away, but when he got there, he found that his crew had disappeared. He walked around the rig while calling out their names. Nothing! He looked in the cab, thinking they might be playing a joke on him. Nobody home! He finally squatted, got down on his hands and knees, and looked under the rig. *Pinches cabrones. ¿Adonde se irían? [Those darn dudes. Where could they have gone?]* he thought to himself.

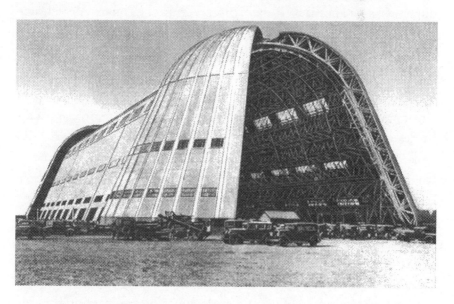

Gavilán stood in the bed of his pickup and did a full 360, looking for his missing crew. He hopped off and started walking toward the only structure in the area—Hangar One. Because he was somewhat of a history buff, Gavilán researched the Internet for the history of the site before he accepted the contract for his current project. As he walked to toward Hangar One, he recalled the *USS Macon* of the early 1930s, the naval airship that the huge structure was to house. At the time it was built, it was the largest freestanding structure with no internal supports and eight acres of floor space. Gavilán imagined what the site must have been like during World War II, when the giant airships served to patrol the coastlines of the United States against submarines.

As he neared the hangar, he looked up at the smooth lines of the curved structure: a collection of arches that reached skyward. And although the future of dirigibles was short-lived due to the many associated tragedies, he appreciated the role that they had played in the history of the naval air program. The fatal final voyage of the hydrogen-filled Hindenburg was the first to cross his mind. But it was the flight of the *USS Akron*, the sister ship of the *USS Macon*, that dominated his thoughts as he approached the hangar. Admiral William Moffet, one of the architects of the Navy's Bureau of Aeronautics, was a passenger aboard that ill-fated vessel, which went down in a storm off the coast of New Jersey. He lost his life that night, but his legacy lives on.

The support for dirigibles died soon thereafter. The future of naval air power was linked to the swift aircraft that could maneuver in air battles rather than lumbering blimps, but the hangar at Moffett Field remains. Gavilán finally reached the foot of the single most noticeable landmark in the South Bay Area, a structure he found much more impressive at close range. Its toxic skin had been peeled away, awaiting a new one to be applied. Gavilán felt he was present at a turning point for the massive structure. Its fate was now linked to Google, its contract with the federal government to lease and improve the property, and Google's ambitious high-tech and space-related plans for the future.

He looked almost straight up at the amazing engineering feat. He gasped for air as it took his breath away. He stared in amazement at the retractable doors of the hangar. In the arches of the doorway, it was like being at the door of a great cathedral. It stirred feelings inside of Gavilán. The grounds at the south end of the bay had been a special place for the indigenous population of the area before the arrival of the Spanish. These were holy grounds for the Ohlone that inhabited the area in centuries past. It was land that ironically had been given back to the Ohlone through a land grant to Lope Yñigo, who, upon his death, was buried on the lands he so much loved. He could feel their presence—the spirits of his northern cousins.

As with many of the native inhabitants who lived in villages in areas where Spanish missions were established, many of the Ohlone in the area were *assimilated*. The Spanish missionaries offered them food and shelter, while the armed Spanish forces represented protection. Although they were a peace-loving people who had survived in large parts of Northern California without outside "protection," many of the Ohlone were convinced by the Spanish that they would be better off supporting the mission. They became dependent on the Spanish, but there was a price to pay. With the mixing of the bloodlines, they lost their identity and became the Mestizos (mixed blood) that kept the missions going.

Cuauhtémoc Gavilán was a sensitive being, and his brain always seemed to be operating on two levels. The focus of his conscious brain was always to take care of the matters at hand, but the workings of his subconscious brain were a marvelous mystery. His subconscious dominated the night in the form of dreams—turning his hopes and aspirations into what seemed reality for an instant and sometimes resolving problems he encountered during the day. But this part of his brain continued to function during the day, becoming more dominant when he was tired.

Out of nowhere, a word emerged from Gavilán's lips: *protection*. When he uttered the word, it was as though he had suddenly come out of a semiconscious state. He asked himself, *Why that word?* He felt a strong presence of visitors from the spirit world. Gavilán knew that like so many of the Native Americans exposed to Europeans, the Ohlone had suffered tremendous losses to the new diseases for which their bodies were unprepared and had no defenses. This was part of the price they paid for "protection"—disease, death, and assimilation of the survivors.

Gavilán had grown up in a family of medicine men, and he was not uncomfortable with spirits from the other side. But he had never felt that a word had been placed on his lips by someone from the spirit world . . . until now. A shiver went up his spine. He reached for a small gold artifact that hung around his neck on a thin strand of leather.

Just then he felt something tapping him on both shoulders. Gavilán gasped as he jumped, turning to see Mike and Danny standing behind him. He was clearly startled.

Danny took a step back, saying, "Steady, big fella."

Mike chimed in jokingly, "I'd say 'get a grip,' but I see you're already gripping your crucifix."

Gavilán let go of the artifact as he took a step back. It wasn't a crucifix as Mike had conjectured. Mike stepped forward, focusing on the artifact. "Where'd you get the gold airplane?" he asked.

Gavilán responded, "Mi abuelo me lo dió." [My grandfather gave it to me.] He had two made—one for me and one for my brother—and he told us to keep them on us for protection. They are replicas of an ancient Mayan artifact, dating back well over a thousand years."

Mike leaned forward and reached for the artifact with his right hand. Gavilán stood still without protest. "Nah, that can't be. This thing bears a striking resemblance to a modern-day jet aircraft, complete with a cockpit. I didn't know the Maya flew airplanes back then. How old did you say that Mayan artifact was?"

"It was discovered with other Mayan artifacts and was dated to be over a thousand years old," Gavilán explained. "My grandfather said that it was one of the vehicles used by *the teachers*. They came to teach us and protect us."

Mike and Danny gazed at each other with incredulous expressions on their faces and then turned to look at Gavilán who interjected, "All right, you guys! You're the ones that are going to need the protection for abandoning the equipment. Let's get back to work."

The three men started back to the pickup, laughing and slapping Gavilán on the back. As the laughter died down, Mike inquired, "No, man, is that interesting trinket you wear around your neck really made of gold, or does it leave green stains on your chest?"

Just then Danny chimed in, "Yeah, just listen to Mike! If he had a cute gold trinket like that, he wouldn't have it for long. It would wind up in the pawn shop!" The laughter erupted again.

This time it was Gavilán who spoke as the laughter subsided. "You know, guys, it's not the gold that makes this artifact priceless." The other two men nodded their heads as they muttered, "Yeah, yeah." Gavilán continued, "Gold was just another medium for their artwork. Besides, *teocuitlatl*, the Aztec word for gold, literally means 'excrement of the gods,' which shows that they didn't regard it nearly as highly as you guys do."

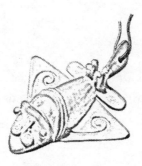

Danny again laughed, commenting, "You're a weird bird, my Mexican friend."

CADMIUM POISONING

FACTS

- The poisons we ingest with the foods we serve on our tables are being spread generously on the fields used to grow most vegetables. In the case of cadmium, it is an element that cannot be broken down, and although some leaves the fields with each growing season in the harvested crops and in runoff, the amount removed is less than what is applied, and consequently, the concentration in the soils continues to increase. Looking at a mass balance of a contaminant, M, on a typical field:

$$M_{(applied)} = M_{(harvested)} + M_{(runoff)} + M_{(broken\ down)} + M_{(accumulated)}$$

In the case of Cd, assuming all things remaining stable from season to season (i.e., amount applied, volume of runoff, etc.):

$$Cd_{(broken\ down)} = 0, \text{ and } Cd_{(applied)} - Cd_{(harvested)} - Cd_{(runoff)} = Cd_{(accumulated)} > 0,$$

and in general, the higher the accumulated concentration in the soil, the higher the concentrations in the harvested crops and runoff. In other words, the problem of cadmium on the dinner table is just getting worse and worse.

- Runoff from the breadbasket of our country contaminates the waters of the Mississippi River, discharging them into the Gulf of Mexico. Cadmium tends to adsorb on surfaces, so that the concentration on suspended solids in the waters of the Mississippi is higher than in the water itself. Because the annual suspended solids discharged from the mouth of the Mississippi is estimated to be an average of 436,000 tons per day, and because suspended solids tend to settle, it is no surprise that shellfish, bottom dwellers like shrimp and oysters, that continuously filter the water that surrounds them bioaccumulate extremely high concentrations of cadmium.

- Cadmium contamination of soils, surface water, and groundwater near mines, landfills, processing plants, and wastewater treatment plants can be problematic, depending on the effectiveness of engineering controls (if any) in keeping mine tailings, contaminated process water, and other waste streams from reaching vulnerable soils and groundwater. Leaching from soils can lead to groundwater contamination, which in turn can discharge to surface water bodies (e.g., streams, rivers, lakes, and reservoirs), either above or below ground surface, depending on site hydrologic conditions.

- Because of the skyrocketing population and associated demand for increased food production, the global increasing trends in mining of phosphate and application of phosphate fertilizers is unlikely to change. However, processes for the removal of cadmium from phosphate fertilizers prior to application have been developed and are being used in a few places like Israel, for example.

Chapter Five

Billy Ruben

The door leading into the lobby from the parking garage opened, and a man carrying an umbrella entered. He walked with great deliberation down the hallway, past the conference room, and into the bullpen, the large room where the cubicles for Sam's department were set up. He worked his way through the maze to Sam's workstation where he found Sam and Ernie reviewing the details of what they had just experienced. Ernie was standing at the opening to the cubicle, and Sam was leaning back in his chair, rocking back and forth slightly. The man walked up behind Ernie and stopped. Sam's eyes shifted their focus from Ernie to the man behind him as he sat up in his chair. When Ernie realized that someone was behind him, he felt a hand grab him firmly on the shoulder. "I want to personally thank you, Ernie, for taking time out from your weekend to help us out with this problem."

Ernie was somewhat surprised, more than anything, by the fact that Dr. Welch knew his name. "Oh, Dr. Welch! No, this is part of my job. I'm happy to help in any way that I can." Ernie stepped slightly to one side.

Dr. Welch also adjusted his position in the restricted space as he tugged at his wire-rimmed glasses. "Hello, Sam, and thank you for letting me know about the problem."

"Well, Dr. Welch, I knew that you have a special interest in the data that I've been compiling for the cadmium project."

Ernie interrupted, "I already released the rest of the crew so that they could enjoy the rest of their weekend, and I guess that I should follow suit. Bye, Sam. Good afternoon, Dr. Welch."

Ernie and Dr. Welch again adjusted their positions, but this time Ernie started down the aisle. Dr. Welch took a step into the cubicle and sat down in the side chair by Sam's desk as Ernie proceeded down the aisle, walking backward with his head tilted to one side, making strange faces, and waving his arms to catch Sam's attention. Sam just smiled.

Cooper came out of nowhere and jumped onto Dr. Welch's lap. He looked at the dog, patted him on the head, held onto his long torso, and said, "Cute." But he didn't miss a beat and continued explaining the significance of the cadmium data. "You see, Sam, it's a project that holds the answers to a lot of questions I have had for decades about the health of my family in New Orleans."

Dr. Welch was a man of moderate stature with thinning salt-and-pepper hair partially covering a shiny scalp. His eyes appeared slightly magnified behind the lenses of his glasses. When he entered a room, his very presence commanded respect. Dr. William R. Welch was one of the *good* good ol' boys at the CDC. He knew how to navigate the CDC political hotbed that dealt with high-paying federal positions, life-and-death issues, and a mixed internal environment that was filled with turf battles and the turmoil they cause. Some of Sam's coworkers aspired to join those ranks, but by and large, dedicated professionals intent on helping their fellow man populated the cubicles in the bullpen.

"I didn't know that you were from Louisiana, Dr. Welch," responded Sam.

"Well, I'm not. I'm referring to my adopted family from when I was attending Tulane University. My dissertation advisor and his family took an interest this good ol' Georgia boy, and they literally took me into their family. After my graduation, it was very hard for me hearing repeatedly about health problems that developed for these wonderful people. They deserve better than what fate dished out—diabetes, cancer, Alzheimer's disease, and countless premature deaths."

Sam was interested but skeptical. He knew the kind of scrutiny that any such claim and the supporting data would be under. Without wanting to sound critical, he asked, "I sort of assumed that the data was for an epidemiological study, but how could cadmium be responsible for all those disease, and how would you ever expect to prove it?"

As he began petting Cooper, Dr. Welch continued, "Well, I ran across a study that turned the light on in the attic. It was an epidemiological study on pancreatic cancer indicating that the consumption of shellfish in southern Louisiana was responsible for that cancer hot spot on the map that caught my attention. And where is the cadmium coming from? The breadbasket of America."

Sam tilted his head and squinted slightly. Dr. Welch recognized the puzzled look and continued with further explanation. "You see, Sam, one of the things that makes this country great is its ability to produce massive quantities of food. We grow enough to not only feed our own but also to have enough left over for export to the rest of the world. But to do this, we use phosphate fertilizers. Sam, for the last seventy years, we've been overfertilizing our farmlands with phosphate fertilizers that are contaminated with cadmium, and the runoff from those field drains into the Mighty Mississippi and flows down to Louisiana. You see, I was already putting some data together on the incidence of diabetes and was contemplating how to test the theory that refined wheat and rice products were responsible for diabetes. In both instances, the consumption of food that contains high concentrations of cadmium is involved. The consumption of seafood that is heavily represented by shellfish including shrimp, oysters, and crabs is part of the Cajuns' culture. Oh, and let's not forget crawfish or the red beans and rice."

A squeamish look came over Sam's face as he blurted out, "I had a shrimp dinner at a seafood restaurant in east Atlanta last night!"

"It's okay, son, you'll live," commented Dr. Welch as he patted Sam on the shoulder. He then continued, "Hispanics share the problem with our Louisiana friends, but they have their *sopas de fidello* [vermicelli], the various rice dishes including Spanish rice, *arroz con pollo* [rice with chicken], and *atole de arroz* [rice pudding], and the delicious flour tortillas that are served at all three meals—breakfast tacos, *fajita* tacos, and served with every Mexican food plate in every Mexican restaurant in Texas. These are all part of the culture, and that's what makes

San Antonio the diabetes capital of the nation. In both instances, the pancreas is involved, and the pancreas is one of the organs in the human body where cadmium is concentrated. This is no coincidence." He began petting Cooper a little more *enthusiastically.* "I started looking at other possible problems caused by cadmium, and I was shocked to find that cadmium is indicated in a host of additional diseases ranging from cancers of the prostate, the liver, the kidneys, the lungs, the bone, and the breast, to osteoporosis, disease of the thyroid, hardening of the arteries and stroke, high triglycerides and imbalance in the high-density and low-density cholesterols in the bloodstream, and indirectly to Alzheimer's disease. Sam, my adopted family was cadmium poisoned. Sam, this is big, and I mean really big. It is probably the most far-reaching and challenging health issue of our lifetimes."

"Yes, sir, I understand," spurted out Sam as he nodded his head up and down. He could sense that the details of the statistical approach hadn't been worked out but that this was a project about which Dr. Welch felt intensely and passionately. He knew Dr. Welch would find a way to *make it happen.*

Cooper jumped down from Dr. Welch's lap and sat next to Sam's left foot. The pitch of his voice rose slightly as though he had just shared the tip of the iceberg with Sam and was frustrated about the magnitude of the problem. He leaned forward in his chair, saying, "There's a lot more to the story, but let's dispense with the 'sir' business. Just call me Billy Ruben like everyone else."

Out of respect for Dr. Welch, Sam bit the inside of his cheek to keep from bursting out laughing.

As Dr. Welch leaned forward, Cooper began to growl in a low tone, and Sam leaned back in his chair, maintaining the distance between them, saying, "Yes, sir . . . I mean Billy Ruben. It's just very unusual for someone as high up the organization as you are to take a personal interest in the collection and analysis of data. I mean, I think that's great, but that's usually left to people at a much lower level, like me, with a statistical background."

Dr. Welch sensed that he was getting a little too intense and that he was pushing Sam out of his comfort zone. He sat back into his chair, took a deep breath, and lowered his voice. "Well, son, I guess I didn't want to just be remembered as the guy that was responsible for making shit brown. Sam, we have data in our possession that can be used to help a lot of people. We need to make something *good* happen."

Dr. Welch continued, "And in case you're curious about my comment, let me explain about my name. You see, when my parents named me Billy Ruben, not to be confused with *bilirubin*, they were just following the pattern that had been set in the family by my maternal uncles and aunts. All the firstborn males were named Billy, with the second name being what distinguished them apart. As you might suspect at this point, my older male cousins include Billy Bob, Billy Joe, and Billy Gene. When my aunt Velma's firstborn was born a female . . . well, she wasn't going to be outdone. She named her daughter Billie Rae. She is truly a unique woman—beautiful, intelligent, talented . . . and then they moved to California. Oh, but I'm getting off track. By the time I came along, I guess all the good names were taken . . . and I was stuck with *Billy Ruben*."

Sam glanced down and saw that Cooper's head was resting on his foot. He decided to follow up with a comment on the discussion just to let Dr. Welch know he was still paying attention. "I guess you got ribbed a lot by other students when you were in school."

"Actually, my grade school buddies never bothered me with the jokes and the madeup singsongs that kids always concoct when there is an unusual name to be made fun of. It wasn't until I was in college at Tulane that my name drew that kind of response from people." He laughed. "It was pretty funny hearing a bunch of drunk twenty-year-olds making up and singing inane limericks about bilirubin, trying to get my goat . . . but I survived."

Sam took Cooper into his arms as he mumbled baby-talk in an affectionate voice, "Is my Agent Cooper doing okay?"

Dr. Welch leaned over and petted Cooper on the head as he reiterated, "He is a cute little fella." Cooper responded by licking Dr. Welch's hand. "Getting back to the cadmium issue, to lay the groundwork for the cadmium project, I sent a memo up the chain, explaining how farmers across this land are concurrently spreading poison with every pound of phosphate fertilizer that they use on their fields. Well, with today's increased sensitivity to vulnerabilities and Homeland Security's concern about the potential for disruption of our nation's food production, my memo got me a couple of invitations to present CDC findings at conferences—one in Houston and another in San Francisco. On Monday, I'll be flying to Houston for the first conference at NASA on Tuesday. The meeting has been billed as an issue of national security. I'm not sure what my role will be yet, but my cadmium . . . no, our cadmium project will probably be discussed. I need for you to brief me on what you've found so far. Sam, pack your bags—you're going to Houston with me."

CADMIUM POISONING

FACTS

- Things that disrupt proper function of the pancreas and/or reduce insulin sensitivity on the cellular level cause Type 2 diabetes—cadmium is one of those things. The insulin-production response of the beta cells of the pancreas is suppressed by cadmium. With the lifestyle and eating habits of Mexican Americans, it is no surprise that San Antonio is the diabetes capital of the nation and probably the world. Common foods and dishes include tortillas de harina [flour tortillas], sopas de fideo [vermicelli], sopa de arroz [rice], arroz con pollo [rice with chicken], and pan de dulce [sweet bread pastries]. Even tamales that are made with corn meal, which is naturally low in cadmium, are suspect. The final product may be high in cadmium because the corn meal is spread on shucks which, along with all the leafy parts of the corn plant, are extremely high in cadmium that may leach out of the shucks and into the corn meal.

- Wheat gluten is added to flour used for making tortillas de harina [flour tortillas]. It helps keep them soft and pliable without adding so much lard. In the processing of wheat, the product with the highest cadmium concentration is the wheat gluten, making flour tortillas even more toxic—a cadmium *double whammy*.

- Today, many people are being diagnosed with gluten sensitivity and celiac disease. Some contend that our diagnostic techniques have improved and that we can now identify biomarkers (i.e., indicators in the blood that point to conditions of predisposition and/or bodily responses to disease or the presence of foreign substances) that had not been defined and could not be identified previously. However, some relatively recent bloodwork results suggest this is not the case. A discovery of intact, preserved blood samples associated with a group of British airmen from World War II offered a unique opportunity to compare bloodwork analysis results with those of a similar group of airmen today. The results indicated a fourfold increase in celiac disease biomarkers in today's airmen compared to the airmen of over sixty years ago. This topic was but a small part of the Gluten Summit, an event that brought together world authorities on celiac disease, held over the Internet in November of 2013. A relevant comment and associated questions and answers regarding the possibility that celiac disease and the disparity in the blood sample biomarkers are a response to chronic exposure to cadmium in the food chain ensued on the Internet, a copy of which is provided in Appendix B at the end of the book. A strategy for recovering from cadmium poisoning is offered in Appendix A.

- Cadmium concentrations in women have increased as they have taken their rightful place in the workforce. But along with the change from the now-antiquated role of housewife came increased incidence of smoking and exposure to secondhand smoke, resulting in an increase in the incidence of lung disease. Women with breast cancer typically have twice the cadmium levels in their bodies compared to the rest of the female population. (They are also generally iodine deficient.)

- Iodine is essential for proper thyroid function and the regulation of many hormones. It accumulates primarily in the thyroid, but it is also found in other tissues, such as the breasts. Iodine also plays an essential role in cancer prevention. Breast cancer has been linked to cadmium poisoning and, therefore, is related to the competition between cadmium (carcinogenic heavy metal in our food chain due to the use of cadmium-laden phosphate fertilizers) and zinc in the body. Most Americans are iodine deficient, and many are also zinc deficient. Iodine cannot perform its normal functions in individuals who are zinc deficient. Iodine is key in the process of apoptosis (scheduled cell death), and cancer cells don't "know" they are supposed to die. Cadmium mimics estrogen in the body, and estrogen inhibits iodine absorption. The following three YouTube videos by Dr. Jorge Flechas provide details and offer insight into the importance of iodine in cancer prevention: https://www.youtube.com/watch?v=EoMfg76gAUo, https://www.youtube.com/watch?v=dcNNKzsUIT0, and https://www.youtube.com/watch?v=ZBM2qWKkFxE.

- Remember to breathe! The metabolism of cancer cells is different from that of normal cells. Cancer cells use glucose rather than oxygen. The process is called glycolysis, and for the equivalent amount of energy production, it consumes 17–18 glucose molecules, compared to 2 molecules when glucose is reacted with oxygen in normal cell metabolism. This is another reason to perform aerobic exercises. Don't create an environment that is favorable for cancer cell proliferation. Several times a day, make a conscious effort to breathe. Take three deep breaths. It will also help relieve stress and reduce cortisol levels in the blood.

- During your research on cadmium, you may encounter brief discussions on estrogen and statements regarding how cadmium mimics estrogen. Some say that estrogen is the only cause of cancer and that other substances labeled as carcinogens are just estrogen enhancers or, as in the case of cadmium, an estrogen emulator. Men and women produce both estrogen and testosterone, but the balance between the two is different, with estrogen being the primary sex hormone in women and testosterone being the primary sex hormone in men.

Chapter Six

Come In, Houston Control

The meeting was to cover a variety of subjects, bringing together respected scientists and engineers from across the nation. The agenda was prepared by top NASA officials and, reportedly, had been expanded by Pentagon officials as directed by the White House. Participants had been hand picked, and no one refused the invitation to participate. The meeting was billed as matter of national security. There was an air of unrest and uncertainty among the participants of the meeting.

Olga entered the auditorium where the first phase of the meeting was to take place. The auditorium was about half full, but because the other four representatives from JPL were still at the hotel breakfast table when she had left, she knew no one in the room. She found a spot toward the front of the auditorium with vacant seats surrounding it, but within minutes the room began to fill. The individual conversations that were discernible when she first took her seat became part of a dull roar that continued to increase in volume.

She glanced to her right and saw two men approaching, working their way toward her to take the two vacant seats to her right. It reminded her of a crowded movie theater at the first showing of a well-publicized Lucas or Spielberg film. She found it rather comical; the two men were obviously stepping on their share of toes and begging pardons as they advanced. The only thing missing was the smell of fresh, buttered popcorn.

The two men seemed nice enough but markedly clumsy. The older of the two finally reached his destination and sat next to her. The younger man kept looking her way, making Olga think there might be someone else to her left that he was greeting. She turned to her left but saw no one that might be engaging him. When she turned her head to the right again, she felt his eyes locked in on her. She looked at his face and was drawn into his eyes.

He stuttered, "We're from the CDC, and I had no idea why I was coming here . . . until now."

His corny line snapped her out of her brief trance, and she responded, "I still don't know why I'm here." *He's very cute*, she thought to herself. *I wonder if he has half a brain.* He began to extend his hand to shake hers, but Olga turned her head to the left, pretending not to see. Just then, the meeting was called to order by a NASA official.

〰〰〰〰〰〰〰〰〰〰〰〰〰〰〰〰〰〰〰〰〰〰〰〰〰〰〰〰〰

Olga felt certain that her sightings in the Sirian heavens had to be the focal point of the conference. Olga had acquired many skills during her research at Stanford University that had continued to develop at JPL. Her access to the Dish, at one time the largest radiotelescope on the continent, mounted atop one of the foothills just northwest of the Stanford campus, had stimulated her curiosity about whether life might exist in nearby star systems. At NASA, she had become heavily involved in the surveillance of the planets of Sirius. She had been directly responsible for developing enhancement software that permitted resolution that was more than three orders of magnitude greater than the current technology used on surveillance satellites. However, the technique required data collection from several vantage points—the greater the number of distinct observation stations, the greater the resolution. For long-distance observations that were of interest to her, Olga had had to coordinate with all the major observatories and owners of satellites that were in fixed orbit expressly for this purpose.

Olga had begun the development of her system, focusing on terrestrial objects. While the capabilities of surveillance satellites were impressive, permitting users to tell whether a shiny new quarter on the sidewalk was lying heads up or heads down, they were dwarfed by Olga's computer-enhanced technology. Olga had combined the technology used with individual surveillance satellites with the simultaneous collection from satellites used for Geographical Information Systems, more commonly known as GISs. Then she went one step further and coordinated data from multiple surveillance satellites. She needed coordinated data collection from four GIS satellites and imaging data from at least two surveillance satellites. With data from six heavenly sources, Olga could not only tell if a quarter was heads up or heads down but could also easily discern the number and dimensions of the tiny bag marks on the surface of George Washington's cheek. The greater the number of satellites available to probe and transmit data, the greater the potential magnification and accuracy of the images produced.

To simplify the data analysis, her software required simultaneous data collection for moving objects. Olga had had to synchronize all participating observation stations on the time of data collection. Subsequent computer analysis of all data could be performed on mainframe NASA OMNI computers as their busy schedules permitted, but simultaneous data collection was critical.

Simultaneous data collection was not so critical for stationary objects, so that a single, mobile data collection station could move about collecting all the necessary data; but to make the data useful, the precise location of each data collection site was needed. For Olga's purposes, her high-resolution digital camera assumed the role of the surveillance satellites, and her programming coordinated the data to produce a three-dimensional image of the stationary object that could be examined from any angle after the data had been compiled.

A man dressed in a gray suit stepped up to the podium, tapped the microphone, and greeted the crowd, "Thank you, ladies and gentlemen, for joining us today at this very important conference. I know that all of you came here after receiving very little information about the nature of the conference, and I thank you for the trust that you have placed in us. I assure you that the theme of this conference is of the utmost importance to our nation's security."

As the NASA official continued with the introduction of various people responsible for organizing the conference, Olga saw her JPL colleagues at the end of her row, making their way toward her. She looked at them and couldn't help but wonder, *Are CDC personnel just naturally clumsier than JPL personnel?* She smiled and glanced to her right, only to see the young man with the captivating eyes looking back at her. She smiled and casually faced forward.

The host NASA official continued, "Before we get started, I have been requested to briefly turn the floor over to Mr. Richard Jones, regional head of Homeland Security. It's all yours, Dick."

Mr. Jones took the speaker's place at the podium. Dressed in a sharp-looking, navy-blue, two-piece suit, he removed a handkerchief from his jacket pocket and announced, "I guess you really have to experience Houston humidity to understand what it would be like to live in a sauna." The comment drew a few chuckles as he continued, "But seriously, folks, you all know that you have been invited to attend this conference in the name of national security."

The audience remained a bit rowdy, and a few conversations could still be heard to be ongoing in several parts of the auditorium. "You must realize," continued Mr. Jones in a voice of a slightly heightened pitch and intensity, "that the topics that we are about to discuss must remain confidential. You are not to divulge the general themes covered or the details of any of the work sessions that are scheduled for this afternoon. This is a matter of national security, and because not all of you have secret clearances, the Homeland Security representatives at the front of each aisle will be distributing your pledges of secrecy." The noise level in the audience dropped significantly. Men in black suits at the front of the aisles started counting out secrecy agreement forms to be passed out at each row.

Mr. Jones went on, "Each of you is expected to identify yourself by printing your name, filling in your social security number, and signing the pledge. If there is anyone who feels that he or she cannot do so, please raise your hand now, and you will be escorted to the front gate by an officer from the Department of Homeland Security [DHS]." The auditorium was absolutely silent; you could have heard a pin drop. Many heads of the members of the audience could be seen to be turning to one side and then the other. Not a word was uttered. "Fine then. On behalf of the Department of Homeland Security, I welcome all of you to what should be a very productive conference. Our representatives will make a headcount of each row to confirm that all secrecy pledges are turned in. Thank you for your cooperation."

The morning session was dedicated to an overview of what was described as *a war against breeches in security on projects of national interest.* The DHS was assuming control of all security measures related to federally funded projects. To that end, the government was assigning a DHS security officer to every government installation and every institution receiving government funding for research and/ or development of sensitive technologies. The DHS security officer would oversee all security measures already in place and implement new measures deemed necessary.

No one was permitted to leave the Johnson Space Center for lunch; instead, all conference participants were to be escorted into a large hall set up as a dining facility. The JPL contingent stood in almost unison, turned, and played follow the leader as everyone started filing out of the rows. As the masses were shuffling down the aisles, Olga heard the young man from the CDC utter, "Uh, oh, excuse me, Dr. Welch." When they reached their dining table in the next room, Olga turned and found an extended hand waiting to greet her. "Hi, my names is Sam Robinson, and I'm very happy to meet you. I'm with the CDC, the statistics group." He stumbled a bit, searching for something else to say, and finally continued "—doing the statistics on the epidemiological studies for the organization. And your name is . . . ?" he ended with a lilt in the intonation of his voice.

"Olga, Olga Ramos," she responded sheepishly as she shook his hand, still stunned from what she saw going on around her. "I'm with the Jet Propulsion Lab in LA. My project is Interstellar Surveillance—Search for Life," she said as she scanned the tables around her, noting that there was a somewhat conspicuous man in a black suit at every table.

A DHS representative was assigned to each table to lead group discussions on security and the vulnerability of government organizations should project security be breached. He was also to collect information about all projects in which the engineers and scientists seated at the table were involved. Each representative was to keep a low profile until the people seated at his table had time to introduce themselves and get comfortable with each other.

The JPL contingent, the clumsy gentlemen from the CDC, and three faculty members from The University of Texas at Austin had assembled at one of what appeared to be about fifty tables. They sat down in their chairs almost in unison. A plate brimming with leafy lettuce and mushroom salad adorned each place setting. A large basket of rolls was passed around, and everyone took a roll except for Dr. Welch and Olga.

The food service personnel tried their best to be good waiters and waitresses, dressed in their neat black-and-white uniforms, complete with black bow ties and cummerbunds for the waiters and short-waisted black vests for the waitresses. They reached over the left shoulders of their dining guests, setting down plates filled with linguini and shrimp covered in Alfredo sauce, and with a few sprigs of broccoli on the side.

Everyone seemed to enjoy the salad and the main course, that is, except for Dr. Welch and Olga who only ate the broccoli. The rest of the food on their plates went untouched.

And then began the inquisition. Just as the first few attendees finished the main course, a man sitting at the table said, "Hi, everyone. My name is DHS Officer Blakey, and I will be directing the discussion on project security. I will also need to have your full cooperation in helping me learn about your government-funded projects. Of course, you know, we have ways of double-checking the information you provide this afternoon, so that your complete and honest responses are expected."

Olga felt like a caged rat being scrutinized by the fat cat in the black suit. Was this Big Brother in action, or was the government just overreacting on issues of security? Where was the balance? Everyone at the table other than the man in the black suit became tense. Their body language was screaming with the indignation they were experiencing, but their voices remained silent.

Mr. Blakey continued, "I know that you've had a chance to chat a bit, but why don't we go around the table, and everyone introduce yourself, give the organization you represent and the name of the government-funded project that you're working on." He motioned to the man on his right, saying, "Why don't we start with you, sir. And oh! If it's okay, I'll just put my recorder in the middle of the table so that I don't have to take notes."

By this time, the food service personnel had begun removing plates and replacing them with dessert: rich devil's food chocolate cake with thick fudge icing, smothered with strawberries in a sugary sauce. A dark Colombian-roast coffee was the featured beverage—the perfect complementary flavor to go with the rich chocolate dessert.

More wasted food, thought Billy Ruben. He had eliminated chocolate from his diet after learning about the high lead and cadmium concentrations that it contains. And chocolate cake! Well, that's a double whammy since it was chocolate mixed with cadmium-rich bleached wheat flour. When he was offered a cup of coffee, he responded, "No, thank you, ma'am. Nothing against Juan Valdez, but coffee is off my diet due to heavy metals."

Olga's ears immediately perked up when she heard Dr. Welch's comment, but it was almost her turn to introduce herself. She took her fork, stabbed the two largest of the large strawberries on her untouched desert, and stuffed the whole strawberries—one after the other—into her mouth just as it was her time to speak. "Ng-ai ng-ayng ih Oga Wah-ngoh, ang I'ng wih guh Gay-Key-Eoh." [My name is Olga Ramos, and I'm with the JPL] *I hope that none of it can be understood on the recording*, she thought to herself. "Ng-ai poai-yec ih

Ing-ah-hey-ah Huh-wa-wengh—Harc foa Ife." [My project is Interstellar Surveillance—Search for Life.] Everyone at the table, including Mr. Blakey, silently stared at Olga in shock and amazement.

⊐⊏

Mr. Blakey's report to Mr. Jones was brief and to the point. "Dick, I had a questionable participant at my table." Mr. Blakey lifted his recorder and pressed the button. The small machine came to life with Olga's garbled voice. "That was her name and government-funded project," said Mr. Blakey in disgust.

"Well, what do you think?" inquired Mr. Jones as he scowled, raising his left eyebrow.

Mr. Blakey's response was damning. "I don't know. She might be Middle Eastern instead of Hispanic, but in any case, she's subversive."

Mr. Jones nodded his head, saying, "Assign Agent Stevenson to her case. Tell him not to let her out of his sight. I want to know where she goes, who she sees, what she does, and when she does it."

⊐⊏

Olga and Dr. Welch looked at each other as they got up from the table. Sam turned toward Dr. Welch, shooting several questions focused on the federal funding of the cadmium project. But Dr. Welch, eyes locked on Olga's eyes, stepped around Sam to Olga's side. In a low voice he uttered, "You've just set yourself up for a tough ride on this bronco. They will scrutinize your project, your background . . . and if they don't like the color of your underwear, they will make it very difficult for you to continue."

Olga responded by whispering into Dr. Welch's ear, "Thanks for your concern, but for the record, my underwear is white, and I use a little bleach on laundry days to keep it that way."

Still in a low voice, Dr. Welch said, "Young lady, don't misunderstand my words of concern. I suggest that we get away from here and go somewhere where we can talk."

Sam watched with a puzzled look on his face. "Dr. Welch, do you want me to go away for a few minutes?"

Dr. Welch turned to Sam and placed his right hand on Sam's left shoulder. "Sit down, Sam," grumbled Billy Ruben as he pushed Sam down into one of the chairs at the dining table. He turned to refocus on Olga.

Olga cleared her throat and began in an inquiring voice, "Dr. Welch . . . [Billy Ruben nodded], I have someone waiting for me when I finish up at the conference. I don't know what you want to tell me, but my friend and I are of like mind, I trust him implicitly, and anything you want to share with me is safe with him."

Dr. Welch leaned toward Olga, again speaking in a low voice. "Well, we can talk about all that when we meet away from here. Do you have any favorite meeting places in the area? I remember a little place over the Kemah Bridge called Two E's, but I'm not sure if it's still there—it's been so long since I was here last."

Olga responded, "Tookie's on 146, just south of NASA Road 1. Meet us there an hour after the conference lets out."

"You got it." Billy Ruben tapped Sam on the shoulder, Sam stood, and the two walked back toward the meeting rooms. Olga watched them walk away and wondered where this nightmare was going.

꧁꧁꧁꧁꧁꧁꧁꧁꧁꧁꧁꧁꧁꧁꧁꧁꧁꧁꧁꧁꧁꧁꧁꧁꧁꧁꧁

It was five o'clock, and the traffic was thick, but Olga's wait outside the Johnson Space Center gates was brief. Following the explicit instructions that he had been given, Gavilán drove up on the north side of NASA Road 1, heading west toward the bustling metropolis of Webster. He saw Olga and pulled off onto the shoulder of the road. Olga quickly hopped in.

"Hola, preciosa," he greeted her. [Hello, precious] "¿Cansada?" [Tired?]

"Naaah, let's just blow this pop stand," she replied, and they were off.

"Now, Eagle Man, your challenge is to turn around and head back toward El Lago, Seabrook, and Highway 146," Olga said with a gentle nudge of the elbow to Gavilán's right arm. She continued, "And if we could make our 180 at the next light, that would be great."

"Right, and are there any other miracles you'd like for me to pull off while I'm at it?" Gavilán turned to see Olga's smiling face, and he said, "I'll see what I can do."

Gavilán focused on his driving. He managed to work his way to the left lane and get to the turnaround located just after the light, and feeling proud of himself for his performance under pressure, he said, "Voila! Seabrook, here we come. So how was your conference?"

Olga responded in a grumble, "I've been sworn to secrecy. If I tell you, I'll have to shoot you."

Sensing that Olga was a bit uptight about the conference, Gavilán quipped, "You can shoot me. Just don't kill me."

"See! That's what I mean! I'm no good at this national security stuff. I'm supposed to kill you, not just maim you. Damn it!"

꙰꙰꙰꙰꙰꙰꙰꙰꙰꙰꙰꙰꙰꙰꙰꙰꙰꙰꙰꙰꙰꙰꙰꙰꙰꙰꙰꙰꙰꙰꙰

Olga and Gavilán got out of their car and strolled into Tookies. The place was decked out in rustic fifties decor. Gavilán kept turning his head as they were escorted to their table, taking in all the sights. Olga noticed and motioned for him to get close so that she could whisper something in his ear. He leaned forward as they walked. Olga raised her hand to her mouth as she leaned toward him and whispered, "Rustic." Gavilán nodded and silently mouthed the word *rustic* back to her.

They arrived at their table, and Olga elected to be seated so that she could face the front of the restaurant. Their young hostess set their menus on the table before them and bade them, "Enjoy your meal." Once they had settled in at the table, Gavilán leaned forward, reaching for Olga's hands. She tilted her head to the left, looking past Gavilán and squinting as she focused on the people at the front door. Gavilán squinted back at Olga and squeezed her hands, whispering, "I've missed you too."

Olga redirected her focus to Gavilán and then scowled as she responded, "What!" Gavilán straighten to a vertical posture in surprise. Olga then continued, "Oh, I'm sorry, I thought that was them."

"That was who?" Gavilán asked with a puzzled look on his face.

"The two men from the CDC that we're supposed to meet here. Sorry, I forgot to tell you," she responded, still focused on the entrance.

"So who are these guys?" Gavilán inquired.

"Two men that I met at the conference," Olga replied. "They, or I should say the older gentleman, has views about food that are very similar to mine."

Still unable to make the connection, Gavilán asked, "So you invited them to share a meal with us so you can compare notes?"

"Not exactly," responded Olga. "The older man, Dr. Welch, thinks I need to hear something about the system. He thinks that I could get blackballed or spied on or both. He thinks that my behavior at the conference may provoke adverse consequences."

"What did you do that was so awful?" asked Gavilán, with tongue in cheek.

"Nothing," answered Olga defensively. "I just refused to play ball with Big Brother. But let's not talk about that. I'm sure you'll get an earful when they get here. Let's talk about the Powwow."

Gavilán sensed that Olga was trying to avoid the entire situation, starting with the current conversation. He was reluctantly accommodating, saying, "Okay, but that's still over a week away, and we'll have plenty of time to make plans on the way."

Olga reached forward, took Gavilán's hand, brought them together at the center of the table, and said, "It's one of my favorite topics, and it brings back fond memories of when we met. Humor me. I don't think we could possibly run out of things to talk about . . . even on a road trip of over two thousand miles."

"Okey dokey," he responded with a goofy look on his face. Gavilán knew he was like putty in her hands, although he tried not to show it.

〰〰〰〰〰〰〰〰〰〰〰〰〰〰〰〰〰〰〰〰〰〰〰〰〰〰〰〰

Olga thought she saw Dr. Welch and Sam walk in the entrance double door. "I think that's them," she said as she poked Gavilán's arm with her eyes firmly focused on the two men at the front of the restaurant.

As the new arrivals began to walk toward them, escorted by their hostess, Olga stood and waved, trying to be relatively inconspicuous. Dr. Welch saw Olga and doublestepped to catch up to his hostess, tapping her on the shoulder. He said something to her and pointed at Olga. They made a beeline straight to Olga and Gavilán's table.

Gavilán stood as they reached the table. The men shook hands, exchanging names, as men always do, but Olga sensed a special squeeze when Sam shook her hand. She instinctively looked at Gavilán and Dr. Welch to see if they had seen anything out of the ordinary in their handshake.

She convinced herself that she must have imagined the squeeze and began with introductions. "These are the two gentlemen I was telling you about, Gavilán, from the conference at the Space Center." Sam's steel-blue eyes were glued on her. As she spoke, Olga thought to herself, *No me equivoqué. Este cabrón me está ligando.* [I wasn't mistaken. This guy is staring at me.]

Getting right to the point of the meeting, Olga asked, "So tell me, Dr. Welch, what do I need to be leery of? Are they going to bug my office, monitor my phone calls, and follow me around like agents of KAOS?"

Gavilán thought to himself, *Get Smart, one of my favorites.*

"Well, Dr. Ramos, let's start by doing away with this 'doctor' formality. Just call me Billy Ruben."

Olga nodded and pointed at herself as she said, "Olga."

Billy Ruben continued, "Today, you have successfully set yourself apart from the rest, and the Department of Homeland Security took note of that fact. You are now being investigated, I am sure, along with everyone involved in your research program."

"But why?" questioned Olga. "What are they trying to extract from us?"

"I really don't know what they were looking for," answered Billy Ruben, "but it was clear that you weren't too eager to play ball."

"Initially, I though that my invitation came as a result of my computer-based observations of anomalies in space," Olga commented, "but I don't think that's the case any more. Why do you think you were invited?"

"Well, at first, I thought it was because of our statistical epidemiological analyses regarding cadmium, but it's obvious they don't give a damn about health issues."

Olga and Gavilán exchanged glances of skepticism.

When Olga again turned to Dr. Welch, he continued, "I'll tell you all about it another time. We'd best keep our visit short. They may have someone watching us right now for all we know. I just wanted to make certain that you knew that you're not alone. I have a strange feeling that our futures are going to be intertwined because of this conference."

The conversation about the conference shifted to more personal themes. Agent Cooper was Sam's fallback topic of conversation. He not only missed his dachshund, but Cooper was also always a great way to break the ice with the girls. *If only she didn't have that Mexican companion*, he thought to himself.

Running out of thing to say and desperate to keep the conversation going, Sam blurted out, "So why is it that I don't detect an accent when either of you speaks?"

Olga quickly responded, "I guess I watched too much TV as a child."

Cuauhtémoc, on the other hand, felt that the questions were getting somewhat insensitive and responded in a deep voice, "Oh, but I do have an accent, one of a Norteño [a person from the northern part of Mexico], but only when I'm speaking Spanish."

Trying to get back into the dog theme, Sam added, "I understand that you people are into Chihuahuas."

Feeling a tinge of jealousy mixed with healthy dose of resentment come over him, Gavilán could not contain himself. "Uh-huh, but my seester, chee has a Ladrador." Olga quickly turned to Gavilán with one eyebrow lowered.

Seeing a chance to correct Gavilán in front of Olga, Sam took the bait, saying, "You mean Labrador, with a *B*."

"No, man, I means La-dra-dor [barker], ju know?" responded Gavilán. "El pinche dog, Esé, hees barkeen all da time."

A repressed grin appeared on Olga's lips as she bowed her head and shook it gently in disbelief. Sam just looked stunned.

Gavilán felt a touch of guilt, knowing that Sam probably was at a disadvantage, not able to pick up the meaning of the bilingual play on words. To rectify the situation, Gavilán continued, "And my aunt, chee has a full-blooded Tearier."

Not realizing he had once again been set up, Sam responded, "Oh really, what kind? A Yorkie, a Jack Russell . . . ?"

Gavilán, in true form, continued, "Nooooh, man . . . a *Tear*ier, man, ju know. The little son-a-ma-beach tears up everyteen. Ju chould'a seen how he tore up my cousin's guitar case, ju know? I guess he wanted to get into music, ju know, Esé?" After examining the glazed look on Sam's face, Gavilán continued but in a low and accent-free voice, "It's a joke, man . . . you know . . . it's a joke.

Dr. Welch had remained silent during the spectacle. At this point, he interjected, "Yes, well . . . it's probably time for us to go back to our hotel rooms so that we can get some rest before the trip back to Atlanta in the morning. You know, I have a conference coming up in San Francisco, and if budget permits, I may drag Sam along, so maybe we'll cross paths soon, and we can talk some more then." He reached over patted Sam on the shoulder with his left hand and, in a low voice said, "Come on, son." He leaned forward to get up from his chair.

Sam, still with a puzzled look on his face, gazed at Olga and responded, "Yes, sir."

Almost in unison, Olga and Gavilán said, "Good night, Dr. Welch." Olga continued, "Thank you for sharing your insight into what lies ahead and your kind words of warning and wisdom."

"I have your cell number," Dr. Welch responded, "and rest assured I'll be in touch."

Gavilán reached over and shook Sam's hand as the two men stood up from the table. "Good night, Sam. It was a pleasure, and I'm sure we'll be in touch."

Olga echoed with a gentle, "Good night, Sam."

As they watched the two men walking away from the table toward the register, Olga asked in a low voice, "Where did you pick that up? You're not a vato from the barrio."

"No, but I'm a quick study, and I've worked with my share of boys from the hood," he responded. "Besides," he continued, "it's a comfortable role for this *homeboy* from down south."

Olga turned to look directly at Gavilán, saying as she gently shook her head, "You never cease to amaze me." The two began to giggle like adolescents who had successfully pulled off a prank.

❑❑❑❑❑❑❑❑❑❑❑❑❑❑❑❑❑❑❑❑❑❑❑❑❑❑❑❑❑❑❑❑

Gavilán wrote something on his napkin and slid it across the table to the right of Olga's plate. Olga read the note. *Don't look now, but I think we have company.* She raised her head and looked at Gavilán squarely in the eyes. He lowered his head slightly, raised his left eyebrow, and glanced to his left, moving only his eyes.

"I feel a sudden urge coming on," Olga said in a low tone. "Excuse me, but I have to go to the ladies' room." Olga slid to the right and out of her chair. She walked up the aisle, trying to be inconspicuous as she looked at the faces of the people sitting at their tables.

She had gone about thirty feet, stopped, and then doubled back and sat down directly in front of her observer. "Hi, I don't think that we've formally met, but I remember seeing you at the conference at the Space Center." She didn't stop to take a breath, continuing, "My name is Olga, and if you want to know anything about me, just ask. That way, you don't have to waste your time sitting there, spying on me in the hopes that I *may* mention something that you *may* want to hear. That will save you a lot of time and save the taxpayers that pay your salary a lot of money." She reached forward, grabbed the earbud from his left ear, and tossed it on the table before him, finishing her thought with, "By the way, transistor radios went out of style decades ago."

The blond-headed young man in the dark-blue suit was totally taken aback and visibly shaken, and he sat in complete silence—stunned.

"What's your name?" Olga inquired.

"S-S-S-S-S-Stevenson. Bob S-S-Stevenson, ma'am." He continued apologetically, "I'm sorry to intrude on your privacy, but I'm just doing my job."

"Well, then do your job right." She leaned over and whispered in his ear, "I'm not supposed to know that you're spying on me." She got up from the table and walked back to where Gavilán sat, smirking at what he had just witnessed.

As Olga sat down, Gavilán said in a loud whisper, "I couldn't hear it all, but I didn't have to. Pobre tartamudo." [Poor stutterer.]

"I think he'll leave us alone now," Olga said confidently. Gavilán motioned for her to turn around, and they both watched Agent Stevenson walk up to the cashier, pay his bill, and leave.

"So what's that all about?" asked Gavilán.

Olga shook her head slowly, saying in a confused tone, "I'm not really sure. But back at the conference—or should I call it an inquisition?—there was a lot of interest in government projects dealing with space travel."

"What? Is our government getting so paranoid that now we're looking for little green men?" Gavilán said jokingly. "I know that the folks at Homeland Security are on the lookout for aliens, but I thought that was the non-U.S. citizen variety . . . [*he automatically switched to his vato alter ego and continued*] ju [you] know . . . da [the] ones from my hood, not aliens dat [that] are from outa dis [this] world." He grinned and looked at Olga as though he were seeking her approval, but she seemed lost in thought, gazing over his shoulder, almost as though she were in a trance. Gavilán slowly waved his hand, palm extended, back and forth in front of her face.

Olga seemed to snap back to the present, saying, "You know, in the years I've worked for NASA at the JPL, I've heard a lot of weird stories, and although some of them were pretty hard to believe, they usually turned out to be true."

Gavilán inquired, "Oh yeah? Like . . . ?"

Olga picked up the ball, continuing, "Like, I couldn't imagine that the people responsible for demonstrating progress on Reagan's Star Wars program would have falsified a demonstration of progress on the project by sending up a rigged plane, one loaded with explosives that were programmed to explode when the trigger was pulled. Reagan's ray gun didn't even have to come close to hitting the mark to have a successful demo that would ensure continued funding."

Gavilán squinted and uttered a wimpy, "What?"

Olga tilted her head slightly as she said, "You heard me." She continued, "And then there's 'aliens.' I've heard my share of alien stories, but some of the accounts about the incident at Roswell, New Mexico, are pretty convincing."

"Are you talking about the alleged crash of an alien spacecraft out in the New Mexico desert in the late forties?" inquired Gavilán incredulously.

"Yep," she answered slowly, as though she were auditioning for a part in a Western. "Having a secret clearance and knowing what I know about the requirements for declassifying secret documents, I can't help but wonder why so many of the related documents that originated from that incident are still classified and unavailable to the public." Gavilán was puzzled, but this was starting to sound interesting.

Olga continued, "What was really taken to Area 51 in Nevada, and what happened within the confines of Hangar 18? You know, I heard that not too long ago, the government even bought two nearby mountain peaks, Freedom Ridge and White Sides, to remove them from public access. I guess they didn't want anyone looking over their shoulder even if it was from who knows how many miles away."

Gavilán could see that she was agitated. He took her hands in his and said, "Just calm down. EGBAR."

"What?" Olga said with a squint of her eyes.

"EGBAR—everything's going to be all right. E-G-B-A-R," Gavilán explained. "Just watch, everything will calm down, and things will get back to normal. You'll see. We need to just go about our business as usual."

Still squinting, Olga responded, "You don't really mean that, do you?"

"Well, we're still on for the Powwow, right?" asked Gavilán. Olga nodded slowly. "Well then, why don't we just swing over to Roswell?

It's not that much out of our way. Heck, neither is Area 51. Let's just swing by Area 51, knock on their door, and ask—"

Olga scowled, saying "Very funny!" as she punched Gavilán in the arm. But the look on her face turned pensive. "We can't just go up and knock on the door, but you know, that may not be such a bad idea. We could go to Roswell and snoop around a little. Then we could drive up toward Las Vegas—"

Gavilán abruptly interrupted, "I'm game!"

"I don't know where this will take us, but I brought my HRDC and my laptop." Olga paused because she saw a querying look come over Gavilán's face. She explained, "HRDC—that's high-resolution digital camera. I know that Area 51 is off limits, but if we could find a few good vantage points, I can take photos with my HRDC, and we can enhance them later. Maybe there will be *something* that will give us a clue as to what makes Hangar 18 such a mysterious place even today, more than sixty years after the alleged crash of an alien spacecraft." She seemed a bit unsure of herself, something Gavilán had never before seen in her. *She* was always the cause, making things happen. But in this case, it was uncharted territory, an area that government and military officials controlled in the name of national security, motherhood, and apple pie.

Gavilán's reassuring tone of voice was resolute. "You get your camera warmed up, and we'll get you those vantage points."

CADMIUM POISONING

FACTS

- The lunch at the NASA conference was a high-cadmium meal. Lettuce and mushrooms along with the dinner rolls, pasta, shrimp, and coffee are all packed with cadmium. Linguini and, in fact, most wheat-based pastas are made with Durham wheat, a strain that is higher in cadmium content than other strains normally used in making flour for baking bread. Broccoli, on the other hand, is high in sulfur, vitamin C, and magnesium, and it is a good addition to any low-cadmium meal.

- The dessert was laden with toxic cadmium. Chocolate, in any form, along with wheat and sugar make devil's food cake with chocolate icing a delicious but highly toxic dessert (appropriately named "devil's food"). The coffee just added insult to injury.

- Making adjustments in your diet doesn't mean that you have to give up all your favorite foods. Quinoa and corn pastas are suitable substitutes for wheat pasta, which is made from Durham wheat. Try quinoa as a substitute for rice: boiled—or better yet, prepared in a pressure cooker. Use it as a base over which you can spread your favorite saucy entree (e.g., Indian dishes). Oat-flour pancakes make a great substitute for flour-based pancakes. Get creative and toss in a mashed banana, chopped nuts, or anything you may have thought of but were afraid to try in the past—as long as it is low in cadmium.

- *Woman's World*, June 14, 2010: "*Earlier diabetes screenings recommended* American Diabetes Association scientists now say anyone with one of the top two risk factors for the condition—being very overweight or having a family history—should be screened beginning at age 30. Early diagnosis and treatment can prevent diabetes-related complications, including heart attacks." Being "very overweight" and "having a family history"—both are potentially linked to cadmium poisoning. When one overeats, the excess calories are accompanied by not only extra pounds, but also by extra cadmium, a metal with a biological half-life of approximately 30 years in the human body. In a relatively recent study, a significant inverse correlation was found between food consumption and life span. The conclusion of the study is correct, but the villain is not food; rather, it is the cadmium that it contains. Furthermore, the impact of cadmium on the thyroid can slow the metabolism, exacerbating the situation regarding weight gain. As for the family history, children who grow up in a family accustomed to a high-cadmium diet are likely to continue with that diet after they leave their parents' home. In other words, *it is learned behavior* (i.e., the food we eat) *more than genetics that causes family history to be a risk factor for diabetes.*

• The predisposition to osteoporosis in women is not genetic either but is rather largely due to the incorporation of impurities like cadmium in the bone structure and set by the late teens. The best thing for young girls who want to avoid osteoporosis in their later years is to stay away from soft drinks, white wheat products, white rice, chocolate, and all high-cadmium foods and beverages.

Chapter Seven

The Ancients

It was early on a hot Treretumian morning that Nivla contemplated his youth as he groomed himself, preparing for a visit with Oleub, his grandfather. Over the years, Nivla and his two brothers had heard many stories from Oleub. Oleub's was a strong personality, and his impact on his grandchildren's lives had been enormous.

Oleub had told his grandsons at an early age that his wish for them was to share an unwavering love of family and an understanding of the universe around them. Oleub had gained peace and serenity through that fundamental understanding and the unquenchable thirst for knowledge that enhanced it. He had always tried to instill curiosity in his grandchildren, knowing it would help them find that understanding by literally reaching for the stars. He felt that only then would progress toward peace, prosperity, and equality be forthcoming for them, for their individual families, and for everyone around them. Because of Oleub's knack for communicating his experiences and views, his grandsons were exposed to many ideas and stories that others of their generation would never hear. His stories stimulated their imaginations, taking them to places beyond physical limits, creating horizons as expansive as the universe itself. Over the years, the three lads had grown into strong Kcalb Clansman, clansmen of whom Oleub was very proud. But now, only two of his grandsons survived.

On this day, Nivla was to pay a visit to his grandfather to make a date—to take his grandfather to the market, a trip he knew Oleub would relish, largely because of the interaction with everyone at this traditional Treretumian meeting place. As he got into his transport capsule, Nivla thought back, recalling one evening when Oleub described the oscillating nature of the universe to him and his brothers . . . .

ᛘᛘᛘᛘᛘᛘᛘᛘᛘᛘᛘᛘᛘᛘᛘᛘᛘᛘᛘᛘᛘᛘᛘᛘᛘᛘᛘᛘ

"Tell us, Grandfather. Tell us about the beginning," requested an inquisitive Nomis, with his brothers, Nivla and Rodoet, at his side.

"Well, all right," responded the old one as he and his grandsons all leaned forward in their seats, preparing for another grand story. "The universe that we perceive is in a mode of oscillation, with the period of this oscillation being many billions of years. It expands, and it contracts, only to begin the cycle anew. With each expansion, the action of gravity slows the expansion to the point that it comes to a complete halt. The continued action of gravity causes the mass of the universe to come together, accelerating toward its center for billions of years. And the result is an era of cataclysmic impacts, explosions, and interconversion between mass and energy, which is how the expansion of our universe started in the first place."

The lads looked at each other in anticipation. "Tell us more about the explosions," blurted out Nomis, the eldest of the three. "One of my friends at school told me about a big explosion."

Oleub looked at Nomis as he slowly raised his left hand, saying, "Patience, my child." He then continued, "The cycle is periodic, predictable, and likely damped. With each cycle, the interconversion between matter and energy becomes so fluid in the shared confines of 'the kernel' that is formed from the accumulating matter and energy of the universe, that matter and energy become virtually indistinguishable. Gravity at the center of the kernel, to which all is being drawn, creates a gigantic black hole from which nothing is able to can escape."

"How can you tell that anything is going on in the kernel if nothing can escape it?" inquired Nivla.

"That's a good question," responded the Ancient One. "No one has ever been through this experience, but we speculate that this will be the case, based on, among other things, black holes that have been studied. You will learn the details of black hole detection methods in your studies at school."

He then continued, "With the decrease in space as the contraction progresses, the outward appearance to the rest of the expansive universe is empty space and darkness—a cold, motionless nothingness. Smaller black holes appear because of nonuniformities in the distribution of mass across the universe, and the proximity of their paths to the center leads them to coalesce, sucking in everything in their paths."

Oleub continued, slowing his speech and lowering his voice as he spoke, "Eventually, virtually all matter and energy, including light and high-energy radiation are drawn in . . . and the space that they occupy keeps shrinking—smaller and smaller."

The three lads were drawn in, leaning forward, getting closer and closer to Oleub and each other. The Ancient One continued in a whisper, "And then . . ."

Oleub jerked back, stomping his foot on the floor, yelling, "*Boom*!" The three startled grandsons jolted backward as he continued in a normal voice, "The Explosion of Conception, a tremendous release of energy—an explosion of sorts that sends the mass of the universe flying away from its center . . . vast distances in a fraction of a second."

Yes, Nivla thought to himself, *my Oleub is quite a story teller.*

ꝓꝓꝓꝓꝓꝓꝓꝓꝓꝓꝓꝓꝓꝓꝓꝓꝓꝓꝓꝓꝓꝓꝓꝓꝓꝓꝓꝓ

Nivla approached the steps of the home of his grandparents. Oleub stood leaning forward, resting his elbows atop one of the twin pillars at the gateway to his property. He was old and wrinkled, as were most of the Ancients, with dark leathery skin that demonstrated his exposure to the elements on their planet. His shoulders slumped forward slightly, and his posture was poor, but his eyes sparkled with the many centuries of experiences that he was always eager to share with his grandsons.

As Nivla approached the top of the steps, his grandfather spoke. "Molahs, oim otein." ["Hello, my grandson."] The old one was decked out in his finest cream-colored hooded robe with a light-tan sash, all of which contrasted against his dark skin.

"Etiam Oleub," ["Beloved Oleub,"] responded Nivla as the two Kcalb Clansmen began a dance, with the two raising their hands into the air, spinning around like planets spinning on their axes. Then Nivla began to circle around his grandfather, coming closer and closer as they continued to spin. Finally, they caught each other in their arms as they came to a complete stop. It was clear that Oleub was exhausted from the greeting, but Nivla's embrace helped to support him. "Come, Oleub, let us go inside." They turned toward the opening to Oleub's home, what appeared to be a dark cave with massive doors at the entrance into the side of a mountain.

֍֍֍֍֍֍֍֍֍֍֍֍֍֍֍֍֍֍֍֍֍֍֍֍֍֍֍֍֍֍

On the agreed-upon day of the trip to the market, Nivla arrived at his grandparents' home to find his grandparents, Oleub and Aleub, sitting on a bench about ten paces behind the two pillars at the gate in front of the entrance to their home—waiting for Nivla's arrival. The couple had shared several bak'tuns (about four hundred years per bak'tun) together, and perhaps their time together had caused a similarity to emerge in their appearances. Both had decreased in stature since their wedding day, slightly hunched over due to their advanced age, to the many physically challenging experiences of their lifetimes, and to their relatively sedentary lifestyle. In part, it was also a sign that they were "tired" and ready to relinquish their responsibilities of guiding their families and community, passing them on to the next generation.

His grandfather, Oleub, was decked out in his finest cream-colored, hooded attire, complemented by a light-tan sash, all of which contrasted against his dark skin. His grandmother, Aleub, was dressed in a pale-green garment with a pastel-yellow sash around her waist. The light colors also contrasted against her skin, which was several shades lighter than her husband's

As Nivla approached, his grandmother rose gracefully as she stepped away from the bench, lifted her hands in the air, and began to turn slowly 'round and 'round. She was tiny in comparison to the two males she accompanied. Nivla followed her example, spinning like a top as he circled around her, stopping with an embrace that seemed to engulf the diminutive female. Their greeting dance symbolized the motion of a star and its planets. The central star was the parent or grandparent that shed light on its offspring, while the more energetic planet orbited the parent star, benefiting from its mere presence. There was joy in the dance between this grandmother and grandson that was very apparent and shone as bright as any star in the night sky.

"She always loved to dance," Oleub muttered.

"Molahs, Aleub!" Nivla shouted enthusiastically and affectionately as his embrace tightened slightly. She responded by wrapping her long arms around his middle, squeezing surprisingly hard, bringing a look of astonishment on Nivla's face as he abandoned his grip and raised his arms into the air. As she loosened her embrace, Nivla took her by the arms and gently guided her back to the bench. "How is my Aleub?" Without saying a word, the tiny female bobbed her head in positive gesture, an expression of well-being. "We are going to the market," declared Nivla. "Aleub, what can I bring you?"

"You should know by now," she said. "Some fruit, of course. Fruit from tall trees."

The massive specimen responded, "Ahhh! Of course . . . fruit from tall trees. Fruit from tall trees because the fruit grows far from whatever contaminants the soils may contain. Indeed, I remember your teachings. The trees serve many functions in our lives, including the filtering of fluids that nourish their fruit, which in turn, nourish our bodies." With great affection, Nivla went on, "Aleub, since my birth, you have taught me so many things. And when my brothers came, you taught us all, sharing your love in every lesson. You taught us well. For that, I am eternally grateful, and you have two grandsons who will protect you over the bak'tuns."

The wrinkled female stepped up to Nivla and pressed the side of her face to his chest. Tears began to stream down her face. "Nivla, I hear your good, strong heart, and I know that you and your brother are concerned about our well-being. But I had three grandsons, and neither my Nomis nor I can rest until his remains are returned home."

"I know, Aleub. Believe me, I have not forgotten," Nivla uttered, consolingly. "The proper time is approaching, and I promise by all that I hold sacred, I will return Nomis home."

Nivla's grandfather had silently observed the emotional interaction between his wife and her grandson, but it was time to change themes and move on. "Somav, Nivla," ["Let's go, Nivla"] he said loudly. "The market will be shutting down soon."

Nivla kissed his grandmother on the top of her head, and as the two slowly separated, he said, "Aleub, all will be resolved soon." He turned and walked a few steps toward his grandfather and reached out with his strong and massive hand as he said, "Somav, Oleub."

They slowly walked to the front of the property. Nivla helped his aging grandfather into his sleek antigravity transport capsule. The capsule was roughly the shape of half a football, sliced in half along its longitudinal axis, with rounded ends and edges. The entire upper portion of the capsule was made of a transparent material. Upon Nivla's command, "open," a panel that comprised half of the middle third of the capsule slid over the other half of the middle third of the vehicle, exposing a large open-top entrance and seats for passengers. After the two Treretumians were seated, Nivla uttered two words: "Destination, market." A voice from the vehicle asked, "Urgency?" and Nivla responded, "Low."

The entrance panel slid closed, seat belts automatically strapped them into their seats, and the vehicle lifted off the ground. It quickly reached the area transport corridor and began to move into the closest transport lane, easily merging into traffic at the speed of the surrounding vehicles. They propelled effortlessly and silently. As with all Treretumian transport vehicles, Nivla's capsule was programmed to share information with the vehicles around it. This enabled coordination and synchronization of vehicles in all transport lanes. The end result: safe, comfortable, collision-free transport.

Not having to focus on the transport capsule, Nivla asked Oleub many questions, trying to gain insight into the current society on his planet. "Grandfather, tell me again about the beginning of the 'New Treretum' events of your childhood."

The Ancient One loved to share stories of the past with his grandsons, but he was a little surprised that Nivla would show interest in the less scientific aspects of their planet's history. Oleub began, "This world in which we and all Treretumians live went through an evolution that included a time of exploration and diversification, a time of great turmoil and internal violence, a time of progress and great change, a time of unification, and a time of growing disparity. This growing disparity represents the beginning of the end of the Old Treretum on which three races—three clans—had evolved. The three were of a single primordial origin, but descendants that took different paths, inhabited different environments, and evolved in different ways to adapt to those environments."

"So the differences we see between say the Kcalb and Drutsab Clans are due to evolution in different parts of the planet," commented Nivla.

"Exactly," affirmed Oleub. "About five and one half bak'tuns [over two millennia] before, leaders of the three ruling clans convened in a clandestine meeting to examine common problems and to piece together a unifying solution, with the various elements of that solution being offered openly without regard to the clan of origin. Several problem topics were discussed that all three clans had in common. They focused on three common goals that truly united them." The Ancient One raised his right hand, extending the three fingers at the end of his hand, one at a time, as he recited the goals, "Control of the masses, extraction of wealth, and retention of power. This common ground led to many accords, including the agreement that this group of leaders would become the rulers of the planet."

"You mean this was the beginning of the Planetary Council?" asked Nivla.

"Correct," responded Oleub. "The foremost challenge for the rulers of the time was the control of the masses. The masses were out of control, doing only things that would bring them immediate gratification. They lacked refinement and were concerned with only the most basic issues such as food, shelter, and procreation in the most primal sense. The masses were of little education. Their primitive ways and lack of foresight caused their society to spiral into turmoil, with no trust in fellow Treretumians, and justifiably so. This was a time of great darkness that pervaded the planet." Oleub was impressed at the great interest that Nivla demonstrated in the history lesson. It was almost like old times with his three grandsons.

"So what did they do?" inquired Nivla.

"The solution that the rulers conceived during that meeting was one that required changing the way of thinking of the masses. The goal was manipulation by consent. *First*, events had to occur that would catch the attention of the masses. Then they had to get them to accept a doctrine—a doctrine that kept them under control. But how would they get them to accept the doctrine? What evolved in that meeting was a doctrine that contained elements to appeal to all three groups, but the control of the masses hinged on three elements—the tyrannical trinity of their doctrine—fear, unquestioning trust, and shame. The doctrine needed to be taught at widespread dissemination centers, built and supported by contributions from the masses."

"You said there were three elements that were required," interjected Nivla, "but accomplishing what you have described already sounds impossible. How could they possibly entice the masses to pay for multiple dissemination centers?"

"Patience, young one. Let me explain." Oleub continued, "Second on the agenda was the extraction of wealth—use of the masses to support the projects that would help the masses but, more importantly, benefit the rulers and the elite of their clans. The support could be in the way of contributed physical labor, contributed items of value, contributed currency—but initially everything had to be contributed. When someone gives out of his own volition, it gives him something to feel good about, something to be proud of, and the best part is that he won't come looking for something in return. And the more wealth that is amassed, the more responsible masses feel for the manifestation of the rulers' continued success. Performing a few well-publicized, beneficent acts encourages more giving.

"In contrast, when a person is taxed, forced to pay, he resents the act and looks for ways of circumventing the required payment. In addition, the forced payment of taxes serves as the seed that breeds unrest among the masses. The dissemination centers would also serve as collection points from which accumulated wealth would be sent to the rulers' governing center. And *third*—"

"Wait," interrupted Nivla. "I still don't see how this would entice the masses to pay and help build the dissemination centers . . . out of the goodness of their hearts? I think not."

The Ancient One responded, "These are pieces of a puzzle. All the pieces had to be in place for the puzzle to hold together. You will see. The *third* element of the plan was retention of power, which came with repeated public announcements and propaganda about isolated beneficent deeds. And with the amassed wealth, they bought the loyalty of a well-trained military force comprised, for the most part, of the young and naive. But propaganda about their good deeds was not enough, so that a control strategy was drafted. To achieve control required acceptance of the doctrine by the masses. The doctrine had to be a composite of the beliefs of the three clans. Some of the teachings naturally would be foreign to many because they would be more akin to those of one of the other clans, so they had to be adjusted and presented in a manner that would be palatable.

"The first element of the control strategy was *fear*. To instill fear in the populace was no simple thing. They had long ago embraced the notion of death and the honor of death for a cause that they considered just so that fear of death was not the answer. Instead, they took advantage of fear of the unknown and the possibility of an afterlife. It was impossible to prove, but it was also impossible to disprove. The process began by selecting three villages, one in each of the planet sectors—they were burned to the ground. When responsible parties were sought, the acts were attributed to Nitas, the evil ruler of the unseen dimension, someone whose existence could neither be proved nor disproved. Targeting groups in all three clans to receive the wrath of Nitas served not only to strike fear in the hearts of the masses but also to offer a great distraction, providing a common enemy against whom they could unite.

"The second element was *trust*. To instill trust, you indoctrinate the young. And for those that are a little older, you start by buying it. The Doctrine of the Protector was introduced through a compilation of stories, each with a moral to encourage the reader to assume the behavior sought by the rulers and, at the same time, strengthen trust in the Protector and his designated keepers of the doctrine. The doctrine included examples of good fortune for the believers in the doctrine and hardship that befell upon those who rejected it. Nitas's role in the maladies was made clear, as was the benevolent role of the rulers. It was important to personify the maladies with evil and treachery and to have a direct link between the rulers and the beneficiaries, placing the rulers in a position of honor and respect.

"The third element of the tyrannical trinity was *shame*. This was a simple matter. To instill shame, again, you indoctrinate the young, making certain that they know what shame is. A great list of Treretumian activities was compiled and categorized. The categories ranged from the *Nis* to the *Yloh*. Behavior that was discouraged was labeled *Nis*, and at the other end of the spectrum, behavior that was encouraged and would directly or indirectly benefit the rulers was labeled *Yloh*. As with the Doctrine of the Protector, the conflict between the Nis and the Yloh was explained through stories. They were interwoven with other stories of the Doctrine of the Protector, with the Protector directly involved in defining the nature of the Nis and the Yloh."

After hearing the additional details, Nivla nodded his head, saying, "I see . . . now I see."

"The wholesale modification of the behavior of a planet's inhabitants was no simple undertaking," continued Oleub. "As I mentioned, key to the success of the project was the indoctrination of the young. Their indoctrination would ensure continued compliance for future generations. Although it took generations to achieve, the unifying effect of the Doctrine of the Protector was largely responsible for the survival of the Treretumians after the invasion of the Muimdac. This event was viewed by many as the moment in the history of Treretum when the clans truly put aside their difference and united against a common enemy. However, it was also a pivotal time in the direction of the leadership of the planet.

"Until then, the rulers had consisted of a council composed by an equal number of members of each of the three clans.

"You mean that members of our clan were partly responsible for the second-rate citizen status that has been imposed on us, at least during my lifetime?" questioned Nivla in a tone of semioutrage.

"Yes, my young one, betrayed by Kcalb Clansmen who were overcome by greed and self-interest," uttered Oleub in a tone of disgust. "What they did not seem to realize was that the other members of the rulers were just as treacherous as they and that loyalty among the group of usurpers was not a prerequisite for membership in their elite group. Because members of all but the Drutsab Clan were reported to have been contaminated by the Muimdac, the Drutsab Clan seized power by having the other rulers hanged and incinerating their bodies. The source of those reports was never identified, and because of the turmoil associated with the invasion of the Muimdac, the actions of the rulers went uncontested. And the Drutsab assumed their self-proclaimed role of the 'supreme race' on the planet."

Just then, their vehicle came to a stop. They had arrived at the market—a bazaar where vendors from far and near sold their wares. They emerged from the vehicle. Nivla pulled a small device from a pocket in his sleeve and pressed a button. The door to the vehicle closed, and the vehicle departed to find a spot in a nearby parking area.

The market was full of movement, full of life, and full of the hustle and bustle of any major commercial area. They walked a few yards and were soon surrounded by colorful products and colorfully dressed vendors and buyers alike. They walked a little further, and Oleub saw one of his old cronies. "Nivla," he said as he patted his large grandson on the back. "You go on and make your purchases for your grandmother while I stop and rest here with my old friend. I'm sure we'll have some stories to exchange."

CADMIUM POISONING

FACTS

- The cancer treatment and diet professed by Dr. Max Gerson focused on fresh raw fruits and vegetables. Films like *The Gerson Miracle* and *The Beautiful Truth* tell the story. One believer of that dietary philosophy who followed the Gerson regimen lived to be 117 years old.

- The comparison of metal content of tissue samples taken from the brains of deceased Alzheimer's patients versus non-Alzheimer's patients showed elevated concentrations of one or more of various metals in the Alzheimer's victims, including aluminum, lead, mercury, iron, and manganese. Present in the normal brain samples but conspicuously absent from the Alzheimer's samples was zinc, a metal that is essential for proper brain function. Cadmium concentrates in other organs, but it competes with zinc, and it is a direct cause of zinc deficiencies. Zinc deficiencies elsewhere in the body rob zinc from the brain, suggesting that Alzheimer's disease is an indirect symptom of cadmium poisoning.

- A general rule that you can follow to minimize cadmium consumption is that foods that grow in the ground or near the ground surface are likely high in cadmium, while foods that grow on trees or long stalks or vines are generally low in cadmium. Of course, there are exceptions to the rule.

- The oceans are an abused medium that was thought to be an inexhaustible pool of natural resources, and infinitely vast repository for our waste. A group of researchers estimated that millions of tons of cadmium are being discharged to the ocean yearly. However, calculations indicated that the rising concentration in the ocean was not increasing at a rate commensurate with the amount being discharged. It was postulated that the concentration of cadmium in the oceans was not rising as would be predicted due to precipitation of cadmium with one or more anions present in ocean water, sending the cadmium-laden precipitate to the bottom of the ocean floor. To test the theory, basic experiments were performed in the laboratory to assess the potential for precipitation of cadmium with carbonates, sulfates, and phosphates. The results indicated that cadmium did indeed precipitate or coprecipitate, not with carbonates or sulfates, but definitely with phosphates. Reading about the coprecipitation of cadmium with, for example, calcium phosphate and the less-than-expected increase in the cadmium concentration in the oceans, I thought about the implications regarding sodium phosphate, calcium phosphate, potassium phosphate, and other phosphate additives to our food supply. Without taking extraordinary measures, phosphate food additives are likely contaminated with cadmium.

- Sugar beets are used in the phytoremediation (removal of contaminants by plants) of cadmium-contaminated soils, with the beet tops having roughly three times the concentration compared to the beets that grow beneath the surface of the contaminated ground. Unfortunately, approximately 56% of our nation's sugar comes from sugar beets, making any product containing sugar suspect as a high-cadmium product.

Chapter Eight

Status and Strategy

Stevenson sat in the air-conditioned office with a view toward the southeast. The office was high enough to overlook part of the downtown skyline and the Gulf Freeway trailing off into the distance. He sat erect, patiently awaiting the arrival of Mr. Blakey so that he could report on the status of his surveillance.

The contrast made between his fair skin and light-brown hair and his sparkling dark-blue eyes seemed accented by the sunlight that poured in through the window, drenching the left side of his head and torso. He would have fit the mold of one of the DHS's fair-haired boys, except his hair was always disheveled. During his childhood, people often called him John-Boy after the character from *The Waltons* because of his hair and the mole on his cheek. There was one more thing about Stevenson that was not apparent at first glance. It was only revealed when he was nervous or agitated, but it was yet another thing that set him apart—he stuttered.

Blakey—dressed in a black suit, white shirt, and red tie—entered the room, walking briskly to the leather, executive's chair behind the desk. Stevenson instinctively jumped to his feet.

"Good morning, Agent Stevenson. Sit down, please," said Mr. Blakey as he took his seat behind the mahogany desk. "What good things do you have to tell me about Dr. Ramos this morning?"

Stevenson responded, "Good morning, sir. Well, Dr. Ramos met with three individuals, two from the conference that joined her and another man. He looked like he might be Middle Eastern, and they talked for a while before the other two got there. I caught part of the conversations, mostly between Dr. Ramos and the first man—they talked mostly about food and a trip to California, but I couldn't get it all."

Blakey leaned forward and lowered his head slightly. "Was anything said that could be construed as a breach of national security?" he inquired in a low matter-of-fact tone.

"Well, sir, I don't think so," responded Stevenson as he began to relax slightly from his rigid posture, "but I'm not sure because they kept throwin' in some Spanish, I think, and something else too." Blakey looked puzzled and wrinkled his brow. The two men looked into each other's eyes as Stevenson said, "Gaw-Vee-Lawn. She used that word in the conversation many times."

"Gaw-Vee-Lawn?" Blakey muttered. Then a light seemed to light in his head as he raised his right hand with forefinger extended, "Gavilán! Eagle! That must be part of some kind of a code."

Stevenson sensed that he was making inroads, and feeling more relaxed, he unbuttoned his suit coat, crossed his legs, and continued, "And another word Dr. Ramos used was Kwow-tem-oak, but not as often."

Blakey lowered his head and shook it slowly, left and right.

In an effort to keep his positive meeting alive, Stevenson impatiently interjected, "Then when two men from the conference arrived, they shared stories about diabetes and astronauts . . . and made dog jokes at the end of their meals. It was strange, almost as though they were trying to cut each other down."

"What!" exclaimed Blakey. "There must have been some embedded codes in those stories and the way they talked to each other."

"The two from the conference left, and shortly after that . . ." Stevenson paused and lowered his head slightly as he raised his right hand to contain a weak, forced cough. He continued in a low voice, "Dr. Ramos detected my surveillance and confronted me."

"*What!*" Blakey jumped to his feet. "Damn it, Stevenson, you blew it!" The young blonde quickly resumed his original rigid stance. Blakey was frustrated, and he could see the tension building in Stevenson. "You idiot! How could you let yourself be detected so easily?" Blakey noticed that Stevenson's neck seemed to thicken, and the veins in his neck began to bulge. This was the same reaction he had seen before when Stevenson was about to go into one of his stuttering episodes. Blakey reacted instinctively, going for the jugular, mocking, "S-S-S-S-Stevenson, you're just plain s-s-s-s-stupid!"

"S-S-S-S-Sir, in all due respect, I was s-s-s-s-spotted because she recognized me from the conference. I was setup for failure. If I hadn't been assigned duty at the conference—"

Blakey interrupted indignantly, "You were spotted because you exposed yourself to the person you were tailing. What about all the high-tech options you had at your disposal?

"But, sir, I thought—"

Again, Blakey interrupted in a roar, "You're not supposed to think. That's not in your job description!" He paused as he slowly walked around to the front of his desk. In a low voice, he continued, "There's a million ways that you can eavesdrop on her without being detected. Did she make any phone calls? Have you had her phone tapped?"

"But I didn't want to infringe on her civil rights," responded the young man apologetically.

"You're just supposed to do whatever it takes to get the job done!" exclaimed the man in the black suit. "For right now, you need to remember two things. One," he said as he shook his right hand, forefinger extended, "in our business, the ends always justify the means . . . *always*! And two"—Blakey lowered his hand and his voice to almost a whisper—"You never heard me say that." Blakey leaned forward to get in the face of the nervous young man. "You have your service revolver and all the resources of the department at your disposal."

Blakey saw Stevenson's brow start to wrinkle and the beginnings of a frown appear on his face. Blakey stood back up and glanced toward the ceiling as he mumbled, "Why can't they just send me all ex-military material?" He turned to Stevenson sharply and glared at him, shouting as he waved his hands, "With the passing of the Foreign Intelligence Surveillance Act, there's very little we can't do in the name of national security. So get your ass out of that chair and go do your job." Stevenson jumped to his feet as Blakey continued, "And I don't want to hear about any more of your pansy screwups!"

"Yes, sir," and out the door went Agent Robert Stevenson, intent on catching up with Dr. Ramos before she left her motel room. He had just gained a new perspective on his relationship with the law. He felt his discussion with Blakey had just lifted the limitations and restrictions he had previously been required to observe.

As he walked to the elevator, he thought to himself, *I've always wondered what that government-issued Ford Taurus could do full out on the highway. I guess we're going to find out as soon as I get on the Gulf Freeway.*

CADMIUM POISONING

FACTS

- Misguided strategies are often responsible for unexpected results. This is the case in many diets (e.g., high protein, low carb) that may show initial promise because they contain elements of a strategy that reduces cadmium intake.

- As with exercise, brain activity and development generates carbon dioxide, which helps to remove the toxins and heavy metals, while lack of use allows them to accumulate. If thinking is not in your job description, get a different job.

- There is growing evidence to support the theory that many of our society's behavioral abnormalities, such as autism and attention deficit hyperactivity disorder (ADHD), are linked to accumulation and/or imbalances of metals in the brain (e.g., zinc deficiency). In the article, "Natural cures for the procrastination disease, The mineral that keeps you calm," in *Woman's World* (Jan. 9, 2007), Meg Lundstrom writes, "It's zinc! It's crucial for helping your body absorb omega-3 fatty acids; plus, studies show that taking it reduces impulsiveness, a common problem for adults with ADHD." Also, some violent crimes are thought to have been triggered by, in part, heavy metal imbalances in the brain (e.g., accumulation of manganese). In a recent statistical study, the violent crime rate in New York City was shown to mirror the concentration of lead in the urban atmosphere due to tetraethyl lead (TEL) in gasoline—both a gradual rise after the use of TEL was initiated and the subsequent decline after it was banned. It is in our society's best interest to gain a better understanding of the link between mental illness and *metal* illness.

- Turmeric, a popular spice used in Indian cuisine, is said to reduce inflammation and arthritis pain when taken at a dosage of a teaspoon of per day. Curcumin, the active ingredient in turmeric, in addition to being a potent anti-inflammatory, is reportedly partially responsible for low cancer rates in a region of northern India (and Pakistan) where the spice is used extensively. (Caution: The characteristic yellow color of these spices can result in permanent staining.) The molecular structure of the spice makes it an effective chelant, binding with heavy metals like cadmium and facilitating their removal from the body. Treating inflammation with curcumin is treating the symptom, but more importantly, it is also treating the cause of the inflammation.

- The other key factor in the low incidence of cancer in northern India is vitamin B_{17}, found in apricot seeds (the kernel within the apricot pit). Vitamin B_{17}, also known as laetrile, was the center of controversy decades ago when people were going outside the United States to receive laetrile treatments because it was not acknowledged (nor is it today) as an acceptable cancer treatment by the established medical profession in the United States. However, stories of successful laetrile treatments abound. Laetrile is also found (but in lower concentrations) in the kernels from peach pits, apple seeds, and pear seeds. The laetrile molecule is composed of two glucose molecules, cyanide, and a benzaldehyde molecule. Reports are that the laetrile stays intact until it reaches a cancer cell, at which point it breaks apart. It was initially thought that the release of cyanide killed the cancer cells, but subsequent studies suggest that it is the benzaldehyde that is most toxic to the cancer cells.

- High levels of both cadmium and zinc have been reported to cause prostate cancer; however, the two metals are competing, and every cell in the body requires zinc. Furthermore, there are control mechanisms (e.g., metallothioneins) that tend to reduce the possibility of overdosing zinc. On the flip side, reducing zinc intake paves the way for further accumulation of the carcinogenic heavy metal, cadmium, not just in the prostate but throughout the body as well.

- In our society, we rely too much on doctors who seem to be nothing more than pill-dispensing representatives of the pharmaceutical companies—dispensing pills for everything from a prediabetic condition to high blood pressure to LDL-HDL cholesterol imbalances—you name it, they have a pill for it. Many of the pills that are dispensed simply suppress symptom of a potentially serious condition . . . like cadmium poisoning, as are the conditions just mentioned, for example. Furthermore, many of the medications have unwanted side effects. Before accepting the "pill solution," consider alternatives that are logical and nontoxic.

- For example, if you suffer from acid reflux at bedtime, consider alternatives including any and all of the following: (1) avoid spicy foods at suppertime; (2) eat an early, light supper (just lying down with a full stomach shifts the contents closer to the stomach inlet); (3) avoid drinking excessive volumes of liquids at the supper table (liquids flow more easily than solids); (4) sleep on your left side (since the stomach is oriented with the inlet on the right side); (5) sleep with your head and shoulders propped up on a couple of pillows (so that the acids from you stomach have to flow uphill); (6) drink a little milk before you retire for the night (since milk tends to sooth irritated tissues in the upper digestive track); and (7) chew a spearmint gum at bedtime (e.g., Eclipse in the green package—it also sooths irritated tissues).

- The human body can survive variations in its environment, changes in the available nutrients, and extremes in the physical demands placed upon it only because it has many self-regulating mechanisms (e.g., insulin synthesis, storage, and secretion; metallothionein synthesis and associated zinc sequestration/release; storage of sugars in the liver and subsequent release; and formation and storage of fat from surplus glucose for subsequent use). Cadmium poisoning is often accompanied by weight gain and difficulty in losing weight. Cadmium impacts the thyroid gland, typically slowing down the metabolism. In addition, synthesis of one of the body's primary fat-burning hormones is likely impacted, since it is generated in the same area of the pancreas as is insulin.

- o Irisin—hormone generated by muscle cells as a result of physical exertion
- o Leptin—hormone directly related to the amount of fat in one's body
- o Amylin—synthesized in the beta cells of the islets of Langerhans of the pancreas

Chapter Nine

Alien Observations

The massive Treretumian slowly but gracefully walked down the curved hallway, stopping at the portal leading to Egroeg's quarters. He was dressed in a loose-fitting robelike garment, maroon in color, with a white sash around his waist. The sleeve of his robe slid down his arm as he lifted his left to knock on the door. He turned his hand to tap the door gently with the back of his hand. In an instant, the door vanished, and he heard a voice from within the room beckon, "Come in, Sucram Suturb. I've been waiting for you."

He leaned forward, breaking the plane of the portal. He looked to the left as he walked. "Sir, I have my first report."

As though he were riding on a great wave, Egroeg entered the room, also in a loose-fitting white robe with a sky-blue sash around his waist, leading his entrance with one arm raised. "Good, Sucram. Please, sit down." Egroeg motioned to one of the larger cubes in the room, which contained numerous cubes of all sizes.

Suturb sat down as Egroeg continued, "One of the important parts of our mission to Earth is to assess the Earthlings, following our previous visits where we assisted their progress on most of the major land masses of their planet—the Egyptians, Hindi, Maya, Inca, and so on. We wanted to see them progress so that they could get to the point of conquering their environment and its impurities. Our ultimate goal is—"

At this point Suturb interrupted, "Yes, sir, I am familiar with our ultimate goal and vision for this planet." Suturb had not forgotten a previous conversation when he was cut off abruptly by Egroeg as he touched on the same topic.

"Well, yes . . . I am sure you have been briefed on the details of our mission," Egroeg responded, as though he were having to readjust his script to get himself back on task with the reason for Suturb's visit. Egroeg continued as he sat down in his favorite chair—a plush, velvety, canary-yellow chaise longue of sorts, made with several cubes as a base "So tell me, Sucram. Tell me of your findings."

Suturb pulled his briefing from his sleeve. It was in the form of a small cube, approximately three quarters of an inch on each edge. He set it on a medium-sized cube that served as a table in front of them and began to speak as a large holographic display emerged from the cube. "These are preliminary findings but appear to be consistent across the planet. Earthling humans are generally kind, trusting, initially inquisitive, protective of their own kind, easily influenced when subjected to stress—whether it is physical, emotional, or financial—and very misguided and misinformed. I have focused on two characteristics that intrigued me and appear to be pervasive—self-infliction of maladies and incomprehensible inconsistency in behavior."

Egroeg lowered his chin slightly as he moved his head back in a gesture that conveyed a degree of surprise and interest. He gestured with his hand as he nodded his head and said, "Go on, tell me more."

Suturb gently motioned at the hologram with his extended palm for a change in screen as he continued, "First, if I may, let me give you some of the subjects' characteristics."

"Yes, please do," urged Egroeg.

Suturb continued, "When the mother takes even minimal precautions to avoid exposure to toxins during her pregnancy, it is most common that her young will be healthy and well prepared to learn about the world into which the offspring is born. The mother's body creates a protective environment in which the fetus can develop. After birth, curiosity is inherent. The humanoid Earthlings learn by observing others, and often, the genuine interest and curiosity that they had at birth is stifled by what they see around them and the placation that they experience when they try to interact. In short, their developing brains are starved for constructive stimulation, and they are starved for nutrients. They are fed many strange products that are void of significant nutritional value and, on the contrary, contain trace concentrations of toxic materials that will harm them in the years to come.

"Before Earth circles their sun ten times, they have been poisoned by their own parents, they have become lazy, and they seek out food that is rich in poison that sends them closer to death each day. They have mastered the art of avoiding work and self-improvement and have joined the world of their elders. It is curious that they are placed in large groups for indoctrination, but the laziness pervades every aspect of their existence to the point that they take pride in how little they can get away with doing. In the process, they reject the opportunity to stimulate their brains . . . and the poison continues to accumulate.

"Their bodies are well designed, having natural mechanisms to fight off infectious disease, heal and repair damaged tissues, break down toxic organic compounds, sequester ingested toxic elements, balance trace nutrients that are potentially toxic at high concentrations, and locally acidify the blood to mobilize toxic elements that do accumulate in their bodies. However, problems arise when specific organs begin to malfunction or cease to function properly, either due to an injury or an ingested toxin.

"The self-inflicted maladies of the society, in general, are manifested in both passive and violent acts and in chronic poisoning of the masses. And this behavior can be seen on the part of individuals and governments alike. On an individual basis, for example, twice each year, on occasions they call Valentine's Day and Easter, they ingest large quantities of a particular dark, brown-colored, poisoned foodstuff they call chocolate, which is made from a derivative of a bean, the cacao, mixed with a sweetener. They usually use sugar as the sweetener, most of which is obtained from a root that is highly contaminated with cadmium. They add it, presumably to mask the flavor of the toxic substances contained in the bitter bean extract, and then mold the mixture into curious shapes. The toxic confections are typically wrapped colorfully and distributed on a large scale."

"How curious . . . Why would they knowingly distribute poisoned foodstuffs among their own people?" muttered Egroeg, almost as though he were talking to himself. "Or perhaps they do not know."

Suturb continued, "It is ironic that the sweets that the humans exchange as signs of love and affection on Valentine's Day are tainted with the ingredients of future pain and suffering. And Easter is even more amazing because humans seem to relish this event, increasing the rate of poisoning of their offspring by feeding them cadmium-laced chocolate in the shapes of eggs and indigenous long-eared rodents."

"Perhaps they do not know," reiterated Egroeg. "Do they always seek out tainted foods?"

"No, they don't. In fact, it is quite the contrary," answered Suturb. "They must know that something is wrong with their food supply," he continued as he paused the progress of his holographic presentation. "Why would Earthlings pay extra for products that *don't* contain certain ingredients rather than what they do contain? For example, they buy products because they are the gluten-free, sugar-free, decaffeinated, low-sodium, or low-fat option. Fortunes have been made selling sugar-free soft drinks, puddings, and other desserts to people who have malfunctioning pancreatic beta cells—they don't secrete insulin in response to increases in their blood sugar. What they may not realize is that they are largely treating a symptom by restricting sugar intake, while the cause of the problem may still be in the sugar-free products."

As he pointed downward, he continued, "Fifty-six percent of sugar in this country comes from sugar beets, a root that is extremely efficient at extracting cadmium from the soil. However, eliminating sugar does not eliminate all of the cadmium that is responsible for the toxicity of many foods and beverages. For example, cadmium is contained in additives such as phosphoric acid in soft drinks. Similarly, cadmium-tainted phosphate additives are used in many food products such as puddings, cheeses, canned milk, and processed meats that they consume daily."

"Interesting . . . Is cadmium the only toxic metal they only partially avoid?" inquired Egroeg as he stroked his chin.

"No," replied Suturb. "Some of those same people with the pancreas problem also avoid high-fructose corn syrup, and others avoid it without knowing why, but they know that there is something in the high-fructose corn syrup that is lethal, and they are willing to pay extra for products that do not contain it. They are correct, but in that case, the toxic metal is the element mercury, a contaminant in the material used to extract the fructose from the corn."

"This is sounding more like a puzzle that they cannot solve," interjected Egroeg. "Please, go on."

Suturb motioned to the hologram cube and continued, "Gluten-free products have become more popular because many people are allergic to some of the cultivated grains, like wheat. They have associated this intolerance to wheat gluten to something they call celiac disease. What they fail to realize is that there is a peculiar similarity between this disease and another intolerance and that they are likely sensitive to an element contained in the wheat gluten that is different from the gluten compounds they avoid. In fact, wheat gluten contains a higher concentration of this element than any other product from the processing of wheat."

"And that element is . . . ?" uttered Egroeg, motioning for Suturb to reveal the mystery element.

"Cadmium, sir. One of the two heavy metals contained in chocolate," Suturb replied.

"Aha! I knew it!" exclaimed Egroeg. "You know, things here are not that different from what they were on our planet a handful of bak'tuns ago."

Suturb's presentation was going well. He had Egroeg's full attention and participation in the presentation. He was touching on things that had occurred early in Treretum's history—problems Treretum was trying to help Earth avoid. Egroeg was engaged.

"Oh, before we leave the subject of chocolate and before I forget, what was the other heavy metal?" inquired Egroeg.

"Lead, a heavy metal that was used extensively in their ancient times to help contain their water supplies and led to the downfall of one of their great societies, the Romans, on another continent from the one over which we are hovering now. It is interesting that the Earthlings seem to be obsessed with foods that are made to taste sweet. In fact, for a time, lead—an element that was already known to be toxic— was used as a sweetener in the form of the compound lead acetate and added to their foods and beverages. More recently, it was used in paints and fuels. It is also interesting that the usage of lead in fuels led to considerable atmospheric contamination in densely populated areas and to an associated increase in violence and crime among the inhabitants." Suturb looked at Egroeg, who seemed puzzled, with his head slightly tilted, changing hands with which he stroked his chin. Suturb continued, "However, its use in paints and fuels has been banned, and there has been a corresponding decrease in the crime rate in the densely populated areas. But I digress, and unless you have additional questions about lead, I should continue."

"Yes, I have one. What have they done to control the lead contamination? It appears that lead is a big contamination problem, and it has been for many bak'tuns. You mentioned it was banned in paints and fuels. How did they get the problem under control?" Egroeg queried.

Suturb replied, "They restricted the use of the metal through governmental legislation—laws that prohibit its use in specific applications that led to widespread contamination of their environment— and they removed it from many places where humans were being exposed. Also, they have governmental organizations that are supposed to protect the public by monitoring and identifying illicit activities and screening proposed activities and new products that could introduce toxic compounds into their environment. The organization that we just probed to obtain our initial data is one of those organizations. But they are not always effective and sometimes appear to just look the other way, ignoring major issues like cadmium.

"Getting back to the characteristics of the individual Earthlings," he continued as he and Egroeg exchanged nods, "they have an aversion for responsibility, perhaps from fear of reprimand should an activity go awry and the intended result not achieved. They want others to be responsible for their actions or lack thereof, to the extent that they have a designated group that is in charge of their health, because they are afraid or incapable of doing so themselves, from all the years of practicing 'responsibility aversion.' The individuals that are in charge of health issues are called *doctors*, and they are protected by a smaller band of their brotherhood that have great influence with the government and power over information that is disseminated to the masses. They attempt to discredit information, individuals, and other health-related groups that are not to their liking.

"Although an oath is not required, and many members take their responsibility of helping their fellow humans in need seriously, just as many members of their brotherhood feel prohibited from identifying those who are not acting in the best interest of their clients. Many members of the brotherhood are competent, but there are many who are not, discouraging their patients from attempting any alternative remedy for their ailment if they did not prescribe it. What they prescribe is often the latest, most expensive drugs from a powerful group of manufactures/distributors that again treat symptoms rather than causes. Together, they appear to be in collusion with organizations that operate facilities where humans go to receive treatment and to die.

"Many of the members of the brotherhood have financial interests in those facilities, and many of the treatments and diagnostic testing prescribed are expensive, unnecessary, and even harmful to the clients. And although it is not the goal of many, the overall goal of the brotherhood and the elite band that directs them is short-term financial gain and to perpetuate health problems among their clients, maintaining status quo with regard to their position in society and enabling them to continue extracting financial resources from the masses in the future. This is a pervasive theme in corporations, but I will delve into that further later in the briefing."

"Interesting," interjected Egroeg. "From what you say, Sucram, it appears that the actions of individual groups are driven by self-interest rather than progress of the entire society. That alone could impede progress of the society as a whole, so that perhaps it is more than just heavy metals that have stunted the progress we were expecting."

"Yes, sir," responded Suturb. "This brotherhood is one of many similar groups they call *professions*, and to some degree, they all appear to have self-serving interests and are guided by elite groups or individuals. Apparently, this dates back to the one that most credit as being the oldest of all the professions on the planet."

Suturb took a deep breath. Egroeg motioned with his hand as he said, "Please continue."

With another hand gesture to the holographic display cube, Suturb continued, "Like their elders, the youth of their society seek immediate gratification in almost everything they do, and the pervading opinion seems to be that everyone has to, as they say, 'party hearty.' There is little interest in finding root causes of problems and there are only few that believe in a phrase that is also commonly used—'cause and effect.' They may even know that something will affect them adversely, but if the impact isn't immediate and severe, it doesn't seem to matter. They will continue the harmful activity, disregarding still another phrase that is commonly used—'delayed reaction.'

"The masses appear to live from one event to the next. The anticipation of the next break is the focus, and the business of true societal progress becomes secondary at best. The events are distributed throughout planet's cycle around the sun, what they call a year, and each event is associated with the spending of money and consumption of foods and beverages that adversely affect their health. It seems that many of these events are planned by a select few to simply extract financial resources from the masses. On Earth, they divide their year into twelve segments they call months, and each month has at least one—but in most instances, two—events. Two that I found particularly interesting were Valentine's Day and Easter, as I noted previously. However, another event that is held at only a few locations and at slightly different times of the year, where the humanoid Earthlings consume some of the most highly contaminated sea creatures on the planet—oysters. They call the event an oyster bake, and the oysters that they consume are what they call bottom dwellers, and they grow in areas where the cadmium concentration in their waters are the greatest."

Egroeg was impressed with the factual material presented but more with the nuances in the local societies that Suturb was able to interpret from the limited data and in the short time frame he was given to prepare his briefing. During the reporting session, Egroeg had become intrigued with Suturb's background. He probed Suturb regarding his position in his clan and his ambitions. He entertained the possibility of taking the Kcalb Clansman into his personal service.

It was evident to Egroeg that Sucram Suturb had put a substantial effort into the research and preparation of the presentation he had just witnessed. It was well done, it showed initiative, and it demonstrated thoughtful analysis by the Kcalb. *This Kcalb could truly be of value in the future*, he thought to himself. *His loyalty could lead to great influence among other members of the Kcalb Clan. I must reward him.*

Out of a pocket within his left sleeve, Egroeg pulled a trinket that one of the members of an earlier scouting party had brought back to demonstrate the primitive technologies that had been and were still being used on Earth. It was a cheap, solid-black digital wristwatch with a wristband made of a rubbery material. It displayed the time, month, and day on its otherwise black face. In a much softer tone than usual, Egroeg began to speak as he extended his open hand with the watch draped over his palm. "Sucram, please accept this as a small token of my appreciation. You have surpassed my expectations, and this is just my way of saying that I anticipate a long and mutually beneficial relationship between us, and you can expect many and more substantial rewards in the days ahead."

Suturb was touched, but he reminded himself of his loyalty to the Kcalb Clan and the welfare of Treretum. "Thank you, sir. I was just doing my assignment to the best of my ability, as any member of the Kcalb Clan would have done."

His response made Egroeg reflect on his own biases. *Have I been misjudging them? Is what my elders taught me correct?* he thought to himself.

"Sir, shall I continue? I have quite a bit of additional material on individual behavior, along with my findings regarding their corporations and governments," Suturb queried with a stroke of his hand, drawing up a different screen on the holographic display.

"No, Sucram," replied Egroeg. "Thank you, but I am tired, and you have given me sufficient information to think about for one day. Let us reconvene later. For now, I need to rest."

"As you wish, sir," responded Suturb as he bowed slightly, taking the hologram cube and placing it in his loose-fitting sleeve. As he turned to leave the room, Egroeg called out his name, "Sucram Suturb," and continued after Suturb turned to look at him, "well done."

Suturb thanked Egroeg, and walked to the door, which evaporated before him and reformed after he had passed through the portal.

CADMIUM POISONING

FACTS

- As mentioned previously, zinc is involved in over 300 enzymatic reactions in the human body; and in addition to being essential for brain function, a healthy immune system, healing, etc., zinc is in every strand of DNA in our bodies. Thus, zinc is required for the development of a fetus. Mothers should take care in balancing their zinc intake. Insufficient zinc ingestion will most likely result in a zinc deficiency in the mother because, as with most fetal building blocks, the requirements of the fetus are met first, potentially draining the mother's reserves.

- In addition, the tissues of the placenta that surround the fetus contain 1,000 times the zinc concentration compared to the rest of the mother's body tissues. This zinc accumulation is possible through a redistribution of zinc from other reserves in the mother's body. The zinc-rich environment in which the fetus develops, coupled with the sequestration of cadmium by metallothioneins, protects the fetus, usually producing an offspring that is virtually free of cadmium at birth.

- A father's semen contains 100 times the concentration of zinc compared to other body fluids of the male. Zinc is needed for neurological development; it surrounds fertilized eggs and remains available in the early days of growth of the zygote.

- Fertility depends, in part, on the presence of sufficient zinc. Insufficient zinc on the part of either the male or the female member of the couple can result in infertility, and zinc therapy may aid an otherwise infertile couple start a family. Thus, zinc supplementation (phosphate-free) is essential during pregnancy.

- Melanoma has been linked to pregnancy (a seven-fold increase in risk of melanoma for pregnant women). To ensure that the placenta has sufficient zinc to protect the developing fetus, the body "robs Peter to pay Paul," leaving the skin and other tissues from which zinc is being drawn zinc-deficient and vulnerable.

- Oysters have high concentrations of zinc, copper, and other minerals, but one of those minerals is cadmium. Oysters have 1,000 times the cadmium concentration in a piece of fish, a piece of chicken, or a cut of beef or pork (not including organ meats).

- Similarly, you've probably been told that you have to eat the potato skins because that's where all the vitamins and minerals are. Don't bite . . . one of the minerals is cadmium.

- Pain due to internal inflammation is often induced by foods in our diets. Most inflammatory foods are directly related to cadmium (e.g., sugar and gluten); however, sometimes it is not obvious. Cheese, for example, is a dairy product, and dairy products are generally said to be low in cadmium. However, a small piece of cheese is made from a much larger volume of milk, and the cadmium concentration is consequently much higher in the cheese. To avoid internal inflammation and the associated pain, avoid cadmium, but also pay attention to your diet and assess how you feel when your diet changes, even a little. Or better yet, keep a diary of what you eat (in general terms), so that if and when you experience pain, and you think it may be related to internal inflammation (e.g., sore joints), you can look at your diary to see what food(s) may be causing it, and you can avoid that food in the future.

Chapter Ten

Invasion of the Muimdac

They arrived in a cloud of cosmic dust that seemed to have come from out of nowhere, engulfing the planet as it sped through the galaxy. An emergency meeting of the Drutsab Egral Security Cabinet was called to brief His Excellency, the Supreme Azteep, on the status of the invasion and Treretumian efforts to combat the invaders.

"This is the beginning of the end of our existence as we know it," mumbled Hsubdab under his breath, just loud enough to be heard by Yenech, the cabinet member standing to his left. "Nothing will ever be the way it was."

"Aren't you being a bit melodramatic," responded Yenech in an equally subdued tone. "You're just concerned about being in the hot seat."

"No! You don't understand this insidious enemy. This invasion has far-reaching implications, and the inevitable consequences will not be know for many centuries," he insisted. The two awaited the completion of the security check on the meeting room just before the cabinet meeting.

The room was octagonal in shape, with a table in the shape of a ring located at its center.

A circle of plush, high-backed chairs mounted on swivel pedestals surrounded the table, equipped with a low-profile control panel at each of the seating stations. Alternate wall panels of the octagon served as screens for the retractable projector that dropped from the center of the ceiling. The rest of the panels were mirrored to discourage concealment. With the same purpose, a low, octagonal structure with sloped, mirrored walls positioned in the center of the ring-conference table, permitted each participant to see the eyes of every other participant. The Treretumians believed that the eyes revealed the truth and that no Treretumian could lie or conceal facts about the topic of discussion without being given away by his eyes.

A door opened in one of the mirrored panels, and the members of the cabinet began to filter in, taking their seats at the table. Momentarily, all seats were filled except one. The Azteep walked in, closing the door behind. The mirrors on the door and wall panel made the door almost disappear. He turned, approached his seat at the table, and spoke.

"In these trying times of invasion and chaos, this meeting is called to order."

The lights dimmed, and each of the members of the cabinet retracted the dark-brown coverings over his eyes, displaying the true eyes of the cabinet members. A glow of light emanated from each of the exposed eyes, and the periodic blinking of the members of the cabinet created the illusion of fireflies in the twilight.

The Supreme Azteep continued, "Members of the Security Cabinet, as you know, our planet has been invaded." He asked in frustration, "How can this be? The invaders are among us—they are everywhere. How could we not detect their arrival on the planet? Hsubdab, what can you tell me of this? You are the head officer of Treretum Security and the Homeland Intelligence Trust, responsible for the protection of our planet from invasion. Did we learn nothing from the invasion of the Yrucrem bak'tuns ago? How could this have happened?"

The young, slender head officer stood. "Your Excellency, our sensors didn't detect the invasion because the invaders are microscopic. There was no conventional spacecraft to detect, and the density of the cloud in which they travel is less than that of most of the other naturally occurring cosmic showers. They travel through space in their cloud of cosmic dust, and during their voyage, the majority of them are in a dormant state. Not until they reach their host and are taken into the body do they awaken, like the spores of a toxic mold. The activated members of their invasion force collaborate, initially impacting the function of strategic organs, leaving Treretumians vulnerable to their further aggressive attack."

The soft-spoken Hsubdab was convincing and effective in explaining away any negligence or culpability on the part of his agency. He had passed the first hurdle, but he still had to field many questions from the Azteep and the other members of the cabinet. "If it pleases the cabinet, indulge me and permit me to bring in a prisoner, a member of the invasion force. What I am about to demonstrate will, I am sure, stimulate the discussion and give you an indication of the difficult times that lie ahead."

Hsubdab motioned to a guard standing by the door. The guard opened the door, and two members of the Treretumian Planetary Guard, dressed in colorful, loose-fitting blue uniforms trimmed in red, entered the room with a prisoner between them. The prisoner appeared to be a member of the Treretumian citizenry, clothed in traditional peasant attire. The guard to his right had a sidearm in hand, and the guard to his left carried an ancient Treretumian battleaxe, a large and ornate broad-edged metal blade mounted on a sculptured, carved wooden handle. It was unusual to see a battleaxe outside formal ceremonial events. "This, my honored members of the cabinet . . ." —the sleeve of Hsubdab's robe hung low as he raised his left arm and pointed one of his long slender fingers at the prisoner—"is our enemy." The members of the cabinet began to talk among themselves, creating a low rumble of disbelief. Hsubdab nodded his head at the guards.

The guard with the sidearm took the hand of the peasant, raised it so that it was outstretched, and pulled back the sleeve to nearly the shoulder, exposing a pale, slender arm. The guard with the battleaxe let go of his prisoner's arm, took two steps in front of the prisoner, and swung the great blade downward, severing the arm from the body of the prisoner. The gasps from the cabinet members resounded in the cabinet room. But the guard's motion continued. He spun around in a single, smooth motion, turning a full 360 degrees with his loose-fitting uniform trailing behind. The motion was smooth, graceful, and swift. He followed through, coming across with the horizontal blade to the neck of the peasant, severing the head from the rest of the body. A second round of gasps emanated from the cabinet members.

The two body parts fell to the ground in succession, but not a drop of blood was spilled. Instead, light and an atomized mist came pouring from the severed arm and neck, streaming from both the severed parts and the body from which they came. In a matter of seconds, a skin formed over the light-emitting surfaces. The body of the peasant remained firm-footed and erect.

Hsubdab stepped forward, placing himself between the body of the peasant and the cabinet members, raising his arm, motioning at the surrealistic body that remained motionless. "This is what we are up against—an enemy that will not die. We know too little about them to effectively combat them. They have not only invaded the planet, but are also now invading our bodies, eventually devouring us from the inside and being programmed to take our form."

The unrest among the cabinet members was evident. The occasional flickering of fireflies had been transformed into a roomful of heads turning from side to side accompanied by a frantic flashing of much higher intensity lights, the effect amplified by the many mirrored surfaces in the room.

Hsubdab continued, "Initially, they need our life systems to provide them with nutrients and to remove their waste. They target specific organs, a quest for conquest on an organ-by-organ basis, and once they have taken control of those organs, the victory is theirs. The rest of the body is assimilated into the Muimdac transform more slowly, with no change in the outward appearance of the victim, and the successful invaders feeding off the remains, multiplying to complete the transformation."

"The biggest challenge for the Muimdac invaders is the disabling of the immune system because it is dispersed throughout the body, and its main functions is to attack foreign objects. Individually—or in groups of up to half a dozen cells—the immune system attack force will fight to the death, effectively ripping foreign cells apart, removing deposited foreign matter, and demolishing damaged host cells to make room for replacements."

"Intelligence Officer Hsubdad, enough of the physiology lesson!" exclaimed cabinet member Yenech, with whom he had spoken at the entrance to the chamber before the meeting had begun. "From what you describe, it appears that this is the beginning of the end of our existence as we know it!" Yenech stood abruptly as the cabinet member around him turned to look at him. "Nothing will ever be the way it was! Now what can we do to eliminate the immediate threat that the Muimdac pose to our society?"

A rumble grew in the room as a dozen side conversations erupted among the cabinet members. Once again taking center stage, Yenech raised his voice, proclaiming, "Let me be the first to offer you my full support in our battle against the Muimdac. We must prevail, whatever the cost!" The cabinet members in the room burst into a unified show of support by rising to their feet and raising their hands into the air. The sleeves of their loose-fitting robes bunched up at their narrow shoulders, exposing their hands, arms, and long boney fingers, which were heavily adorned with rings. Their fingers clinked as the rings hit each other. The small mouths of the Treretumians all opened wide, and shrill, screeching, pulsing tones, interspersed with clicks and snaps, came forth, filling the room with an almost unbearable sound.

Hsubdab's and Yenech's eyes locked on each other in the midst of all the noise and commotion. This was the end of the existence that they had known, but it was the beginning of another era. Each knew the skills of the other, and both were opportunists. Each slowly developed a confident smile—almost a smirk. It appeared that the two were destined to lead Treretum through the time of turmoil that lay ahead, and each was thinking about the personal gain that could result during their command.

CADMIUM POISONING

FACTS

- A conflict within our bodies involving cadmium takes place every day, similar to invasion of the Muimdac inside the bodies of Treretumians. The Muimdac take over one organ at a time—in organs equivalent to our liver, kidneys, lungs, pancreas, and bones. Battles involve body response to the invasion. Imagine, if you will, that you are overhearing a briefing taking place within the body of one of the first Treretumian victims of the Muimdac invasion. The captain of the Principal Attack Force and his direct superior, the commander of the victim's Systemic Invasionary Forces, share in the following exchange:

"Captain, you have had enough time to execute your conquest plan, run reconnaissance, and prepare a briefing on the status of the assumption of control of our host Treretumian. I want to hear your briefing. What have you accomplished thus far?"

"Commander, we have successfully assumed control of the hepatic function of the Treretumian. Our troops that reach the detoxification chamber will be safe."

"Good! What is the status on the liquid waste elimination plant?"

"The plant is partially occupied, and its function is compromised. It is passing protein and work on completely incapacitating the organ is in progress. If we choose to take the work on this organ to completion, the Treretumian will require outside purification of the bloodstream to survive."

"Well, then perhaps we had better slow down the shutdown until we are ready to take control of the entire body. Good! And what about the pancreatic function that activates food absorption throughout the body?"

"Commander, the specialized cells on the topside of that organ have been deactivated—they no longer respond to changes in the blood. Now when the Treretumian consumes food to fuel his body, the food—in the form of an easily digestible sugar—will simply circulate in his bloodstream. His body will be unable to absorb it, and the more he eats, the higher the sugar concentration in his blood will rise. Before too long, he will have sugary *syrup* flowing through his veins. And the best part is that his cells will actually be starving."

"Good! And what progress has been made on the support structure?"

"All is proceeding as planned. We have implanted agents throughout the skeleton, and we plan to let the Treretumian's own defenses render his support compromised. When we reach a sufficiently high concentration, the pain will begin. At the same time, his body will send out cells in the bloodstream to eliminate the 'impurities' by dissolving the surrounding bone. Soon the support structure will begin to slump, and if we choose to have a sufficiently high population infiltrate into the skeleton, the Treretumian's own defenses will make the bones so weak that they will be unable to support their respective parts of the body."

"Good! And tell me, what are you doing to keep the oxidant from being available for reaction with the food consumed?"

"Sir, this is an interesting situation where we began by concentrating our efforts on the organ that is the point of entry for the oxidant. Without this oxidant that they absorb from their gaseous surroundings, they cannot function, collapse, and die. We found that the Treretumian was particularly vulnerable at this location. About half of our troops were successful in entering at this point, compared to only one in ten through the digestive system. We found that a large fraction of the bloodstream was sent directly from the circulatory mechanism to pick up oxidant for distribution throughout the body, and thus, this point of entry served our needs well. We sought out the control of the metabolism and found it in an organ in the throat of the Treretumian. Furthermore, we have impacted the cells that carry the oxidant. There are now fewer of them, and they are smaller, having lower carrying capacity."

"Good! Good! It sounds as though you have things well in hand, and the total collapse of this Treretumian's natural body functions and our assumption of complete control are imminent. Is there anything that you foresee that could impede our progress?"

"Yes, Commander. Right now, our primary nuisance is a group of mobile cells they call their immune system. It's ridiculous! They think that their body is immune and attack us as though we were bacteria, not realizing that we are made of a different mettle. Most of our targets are stationary organs, and all fall easy prey when we amass sufficient Muimdac to impede their function. There is one thing though. It appears that we are competing with an adversary element in the body that works in ways very similar to our own. Right now, we can gradually drive him out, but occasionally he and his reinforcements arrive in mass, and we suffer temporary setbacks. However, they never stay for very long, and when they leave, we can quickly regain lost ground."

"Captain, you must do everything that you can to expel this adversary element from the body so that we can assume control without delay."

"Yes, Commander. We will continue to try our very best."

- Don't overeat—not just because you don't need the extra calories; you don't need the extra cadmium. Eat to live, not live to eat.

- Take zinc with meals especially if cadmium is known to be present in higher-than-usual concentrations. Studies have shown that the assimilation of cadmium is greatly reduced when zinc is taken concurrently. That is why bread made from whole grain wheat is less harmful than white bread. The zinc in a grain of wheat (or rice) is concentrated on the outer part of the grain—the dark outer portion that is stripped away during processing.

- A common practice among chicken producers has been to include roxarsone or some other arsenic-containing additive to chicken feed to combat digestive tract infection. The chickens assimilate much of the arsenic. The toxic metal accumulates in various chicken parts, especially in the skin. Thus, it is best to avoid eating the skin of the chicken unless the chicken's arsenic-free dietary history can be confirmed. While many of the nation's major producers have announced the elimination of arsenic from their operations, arsenic persists in chicken on the market, with the widest range of concentrations found in the fast food industry.

- Arsenic is also found in eggs that are brought to market. Studies show that the highest arsenic concentrations are found in chicken eggs approximately four to five weeks after arsenic is initiated in the laying hens' diets. The concentrations tend to level off at a relatively low concentration, with the smallest eggs tending to contain the highest concentrations.

- Mercury poisoning has received a great deal of publicity due to its concentration in large fish like the tuna. However, it is a contaminant in coal used as fuel at power plants primarily in the northeast. Champions like Robert F. Kennedy Jr. have helped to inform the public about the hazard of mercury poisoning in our food supply and other environmental media like streams and the air near power plants. However, mercury may also be in an unexpected part of your diet. Mercury may be found in high-fructose corn syrup (HFCS)—in ice cream, soft drinks, maple syrup, canned fruits, and many sweets. Extraction of fructose involves a process that uses caustic (sodium hydroxide) made in mercury cells. Trace amounts of mercury are transferred to the HFCS product.

- In addition, "silver" fillings that you may have in your mouth are more mercury than silver. They are made of an amalgam of mercury and silver, with over fifty percent being mercury. Slowly, with exposure to saliva and acidic beverages, traces of mercury enter the bloodstream and accumulate in various parts of the body. The biological half-life of mercury in the body varies, depending on the form of the metal and what organ is involved. However, mercury is capable of crossing the blood-brain barrier, and its half-life in the brain is approximately 20 years.

Chapter Eleven

Area 51

The drive began early because there was a lot of Texas to cover before they would get to the New Mexico border. It was a brisk April morning, and the early spring temperatures had lingered a few weeks longer than usual. The last noteworthy cold front had just blown through, and although summer was just around the corner, it had not yet had a chance to get its grip on Texas. The cool winds from the north had dropped the humidity a long way—like a penny off the top of the Empire State Building. It was a pleasantly different from the warm, sultry evenings and early mornings for which Houston, the city noted for being an outdoor sauna, is famous.

They had decided that Gavilán would drive first since the conference had been more of a strain than Olga had been willing to acknowledge the previous day. Olga was looking forward to the long drive, anticipating that it would be one of those relaxing drives with interesting scenery, good music, lots of chitchat, and an occasional catnap. It would be particularly interesting to drive through San Antonio, her hometown, to see how much change in the city she could see from the highway. There would be no time to stop and explore. Their destination—Roswell, New Mexico, the closest city to the site of the famous UFO crash, out in the middle of the New Mexico desert. The expedition would first focus on Roswell and the Army Air Station

(AAS) that, in 1947, fielded the original call regarding the crashed spacecraft.

They left their motel on NASA Road 1 and started north toward downtown Houston on IH-45, the Gulf Freeway. Because the conference was held on a Friday, the Saturday morning traffic was relatively light, making the drive through Houston much more bearable. Not much was said in the first few miles, and at first, Gavilán chalked it up to the early departure and lack of coffee.

Gavilán broke the silence. "Want to stop and catch a bite to eat, or would you prefer to just catch a cup of coffee when we tank up?"

Olga leaned back, stretched out her left arm with her palm toward Gavilán and fingers pointing to the sky—almost as a reflex—raised her left eyebrow, and said emphatically, "Thanks, but no coffee for this lady. I'll reserve my cadmium intake for other things . . . like food."

The simple question evoked an unexpected response. Gavilán was both surprised and curious. He thought to himself, *What could rechargeable batteries have to do with food and coffee? And maybe coffee's not a good idea for her right now, anyway.* He was sure there would be plenty of time for food and conversation during the trip. And if the topic didn't come up by the time they reached the New Mexico border, he may just have to bring it up before they reached Roswell or, better yet, just let it slide. But for right now, he thought it best to let sleeping dogs lie.

The flatness of the Houston terrain made its urban sprawl seemed endless, extending westward to Katy and beyond. Gavilán sensed that Olga was tense and that her experience at the Houston conference didn't turn out the way she had expected. Olga needed something to break the tension, and he would have to do his best to do just that. "Okay, Dr. Engineer . . . you should appreciate this story. It's a story about a balloonist and an engineer. Okay, there's this balloonist, and he's flying around, but he realizes that he's lost, so he decides to drop down to ask for directions. He catches the attention of a woman below and shouts down to her, 'Excuse me, but I've apparently gotten off course. I was supposed to meet someone about an hour ago, but I'm lost. I don't know where I am. Can you help me?'

"The woman wants to help by starting with his current location. She responds, [*Gavilán changes voices to a shrill falsetto to make it obvious that it was a woman speaking*] 'You're hovering in a hot-air balloon about thirty feet off the ground. You're at exactly, uh . . . .'" There was a pause because Gavilán realized that the only coordinates he knew by heart were those of the house where Olga had grown up in San Antonio. He remembered them from a conversation they'd had during her senior year when Olga was taking a GIS class to finish off the breadth requirements for her engineering degree. He continued by rattling off the coordinates, thinking that Olga would never make the connection, "Uh, 29 degrees, 31 minutes, and 21 seconds north latitude, and 98 degrees, 29 minutes, and 33 seconds west longitude."

Gavilán coughed from the strain of the falsetto voice. He cleared his throat and recovered his normal voice. He looked at Olga, and the tension and concern in her face was all but gone, replaced by a big smile. She tilted her head slightly to the right as he continued, "The balloonist is amazed that she would know the exact coordinates of their location, so he leans over the side of the gondola and shouts, 'I'm very impressed with the precision of your response. You must be an engineer.'"

Again in falsetto, Gavilán continued, "'Why, yes, I am. How could you tell?'"

This time the recovery from the falsetto went smoothly. Gavilán added, "This is where the dude shows his true colors, the colors of a condescending jerk. He responds, 'Well, to me it seemed fairly obvious. Everything you told me is probably technically correct, but I can't use any of it. I'm still totally lost. I don't have a clue as to where I am or how to get to where I need to go. You haven't helped me in the slightest. On the contrary, all you've done is made me later than I already was.'"

Gavilán had Olga's undivided attention, and he was loving it. He continued with the story, "The woman paused for moment, shaking her head. Then she looked up at the man and said, 'You must be in management.' The man thought he was a really bad vato [dude] and his chest puffed up as he proudly said, 'Why, yes, I am. How did you know?'"

At this point, Olga could sense that Gavilán's final falsetto performance would contain the punch line. With a big grin on her face, she looked at him in anticipation. Gavilán continued, "So this was the woman's chance to really let him have it. After all the grief he had given her, it was her window of opportunity that had just opened."

Unable to contain herself, Olga interrupted him and gestured with a reciprocating motion of her hands, palms up and fingers spread, for him to hurry up. "Come on, come on—what did she say?"

In falsetto, Gavilán finished the joke, saying, "'Well, to me it seemed fairly obvious. You don't know where you are or where you're going. You've attained your current position by and large because of a lot of hot air. You've made promises that you can't keep, and you want people beneath you to solve your problems for you. In fact, you've made no progress toward your destination since before we met, and somehow, now it's my fault.'"

In full laughter, Olga tugged at the shoulder of Gavilán's shirt, leaned over, and planted a big kiss on his right cheek. "¡Estás loco!" [You're crazy.] The laughter stopped, the two looked at each other for a moment, and then Olga whispered, "Thanks."

〰〰〰〰〰〰〰〰〰〰〰〰〰〰〰〰〰〰〰〰〰〰〰〰〰〰〰〰〰

All was quiet, and the murmur of the engine had lulled Olga to sleep a few miles back. Gavilán glanced at Olga several times as he drove. She had raised her feet onto the seat and had fallen asleep hugging her knees and leaning against the door in a fetal position. The signs said they were approaching IH-410, the inside loop around San Antonio. "Loop 410," Gavilán said in a low voice, but it was like an alarm clock for Olga.

She awoke in an instant, straightened up in her seat, and instinctively began giving instructions as she rubbed the sleep from her eyes. "Don't get into the right lane because the cutoff for IH-37 and Highway 281 is an exit-only lane, and that would take us way out of our way. This lane is okay, but it would be better to move over one more lane to the right because this lane goes to the lower deck when the highway splits into upper and lower, and the cutoff for IH-10 West is off the upper deck only."

With that, Gavilán broke into a chorus of "You take the high road, and I'll take the low road, and I'll get to Scotland before you."

Olga gave him a puzzled look, paused, and then responded, "Okay, I get the hint . . . but I was just trying to help. I forgot you're a Stanford grad, so you know how to read."

Gavilán just said, "Yep."

Olga gazed out the window as they started west on IH-10 after having successfully navigated through the various interchanges and cutoffs. In a low voice, she said, "Tío Pepe went to Roswell Air Station back in the '50s. It was a short-term assignment, taking him from his regular job at what was then Kelly Air Force Base here in San Antonio, and when he returned, he didn't talk much about his experiences."

Gavilán remained quiet for a moment. He remembered hearing Olga speak of Tío Pepe several times before in the context of his painful battle with kidney cancer and premature death. Images of a mischievous young man caught in the act by his father were vivid in Gavilán's mind. When confronted behind la caballerisa [the stable] about smoking at the tender age of fourteen, the young man, standing erect with his hands behind his back denied having started smoking, but his denial was contradicted by the sinuous, telltale trail of smoke that rose behind his head. Feeling compelled to respond, Gavilán asked, "Was this the same Tío Pepe that died of kidney cancer because of what you thought might have been overexposure to chlorinated solvents at Kelly?"

Olga turned to Gavilán in amazement. "You remember my comment from so many years ago?"

Gavilán locked in on Olga's eyes, saying, "I pay close attention to everything that you say. You and everything that you say and do are very important to me."

Their gaze seemed to draw them closer to each other. Olga felt the *pull* of his dark eyes. But Gavilán was driving, and he had to sneak an occasional glance at the road. Feeling half mesmerized, she thought to herself, *¿Como puede hacer esto este cabrón?* [How can he do this?] She took advantage of the next glance at the road to sit up in her seat, uttering, "Uh, well . . . the chlorinated solvents probably contributed to it, but I heard some things about cadmium, did a quick Google search, and now I believe that it was probably a combination of the two that caused his demise. The reason I believe that cadmium poisoning is at least part of the cause is that he was also diabetic, and the symptoms of Type 2 diabetes can be induced by elevated cadmium concentrations in the pancreas."

Disappointed but understanding the impossibility of the moment, Gavilán looked at Olga in puzzlement. It took him several seconds to snap out of it. Now he had to replay in his mind and digest what Olga had just said. The pause caused Olga to look at him, tilt her head, and query, "Are you okay?"

"Yeah," he responded, "I was just thinking about what you just said." He pulled himself together, asking, "You mean that cadmium poisoning can impact several organs in the body at the same time? And cadmium is the bad boy that you say is in coffee that you now avoid like the plague."

"Yes, exactly!" she exclaimed. "Did you hear about the big chocolate class action suit they had in California against all the big companies that manufacture and sell chocolate products . . . to make them list the cadmium and lead content on the labels of their products?"

"No, but I guess that would probably make a lot of mommies put fewer chocolate bars in the kiddos' lunches," he said almost apologetically.

"And that translates into fewer of those big bucks for the chocolatiers. And see . . . you're a pretty well-informed individual, but you hadn't heard anything about health issues related to cadmium, had you?" asked Olga in a tone of frustration. She continued, "No one seems to know or care about its monumental implications on the health of every man, woman, and child on the planet."

Gavilán could see that the intensity of the conversation was steadily rising, and that wasn't good for either of them. "So help me out here," he said jokingly. "How does it get from rechargeable batteries into coffee and chocolate?"

"Okay, wise guy!" she said as she did an intensity check and subsequently lowered her volume a few decibels. "It's everywhere—cigarette smoke, soft drinks, tortillas de harina [flour tortillas], even lettuce. But nobody knows about it or talks about it, much less does anything about it."

"Somebody must be doing something about it," replied Gavilán in disbelief.

"I would have thought so too, but it doesn't look like it to me." Olga paused, turned to gaze out the window, and muttered, "People need to know." Then, in her characteristic *I-need-to-be-prepared* manner, Olga announced, "Well, I guess I'd better do my homework and get the layout of the Roswell Air Station."

"And just how are you going to do that?" Gavilán inquired with a pronounced tone of skepticism in his voice.

Olga reached down and lifted the laptop case from next to her feet. She placed it on her lap, slowly lifted her head, turned to Gavilán, smiled, and said, "My computer has a long-range, roaming broadband Internet connection . . . and Google knows all."

"Well, before we get out of San Antonio, the only place in Texas that has a taco stand or a panadería [bakery] at almost every corner, how about we stop at the next panadería that we see."

"No thanks, I've been eating too many things with too much cadmium in the last few days," Olga responded.

In a whining tone, Gavilán pleaded, "Andale, una piesa de pan de dulce con un cafecito." [Come on, a piece of sweet bread with a cup of coffee.] He paused briefly and then continued very nonchalantly, "Una vez al año no hace daño." [Once a year does no harm—in rhyme.]

His almost flippant attitude made Olga react. "¡No, cabrón! A mí no me haces eso. Es que tú no has visto el sufrimiento . . . ¡ni has sufrido tú mismo!" [No, dude. You're not doing that to me. It's that you haven't seen the suffering . . . nor have you yourself suffered.] Olga thought to herself, *Boy, did he step in it this time,* but then she caught herself. She realized he meant no harm; Gavilán would never intentionally do anything to hurt her. And rather than lighting into him, she needed to enlighten him. She took a deep breath and explained, "Gavilán, you see, I have a vivid imagination and an excellent memory. I know what all that is about, and I'll be the first to admit that I enjoyed that whole experience with friends and family members many times. But I also remember how my dad, shortly before he died, suffered from lower back pain one night and the whole next day by just once falling off the wagon and indulging in a high-cadmium supper. The impact of cadmium is cumulative. Thanks, but no thanks. The pleasure that it would give me would be very real, but potentially, so would the painful consequences. I probably have a couple of signs of cadmium poisoning already, and I don't want to reach any thresholds any faster than I have to."

Gavilán took a deep breath, exhaled, and gingerly said, "Okey dokey," as he turned his head forward to focus his attention on his driving.

ꙮꙮꙮꙮꙮꙮꙮꙮꙮꙮꙮꙮꙮꙮꙮꙮꙮꙮꙮꙮꙮꙮꙮꙮꙮꙮ

About an hour had passed, and hardly a word had been said. Gavilán had been looking straight ahead, occasionally letting loose with a sigh and glancing out the window to his left. Olga too had been occasionally glancing to her left, but without so much as a sound, she returned her eyes to the road, almost as though she were driving. She could tell that her outburst had probably unintentionally bruised Gavilán's ego. It was apparent that her explanation had not soothed the impact.

All of a sudden, Olga turned toward Gavilán and said, "Una vez al año *sí* hace daño." [Once a year *does* do harm.]

Gavilán turned in surprise and asked, "Where did that come from?"

She responded, "An ounce of prevention is worth a pound of cure."

"Now you really have me confused," he uttered with a baffled look on his face. "You'd never called me cabrón before." His look went from baffled to hurt.

Olga responded, "Look, Eagle Man, I'm sorry—"

"Ah, the magic words," he quickly interjected, keeping her from finishing her thought. Gavilán continued with a touch of indignation, "Know here and now that I am not trying to hurt you—never have, never will. If I say something that seems out of line, consider the source. If it came from my lips, it was not intended to hurt, harm, insult, embarrass, intimidate, malign, or deceive you. I always speak to you from my heart."

"Peace?" asked Olga apologetically with a sheepish half-smile on her face.

"Peace!" he replied. He reached over to take hold of Olga's hand. Alternating glances between the road ahead and Olga's big, tearful eyes. "Consider the source," he reiterated slowly in a low voice as he gave her hand a squeeze.

"Tienes razón. Perdóname por favor." [You're right. Please forgive me.]

⊓⊔

The stop in Roswell was relatively uneventful. There was all the UFO hype they both expected—displays, museums, and larger-than-life personal accounts of the aftermath of the crash scrawled on walls. The trouble was that they had both seen so much related non-factual material on the Internet, and it made all of what they saw before them seem contrived and invalid. In short, although it was very entertaining, it was a little disappointing. It had turned out to be little more than an interesting side trip on the way to the Powwow. Next stop: Albuquerque.

⊓⊔

Gavilán and Olga arrived at the address written on the back of the section of a Corn Chex box top that Gavilán had pulled from his shirt pocket. Their vehicle slowed to a complete stop in front of the building. It was a large metal building with a "For Lease" sign at the front door. Olga looked at Gavilán with a puzzled look on her face.

"I'm as much in the dark as you are," Gavilán said in an emotionless tone as he continued to stare at the sign. "For Lease," he muttered.

He pulled his cell phone from his shirt pocket and was quick to find a number to dial. After a brief pause, he exclaimed, "Orville, what gives? We're at your building, but it's for lease." After another brief pause, Gavilán continued, "Yes, it's the same building that I went to during the Balloon Festival a couple of years ago."

Olga inquired in a whisper, "What's going on?"

Gavilán responded with an extended vertical forefinger of his right hand as he continued, "Yes, we're in Albuquerque!" Gavilán was starting to sound a little annoyed. "Minor detail." Again, Gavilán paused for several seconds and then continued, "Yeah, I got it. Okay, we're on our way."

Gavilán looked at Olga apologetically. He again raised his forefinger, this time in front of his nose, and said, "Slight detour. Please have patience, and trust me. It will be well worth it."

Olga raised both eyebrows and didn't say a word.

ꖦꖦꖦꖦꖦꖦꖦꖦꖦꖦꖦꖦꖦꖦꖦꖦꖦꖦꖦꖦꖦꖦꖦꖦꖦꖦꖦꖦ

After miles and miles of dirt roads, out in the middle of nowhere, they had finally arrived. The modest warehouse didn't look like much. In fact, it looked more like an old barn in desperate need of a coat of paint, but Gavilán assured Olga that he was a man of his word and that she would not be disappointed.

Gavilán turned off the engine, and they waited for the dust to clear a bit before getting out of the car. They slowly approached the only visible door to the building, looking around them as they walked, until they reached the door. It was a sliding door with a large padlock attached to the open hasp.

The sliding door opened a crack, and out popped the head of a man who looked as though he had just awakened and was recovering from a long night with a wine bottle. His hair was disheveled, and it was clear he hadn't shaved in several days. When he realized he had company, he said, "Oh, you must be the folks coming in from Houston." The door opened a bit more, and out walked this more-than-middle-aged geezer, dressed in coveralls.

Gavilán took the lead and introduced himself. "Hi, I'm Cuauhtémoc Gavilán, the one who called from Houston about renting a hot-air balloon. I don't know if you remember me, but I've ridden with you before." Olga was stunned. Now it all began to make sense: the comment about getting the multiple vantage points for the high-resolution photographs and, to top it off, the joke about the balloonist and the engineer. She looked at Gavilán in amazement as he introduced her. "And this, my good man, is Dr. Olga Ramos. We'll only need the balloon long enough to get to Area 51 and back." Parenthetically, he added in a subdued tone, "She's never been in a hot-air balloon."

The man seemed neither impressed nor concerned. He shrugged his shoulders, glanced at the ground to his left momentarily, and said, "Oh well, you can just call me Orville . . . you know, like one of the Wright brothers." The man shuffled around a bit and then turned around abruptly, looked Gavilán in the eye, and said, "You do realize that Area 51 isn't just around the corner. In fact, it isn't even in this state!"

Gavilán just nodded.

Orville grunted, "Hmp." He gave Gavilán and Olga a scowl that was full of disbelief and amazement. After a pause, he continued, "I think we'd better pack our balloon and drive most of the way." He shook his head as he looked to the ground and started walking away, again in a shuffle. He motioned for them to follow him as he walked, grumbling, "Damn good thing that I have friends in Nevada."

This was to be Olga's first balloon ride. Although Gavilán had enjoyed the experience of riding in a couple of balloons during the Southwest International Balloon Festival a few Octobers past, he'd never been responsible for flying one. Neither he nor Orville could afford for anything to go wrong with the flight, so the grubby but experienced gentleman in coveralls was the default ace aviator for the flight.

"I hope you brought your grubbies, son," grumbled the old codger, "'cause we have some packing to do before we leave in the wee hours of the morning."

ꙮꙮꙮꙮꙮꙮꙮꙮꙮꙮꙮꙮꙮꙮꙮꙮꙮꙮꙮꙮꙮꙮꙮꙮꙮꙮꙮꙮꙮꙮ

Everything was loaded into the twin cab and trailer, and it was time to get started on the great adventure. Olga and Gavilán piled in on the passenger side, and Orville took the driver's seat. He gently eased the pressure off the clutch pedal, raising the pedal and his foot away from the floorboard. The increased tension between the pickup and the trailer was felt with a slight jerk, and the loaded vehicle was in motion—a twin-cab pickup with balloon-toting trailer in tow.

Orville dialed ahead to a friend on the outskirts of Las Vegas. "Hi, Bill. Get ready for us, 'cause we're on our way." Orville placed his hand over his phone and spoke to Gavilán and Olga, "He has a warehouse, loading docks, and plenty of open space."

He uncovered the phone and continued his conversation. "We'll be there when we get there." He paused and then continued, "I know, Bill, but I've got a balloon in tow, and that's the best I can do." After another pause, he ended the call with, "Your guess is as good as mine!"

The geezer hung up the phone and tossed it on the dash. No one said a word.

〰〰〰〰〰〰〰〰〰〰〰〰〰〰〰〰〰〰〰〰〰〰〰〰〰〰〰〰〰〰

They approached the outskirts of Las Vegas but took the loop around the main strip to the northwest side of the city. After exiting the highway, they turned on a side road that seemed to take them to nowhere. Eventually, the paved road ended, but the pickup continued slowly on the pothole-ridden dirt road. Even though they seemed to be advancing at a crawl, the pickup kicked up a cloud of dust around them.

Although the windows were rolled up and the AC was on, Olga could taste the grit in her mouth. "How much further?" she asked. She peered forward through the windshield, but her field of vision was obstructed by dust. She and Gavilán looked at each other as she gently and shook her head with frustration visible on her face.

With his eyes glued straight ahead, Orville mumbled, "We're almost there. The cutoff is just ahead." Their crawl slowed to a halt as the cloud of dust that had surrounded them continued moving forward. As the haze dissipated, a large warehouse materialized a couple of hundred yards behind a large open gate with a tall arched threshold off to their left. "There it is. We have arrived," Orville uttered with a sigh as he proceeded to get the vehicle and trailer into motion.

Orville pulled his cell from his shirt pocket, pressed a single key, waited for a few seconds, and said, "We're here. We're pulling in right now." They were soon at the large structure. It had a loading dock to the right and a set of sliding doors to the left, which started to open as they approached. They entered the warehouse, which seemed reminiscent of an aircraft hangar with an expansive, sealed concrete floor. Overhead lights reflected off the clean concrete.

"Wait here," Orville instructed the silent duo as he emerged from the cab of the pickup to meet the man who approached. They met about ten yards in front of the pickup and shook hands, pulling each other into an embrace that was accompanied by several strong pats on the back.

Olga and Gavilán just gazed out the front windshield, looking at the two men. "That must be Bill," Olga said.

Gavilán responded with a simple, "Yep."

The contrast between the two men was stark. Bill's appearance was squeaky clean: short haircut; pressed jeans; a starched, light-blue, short-sleeved shirt; and white tennis shoes. Even from a distance, it was clear there were strong ties of friendship and respect between the pair.

After a couple of minutes of talk and hand waving, the two men approached the cab of the pickup. Gavilán opened the door and got out of the truck, and Olga slid over to the open door. After the introductions were made, Orville announced, "Bill and I have known each other it seems like forever. We served together many years ago." Orville took a step to the side, looked at the trailer, and then looked at Bill. "Ya think we can get this bucket in the air."

"I do believe so," Bill responded. "As I recall, we managed to get many an aircraft airborne years ago. This should be a piece of cake. Let's get inside so you folks can get cleaned up and rested before the morning. The sun rises pretty early around here." They all grabbed their light travel bags and followed Bill into the sectioned-off portion of the warehouse where he lived.

ꙴꙴꙴꙴꙴꙴꙴꙴꙴꙴꙴꙴꙴꙴꙴꙴꙴꙴꙴꙴꙴꙴꙴꙴꙴꙴꙴꙴ

The foursome stepped out of the building but kept walking on the expansive concrete slab to the area where Orville and Bill had already unloaded the trailer. The large folded balloon, fan, burner, and gondola were all sitting on one edge by a small boarding platform at the end of the slab.

Orville announced, "Yep, we had a real turd-floatin' gully washer day before yesterday back in Albuquerque. It rained so hard I thought the roof on my warehouse was going to cave in. We had several RVs that got washed away with the flash flooding that came with it. But you know, Bill, that really cleared the air, and now the atmosphere has really calmed down. Too bad we couldn't fly out of Albuquerque."

It was obvious he was trying to give this, Olga's first balloon ride, a touch of *local color*. With tongue in cheek, Olga responded in a convincing Texas drawl, "Damn, if I didn't know better, I'd-a thought you were from Texas, bragging about that downpour and all."

He took it in stride, saying, "Why, thank you, ma'am. I do appreciate the compliment. But now we have to get ready for the liftoff."

Olga looked at Gavilán with eyebrows raised in amazement.

Orville motioned to a bench that was off to the left as they walked. "Y'all wait over there." He turned and tapped Bill on the arm. "Come on, Bill, let's get this old bird in the air."

The two men walked over to a large burner and fan. "You get the fan and burner going, and I'll check the tethers."

Bill turned on the equipment as Orville checked the tethers and began unfolding the huge balloon. The burner and fan were placed on idle. With the flip of a switch, the large fan blade would shift to high speed within the cowling that directed and focused the flow of air. After placing the fan in front of the opening at the bottom of the balloon, the two men unfolded the rest of the balloon, placing it flat on the ground. They walked around to the fan, and Orville lifted one edge of the opening of the balloon and gave Bill a nod. He flipped the switch on the fan, and the force of the huge blade began to push air into the balloon. The huge balloon began to inflate, coming to life and moving like a lumbering giant awakening from a long sleep. The fan hummed loudly with a high-frequency pulsing as it continued to force air into the skin of the balloon. This continued until Orville gave Bill a second nod as he moved back to the edge of the opening.

The flame of the burner shot out directly into the opening. The roar of the burner was almost deafening. The heat from the burner expanded the air within the balloon, and the balloon began to rise from its former resting position. Orville motioned for Olga and Gavilán to come toward them to the boarding platform. It was clear that these two men had prepared balloons for flight many times before, but Olga was still a little apprehensive about putting her life in the hands of the old geezer, despite the fact that his name was linked to aviation history.

Gavilán placed his backpack next to the gondola by the boarding pad. Olga had just set her computer down next to her backpack and a large ring onto which was tied one of the basket's three tethers. She turned, saw Gavilán's backpack, and instinctively picked it up to put it with her computer and backpack.

Gavilán laughed and said, "Yo lo coloco, y ella lo quita." [*I place it, and she removes it*. The phrase is a play on words.]

"What?" Olga responded in a loud voice as she squinted and wrinkled her nose. "I can't hear you."

Gavilán laughed and said, "Yo loco loco, y ella loquita." [*I'm crazy crazy, and she's a little crazy.*]

"I still can't hear you!" she said as she shook her right arm with the palm of her hand facing up to the sky.

Gavilán laughed more loudly, saying, "I'll tell you when we get in the air," as he pointed into the sky with his hand bouncing up and down in front of his face.

Olga glanced at the less-than-graceful man in coveralls bending over and tugging at one of the tethers to a large ring anchored in a concrete slab. She took Gavilán by both sides of the collar and pulled him toward her until they were looking at each other eyeball to eyeball. "Are you sure this guy knows what he's doing?"

"Oh yeah," responded Gavilán, bobbing his head up and down as he recovered from the neck strain his nervous friend had induced. "I've ridden with him before. He's a veteran! Actually, he was an Air Force pilot in Nam who got to the rank of lieutenant colonel before he decided to pull the plug. He lived for the flying, not the killing, and wanted to slow down the pace—change the direction of his life."

"You sound like you're old buddies," said Olga in a slightly less apprehensive tone.

Gavilán smiled, saying, "Let's just say that I understand where he's been, and I am in harmony with the song he currently sings."

"All aboard!" shouted Orville as he throttled the fuel to the burner. Bill went over to the platform to help with the boarding of the gondola. The roar attenuated to a rumble, but Orville continued in the same loud, gruff voice, "Please make sure that all seat backs and tray tables are locked and in their upright positions and that all carry-on baggage is properly stoed in the overhead bin or below the seat in front of you." His voice dropped a few decibels as he continued, "Oh, I forgot . . . we don't have any overhead bins on this flight."

Olga again looked at Gavilán in disbelief. Not a word was uttered, but communications were flowing. Gavilán simply raised his eyebrows and took a deep breath.

Olga walked over to the boarding platform and climbed the steps. Bill extended his hand, and Olga took it as she stepped over the wall of the basket. She lowered her head as she stepped down into the gondola.

Gavilán hopped over the basket wall right behind her, and Orville brought up the rear. He reached up and pulled a lever, sending more propane to the burner and increasing the tension on the tethers. He waved at Bill who then pulled the ends of the three tethers, releasing the slipknots that had secured the gondola to the earth earlier. The gondola creaked as the balloon slowly lifted away from the boarding platform. Bill waved and yelled, "Bon voyage!"

Gavilán muttered, "Up, up, and away."

Orville picked up on the few words and broke into song, "Would you like to ride in my beautiful balloon?" Then, looking directly at Olga, he asked, "Wasn't the Fifth Dimension just the greatest?"

Patience and tact not being Olga's strong suits, she blurted out, "Let's cut the crap. What are *you*, an old man who's already retired at least once, doing out here in the middle of nowhere renting out a hot-air balloon?"

Orville looked at Olga in amazement, glanced at Gavilán who was apparently just as stunned as he, wiped his lips on the collar of his coveralls, and said, "Well, I got very tired of the impersonal way that I was killing people in Viet Nam." His somber tone was deep and subdued. "My head was full of all these idealistic, somewhat romantic ideas of how things were supposed to be and how it was the responsibility of the United States to give the people of Viet Nam a chance at democracy, liberty, happiness . . . motherhood, and apple pie. I had a healthy dose of reality in Viet Nam, and I came to the sobering conclusion that you can't force happiness on someone by killing his family and friends. For me, most of my killing was very impersonal, thousands of feet removed. Puffs of smoke as the bombs hit their targets on the ground. I didn't hear the screams of the women or the horrified cries of the children as their world exploded around them. You know, the crew in the tail section of the bomber always complained that the ride back there was bumpy, but that was nothing compared to the ride we delivered to the people below. We were told that *Charlie* was occupying some of the deserted villages that we targeted, but the follow-up ground photos of our work said something different. The villages weren't deserted. We were lied to every step of the way, and the lies came from every level, all the way up to the president."

"I'm sorry—I shouldn't have verbally attacked you," Olga said. She could hear the pain in his voice and see the anguish in his eyes.

"Well, now you're going to have to hear a little more," he said as he looked over the wall of the gondola and the ground below, "unless, that is, you'd prefer to jump. Today, I work with hot air, not too different from what my superiors were doing back in Nam. I stayed in to get my comfortable retirement and hated myself every minute. Now, I try to keep my nose clean, keep a low profile, and live with myself and what I was involved in, in the name of democracy and preservation of the American way of life."

Gavilán interjected, "And not to change the subject, but how high do we need to go, and where are we going?"

"Holy guacamole!" exclaimed Orville. "I'm sorry, folks." It was like someone had flipped a switch. It was strictly business. He began making adjustments, lowering the burner setting, and pulling a cord to open the parachute valve at the top of the balloon. The balloon began to gently descend. Their direction seemed to change as they picked up a different wind current at the lower elevation.

They were on their way, drifting, weightless in a sea of invisible fluid. The air was crisp and dry, and the panoramic view was breathtaking. But Olga was still visibly bummed about the Viet Nam story, or was it that she was realizing she shared some of the views of this old relic from a different age, a different war?

Gavilán was intent on snapping her out of it. He leaned over and said, "What I said earlier, down on the ground when you picked up my backpack, was 'Yo loco loco, y ella loquita.' Or did I say, 'Yo lo coloco, y ella lo quita?'"

"What?" Olga responded in a lilting *say-it-again* tone of voice.

Gavilán remained quiet and watched the light come on in Olga's eyes when she realized what he'd said. She began to laugh, and Gavilán's efforts at distracting her were again successful. The laughter grew in intensity, and Olga leaned toward him, gently hit him on the left shoulder with her open palm, and affectionately said, "Pendejo." [Dummy]

Now she felt it was her turn. "That reminds me of a story Tío Pepe loved to tell. It's about Ramiro and Margarita, this little rancherito [rural—little ranch type] couple. They were young and innocent, and they lived in very humble surroundings, but they had a few chickens, and Margarita had some very nice potted plants in some pretty pots they had brought up from Mexico."

Gavilán leaned forward with his elbows on his knees, intent on hearing every word. Olga took center stage as she continued, "They were a very traditional couple, and they were both comfortable with the fact that Ramiro wore the pants in the family. Ramiro worked in a job that occasionally required him to be out of town a day or two at a time. Their first winter together, when the first cold snap was about to hit, Ramiro was out of town and called his wife, 'Margarita, va estar muy frío a la noche. Por favor, mete las gallinas y las matas.' [Intended meaning: It's going to be very cold tonight. Please bring in the chickens and the plants.]

"The next day when he arrived home, he found that all the plants were still outside—frozen. He went inside only to find feathers scattered everywhere. His wife had slaughtered all the chickens. A bit distraught about the situation, he exclaimed at his wife, '¡Margarita! ¿Que hiziste?' [What have you done?] In tears, she responded, 'Pues no sonó bien, pero no mas hice lo que me dijiste.'" [*Well, it didn't sound right, but I just did what you told me to do.* Alternate and incorrect interpretation of what she was told to do: Please bring in the chickens and kill them.]

Gavilán laughed as he lower and shook his head. Olga wrapped up the story with, "I guess there's a moral to the story . . . that sometimes unquestioning obedience can lead to disastrous results."

Gavilán looked up toward Oville, and Olga's head turned to see what he was looking at as he responded, "I think that everyone present would agree with that."

ㄖㄖㄖㄖㄖㄖㄖㄖㄖㄖㄖㄖㄖㄖㄖㄖㄖㄖㄖㄖㄖㄖㄖㄖㄖㄖㄖㄖㄖㄖㄖㄖ

Area 51 came into view as they drifted closer. The characteristic runway that is present at every air station and Air Force base was unmistakable on the horizon. Their approach was relatively silent and graceful in comparison to other aircraft that frequented the area runway.

"We won't be able to get too close," stated Orville authoritatively. "These folks are pretty serious about protecting their airspace."

Olga responded, "That's okay. As long as I can identify Hangar 18 and snap about a dozen photos of it from different locations, we're set. How stationary can you hold our position while I take the photos and get the corresponding GIS positions?"

"Area 51 is part of the Nellis Bombing and Gunnery Range," commented Orville, "but we're in luck because it is on the western edge— by a corner of the facility boundary. That'll allow us to get fairly close."

Olga looked at Gavilán who simply raised his eyebrows and shrugged his shoulders. Orville had pulled out a pair of binoculars and responded as he adjusted the focus, "It all depends on the wind. I'll do the best I can. I can deal with steady breezes, but sudden gusts could cause a bit of a problem. Fortunately, the atmosphere seems pretty calm."

Olga opened her backpack and pulled out a digital camera attached to a lens cluster approximately a foot long. She aimed, holding the large lens in the upturned palm of her left hand, and the image appeared on the rectangular screen on the backside of the camera. She nudged Gavilán and said, "You're awfully quiet."

He responded, "I just came along for the ride."

She gave him an affectionate scowl.

Gavilán continued, "You know, I could be getting the GIS positions while you take the photos. You have an extra set of hands at your disposal."

"Sounds like a deal." Olga pulled the handheld GIS position-logging unit from her backpack and gave Gavilán the simple instructions.

They continued drifting toward Orville's ill-defined boundary until finally, Orville said, "Okay, folks, it's showtime."

Olga focused the camera on a hangar at the end of the flightline and said, "Is there any way we can get closer?"

"Yes," responded Orville, "but we want to remain as inconspicuous as possible. Let's take a few shots out here, then we'll drift in a little closer." They slowly began to circle the air station. If anything related to the alien aircraft was exposed near the hangar, they would know soon.

ᴜᴜᴜᴜᴜᴜᴜᴜᴜᴜᴜᴜᴜᴜᴜᴜᴜᴜᴜᴜᴜᴜᴜᴜᴜᴜᴜ

"You're awesome, Orville!" exclaimed Olga.

"I didn't think we'd be able to get in this close," added Gavilán.

Just as they were finishing the photo/GIS set, Orville said, "That was our last photo, folks. The jig is up."

The flashing lights of a military police squad car below, racing toward them on State Highway 375, the Extraterrestrial Highway, caught Gavilán's eye. "Now what?" he asked. He didn't have long to wait for the answer to his question. The squad car came to a screeching halt. A short man in a black suit jumped out of the passenger's side, pointing at the balloon as he yelled something at the driver.

Olga raised her camera and peered through the lens to see the action up close and personal. "Damn, it's Stevenson!" she exclaimed.

Gavilán followed, speaking very deliberately, in a lower tone, "Pinche tartamudo." [Darn stutterer.]

Orville tapped Gavilán on the shoulder and said, "More bad news, I'm afraid," as he pointed toward the complex of buildings they had just been photographing. A black Huey helicopter was rapidly approaching.

Below, an MP emerged hastily from the vehicle, raised a gun, and fired a flare that came within twenty feet of the gondola. Orville didn't flinch. He wiped his mouth on the sleeve of his coveralls with a single stroke of his right arm, saying, "I think that was the equivalent of firing a volley across the bow of an unwelcomed ship. That's our cue to head home, and hopefully we won't be followed." Orville proceeded to make the appropriate burner, sandbag, and fan adjustments. By that time, the Huey had reached them and buzzed just past them, making a sharp left turn at full speed as he passed.

"That idiot!" exclaimed Gavilán. "Does he realize how close he came to slicing open the skin of this balloon, sending us plummeting to our deaths?" The helicopter stabilized and hung there at the elevation of the gondola, a hundred feet back toward Area 51. Armed personnel and a gunner at the machine gun mounted at the helicopter's door were clearly visible. Gavilán looked at them and said, "Uh . . . I guess they were trying to tell us something too."

"Now, folks, just stay calm," Orville said. "The party's over, but this balloon hasn't gone into restricted airspace, so we should be okay." Orville waved at the Huey and pointed at the impeller that was slowly pushing the balloon, gondola first, away from the site.

After they drifted away from Area 51 for a few minutes, the Huey slowly retreated backward toward the complex. Soon after that, the men below got into their squad car and sped away toward Las Vegas. Orville let out a big sigh. Gavilán looked at him and put his hand on his shoulder. Orville uttered in a low, slow, deliberate voice, "I think we're okay."

The trip home proved uneventful except for the beautiful southwest sunset as they approached their final destination, Orville's friend's warehouse. As the burner throttle choked the capacity to stay aloft out of the balloon, Orville turned to Olga, saying, "Dr. Ramos, Gavilán didn't tell me much about your project, but I have a feeling that it might have something to do with making our government tell the truth about Roswell. If anyone inquires about our little day trip, well, I just got off course and accidentally drifted too close to the air station. We never violated their airspace. Your name won't be in my records, and Gavilán's forethought about paying with cash makes it an easy matter. And by the way, my balloon is my escape from my past. Sorry if I overdid it at the beginning of the flight."

Olga responded, "Forget it, mister. I couldn't have had a better flight, and I am in your debt."

CADMIUM POISONING

FACTS

- This morning, I had a choice to make regarding the cereal I had for breakfast. Knowing that wheat products are loaded with cadmium, wheat-based cereals are not in the pantry. The theory is that corn- and oat-based cereals should be low in cadmium because corn and oats are naturally low in cadmium. So what was the decision about? The question was "What poison do I want to put in my body—cadmium or mercury?" The oat cereal contained sodium phosphate, and on top of that, it was sugar coated; while the corn cereal contained high-fructose corn syrup (HFCS). Cadmium is contained in the added phosphate and the sugar (absorbed from the soils by sugar beets), while trace amounts of mercury are contained in HFCS from the sodium hydroxide used to extract the fructose from the corn. (Many processed foods, such as cereals, cheeses, evaporated milk, processed deli meats, and puddings, as well as non-food products such as vitamins and supplements, contain phosphate additives. Always read the labels, and avoid cadmium by avoiding phosphates.)

- I recently saw a product made from beets for treating diabetes. Beets could be part of a treatment for diabetes but only if they are cadmium-free beets. You see, cadmium is a carcinogenic heavy metal that is a contaminant in phosphate fertilizers used in growing almost all farm products. Cadmium concentrates primarily in the pancreas, kidneys, liver, lungs, and bones, and to a lesser degree in the thyroid, prostate, and other organs. When it reaches a certain threshold concentration in the pancreas, it results in Type 2 diabetes. On the average, cadmium has about a 30-year biological half-life, compared to about 78 days for zinc, which is an essential mineral for proper brain function, a healthy immune system, and healing in the human body. It is normally found in every strand of DNA and slowly but surely gets pushed out of the body by

131

cadmium. Beets are very efficient at absorbing cadmium; therefore, they are used in the phytoremediation of contaminated soils. Since approximately 56% of the sugar production in the United States is from sugar beets, sugar consumption is accompanied by cadmium consumption/poisoning. If you *know* that the beets you consume were grown in a cadmium-free environment, they could help with diabetes. However, if they were grown with phosphate fertilizers in contaminated soils, you would be shooting yourself in the foot by eating beets, since you would be ingesting large quantities of cadmium, adding to the cause of your Type 2 diabetes.

- Phosphate deposits always contain cadmium, and they are mined to produce phosphate fertilizers and additives (with minimal processing), so if you see *phosphate* on a food label, it is probably accompanied by cadmium. Phosphates are usually added to bacon so that it retains water. That way, they can sell water and rocks for the price of meat.

- Just last night I had to make a similar decision. "What poison do I have for supper—mercury or arsenic?" I was debating between tuna fish and chicken, respectively. I find having to make this kind of decision distasteful (more like utterly disgusting!).

- Many of the mentally ill in this country are turned out onto the streets because there is no room in our country's asylums. Approximately 10% of the mentally ill are violent. While mental illness is strongly linked to poor diet and imbalances of metals in the brain, manganese accumulation and zinc deficiency are implicated in the violent behavior. And zinc deficiency in the brain is strongly linked with the accumulation of cadmium in the rest of the body.

- People who are suffering from cadmium poisoning (and most people are) should avoid x-rays and all forms of ionizing radiation. DNA that is damaged by ionizing radiation in individuals suffering from cadmium poisoning (and consequently zinc deficiency) is less likely to be repaired, and the affected cells are less likely to be dismantled due to the likelihood of a zinc deficiency and impaired immune system. Therefore, propagation of cancer cells that originate from altered DNA due to radiation damage is more likely in individuals suffering from cadmium poisoning. (I don't even let my dentist take x-rays!)

- The FDA, its regulations, and its requirements do not always protect the public. On the contrary, at times they appear to favor special interest groups such as agribusiness and pharmaceutical lobbies. In an article titled "NRDC Scores Major Court Win to Limit Antibiotic Use in Livestock," Natural Resources Defense Council (NRDC) attorney Avinash Kar is quoted as saying "It's time for the FDA to start protecting the American people instead of powerful special interests." The article appears in the June/July 2012 edition of *Nature's Voice*, a publication of the NRDC.

Chapter Twelve

The Encounter

The three adventurers were at the door of Orville's warehouse, exchanging their goodbyes. Olga's first impressions had been completely turned around. She had found that the old geezer had his good points, and her departure was accompanied by a warm feeling of admiration. Gavilán shook Orville's hand, passing a small roll of cash in the handshake. Orville looked down at his hand and back up to Gavilán's face in puzzlement. He had already been paid generously, in cash, for his time and services. Gavilán raised his left hand, almost touching his fingertips to Orville's lips. Not another word was said.

They turned and walked back to the car, Gavilán taking the driver's side and Olga the passenger's side. They simultaneously opened doors and slid into their seats. The taillights came on, and the sound of the engine cranking momentarily broke the silence of the early evening. A puff of dust appeared on the ground beneath the exhaust pipe, and Orville watched them drive off in a cloud of dust.

Olga was very pensive. She was thinking about all that was happening: her sightings in the Sirian heavens, the increasing clarity of the images that appeared to be approaching Earth when they weren't consumed by the brilliance of the star that served as their backdrop, the NASA conference, and now, her clandestine surveillance of a hangar that reportedly contained the remains of an alien aircraft and at least one of its crew members. Were these events related? Was the government trying to hide something? Or was she just becoming preoccupied with the possibility of life elsewhere in the universe? It was all very confusing, but somehow, she *felt* that it was all related.

Olga raised and turned her head slowly toward her devoted Mexican companion and inquired in a soft, low, but deliberate voice, "Gavilán, you know, we've talked about your religious beliefs and my perpetual skepticism before, but do you think that we might not be so unique and that there might be life on other planets?"

"Yes, I think so," came softly from the back seat. Olga and Gavilán looked at each other with puzzlement that quickly turned to astonishment and apprehension when they realized the response was not uttered by either of them. In unison, they jerked their heads around and looked to the back seat. Olga screamed, they both spun around to face forward, and Gavilán slammed on the breaks.

The tires screeched, and before the car had come to a complete halt, Gavilán had killed the engine and removed the key in one smooth stroke. Olga and Gavilán swung their doors open in unison in a cloud of dust. They ran around to the front of the rental car, only to see the being that they had seen in the back seat now sitting on the hood at the front of the car. Gavilán grabbed Olga's hand, and they began to run.

"Wait, please, I mean you no harm," he stated. He spoke flawless English with no discernible accent. "My name is Nivla, and I need your help."

They ran with all that they had in them for about half a minute, but then Olga began to slow down, tugging at Gavilán's arm. She turned as they ran to look at Nivla who seemed very serene, sitting on the hood of the car. Gavilán turned to see why he was having to pull so hard. They both slowed down and came to a stop when they realized the alien was not in pursuit.

They looked at Nivla from a distance, and Olga couldn't contain herself, saying, "What am I doing? All this time I've been searching for alien life-forms, and now . . ." Gavilán heard her speaking but was too stunned to react. Then Olga finished her thought. "I'm going back."

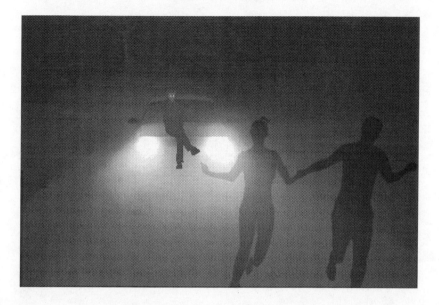

As they approached the vehicle, they could see the creature slowly blinking his large, dark eyes. When they got within fifty feet of the car, Olga asked in a loud voice, "How did you get to the front of the car so fast?"

His small mouth and pointed chin moved slightly as Nivla responded, "I took a shortcut."

Gavilán felt they were getting too close. He grabbed Olga's arm to slow her down as he mumbled, "Oh my god . . . a wise-ass alien!"

Nivla saw that the answer he had given was not very satisfying for the curious Earthlings and continued, "The space that you perceive is like a large piece of fabric. You see it as uniform, but I see the wrinkles in the fabric. When the wrinkles are sufficiently large, the fabric folds back onto itself, and the straight-line distance between two points on the fabric is less than the distance between the two points by following the fabric's surface. I saw the wrinkle and just stepped through the fabric into another dimension and back out at the other point on the fabric while you scrambled about on the fabric's surface.

Gavilán asked in a firm voice, "Who are you, or what are you, and what do you want from us?"

"Nivla is my name, and I mean you no harm," the creature answered. "I come from the planet Treretum that circles a neighboring star system—the star you call Sirius, the Dog Star. And I need your help to recover the remains of my brother."

Olga immediately connected the creature's statement with her sightings. "So tell me. In your travel, do you proceed in a *straight line*, or do you follow the surface of the fabric?" she inquired.

Nivla was pleased to see that the Earthlings had made some sense of the simplistic explanation he had given. "We travel in a straight line," he responded.

I knew it! Olga thought to herself as her face lit up. *That's why the sightings were intermittent.*

ꊐꊐꊐꊐꊐꊐꊐꊐꊐꊐꊐꊐꊐꊐꊐꊐꊐꊐꊐꊐꊐꊐꊐꊐꊐꊐꊐꊐꊐ

They stood in front of the hood of their rental vehicle, headlights still burning, illuminating dust particles that traversed the beams of light. And the creature sat calmly on the hood, listening to Gavilán. The initial apprehension Olga and Gavilán had felt was fading. "Why us?" asked Olga.

The creature replied, "Your profile was one of several that indicated your natural curiosity would allow you to overcome your initial fear and that you might be sympathetic to my honorable mission. My appearance before you is unauthorized by my superiors, but my brother's remains are needed by my family to be able to continue without him."

Gavilán interrupted, "You mean that this encounter has nothing to do with me, right?"

Olga put one arm across Gavilán's chest to regain control of the conversation, asking the alien, "Whuh, what makes you think that I can do anything to help you?"

Paying no attention to Olga's gesture, Gavilán again interrupted, "I never imagined that I would be the one to actually meet one of *the teachers*." His comment caught Olga's curiosity, so she remained silent to let her companion go on.

Gavilán continued, "My grandfather was a storyteller, a historian of the Socolsotav tribe. He was charged with the responsibility, as were his grandfather before him and his grandfather's grandfather before him, of learning the stories that were passed down by our ancient Mayan ancestors. Each grandfather and grandson spent many months living together passing on the details of the many stories, followed by countless evenings of reviewing the details until the day that the elder's spirit left his body to join the Great Spirit. My brother, León, was the chosen one of my generation to be the storyteller, but I remember many of the stories that I heard my grandfather tell." Gavilán looked at Olga, and then they both looked at the pale creature with the large brown eyes as he gazed at Gavilán, showing no expression in his face. Gavilán grabbed the leather strand that went around his neck to pull the gold artifact from under his T-shirt. He placed it on the palm of his right hand and extended it toward the alien.

Olga asked, "Do you understand what he is talking about?"

The creature responded by opening his small mouth, uttering a single word, "Yes."

Gavilán continued as he tucked away the artifact, "It was when I was an undergraduate at Stanford, taking a course in comparative religion, that I first had a strange feeling that there was a bigger picture of which we were only seeing a small piece. I was doing research for a paper that I was doing on the Hindu religion, and I ran across some passages from an ancient tale of *the teachers*. These were beings of great intelligence, knowledge, and wisdom that provided guidance on construction projects, on matters of health, and interpretation of the movement of the stars. They floated over the Earth that they traversed, and they rose high above the Earth in winged chairs and flying machines. These were the same stories I had heard my grandfather tell of *the teachers* that guided the construction of the great pyramids and observatories of the Yucatan. The legends say that *the teachers* would return one day. Nivla, does any of this make sense to you? Can you shed a ray of sunlight on this shadow that has been troubling my soul for the last twenty years?"

"I do not have firsthand knowledge," said the creature, "but I heard my grandfather tell stories of his trips to planets of our nearest neighboring stars, a star you call Epsilon Eridani and your sun."

With a puzzled look on his face, Gavilán tugged at Olga's sleeve as he leaned toward her, asking in a low voice, "Isn't that where Spock was from? Yeah, the planet Vulcan."

The creature continued in the tone of an instructor, "Epsilon Eridani is closer—a little over seven light-years from Sirius, compared to the 8.6 light-years to your sun. But I remember my grandfather talking of his experiences and those of his grandfather before him, and the most interesting stories were about their interactions with the inhabitants and the guidance they provided at several locations on the third planet . . . I think that they were referring to their visits to your planet, Earth."

Doubting that there could be a connection, Gavilán said, "But no, this would have happened several thousands of years earlier."

"My grandfather died not long ago, when he was nearly six bak'tuns old," interrupted Nivla. "In terms that you will understand, he was more than two thousand of your Earth years old. And both he and his father were the youngest in the family of each of their generations."

Gavilán and Olga turned to each other with looks of astonishment. Olga slowly turned again to Nivla with her head tilted slightly to the right and asked, "Nivla, how old are you?"

Nivla tilted his head slightly to the left in response to Olga's head mannerism. "I am a middle-aged Treretumian. I have lived almost three bak'tuns, more than one thousand of your Earth years."

Gavilán stared at Nivla as he muttered, "Pinch me, Olga. I think I'm dreaming the craziest dream I've had in a really long time."

ꛯꛯꛯꛯꛯꛯꛯꛯꛯꛯꛯꛯꛯꛯꛯꛯꛯꛯꛯꛯꛯꛯꛯꛯꛯꛯꛯꛯ

"Nivla, can you tell me anything about the ancient Rishi City of Mohemjodaro in India which appears to have experienced three nuclear blasts several thousand years ago? This issue has also bothered me for far too many years," Gavilán admitted openly. "The ruins were unearthed by archaeologists in the last century when the high radiation levels were detected. Radioactive skeletons of people holding hands were uncovered, lying in street, as though they were running from something but were overtaken."

Olga's jaw fell, and her eyes opened wide, staring at Gavilán. "You never told me about any of this." Gavilán raised one hand, palm extended outward, and motioned with the other hand for her to stop as he continued to focus on Nivla.

Nivla responded almost apologetically, "It was never intended to happen."

There was a long pause. Olga and Gavilán looked at each other and then back at Nivla.

"You mean that the Treretumians attacked the citizens of Mohemjodaro with nuclear weapons?" asked Gavilán, with Olga interjecting as an afterthought to complete the sentence, "But you meant them no harm, just like you mean us no harm."

Nivla looked at Olga and then turned his head toward Gavilán without saying a word. It was clear that both had become more unsettled. Finally, Nivla spoke. "The mission was to aid in the advancement of civilization on your planet—to assist with the advancement of your technology—to help Earthlings in the recognition of problems associated with the environment and lend support in its conquest."

"Conquest?" exclaimed Olga, almost as a reflex to what she had just heard.

Gavilán, having been intrigued in his earlier years by ancient reports of the blasts, responded with more composure. With great deliberation in his speech, he inquired, "You mean that the ancient epic Hindu tales that describe flying machines, flying multistory structures, and terrible battles raging across the skies, culminating in the detonation of what now appears to have been several nuclear devices that were described as 'a column of energy that had the intensity of a thousand suns,' were all based on fact?"

"Please, let me explain," Nivla implored. "We were under attack."

"Oh right, by a band of spear-hurling Neanderthals," Olga said, sarcastically.

A bit disturbed, Nivla said in a controlled but stern tone, "No. You wanted to know, and you asked the question—now please be so kind as to listen to the answer."

It was as though she had been corrected by her third grade school teacher. Olga and Gavilán were both silent and attentive.

"Those were difficult times on Treretum," Nivla stated softly. "The invasion of the Muimdac had been thwarted, and it was time to plan ahead and prepare for the future. As in any civilization that has survived a war that could have ended its existence had the outcome been slightly different, Treretum and its inhabitants needed to heal, to recover from the massive loss of life experienced and the disruption in progress that every war creates. The population began to increase, and soon it was predicted that our planet would be overrun."

"You mean that your planet would not be able to support the needs of the population?" asked Gavilán.

Nivla responded, "Yes, it became clear that with the technologies of the time, Treretum was incapable of generating sufficient food for the masses. There was insufficient space for us to adequately capture energy from our suns to generate the food necessary to sustain us. We had difficult decisions to make. Emphasis was placed on our interplanetary exploration efforts and, of course, birth control."

Olga was amazed to hear this creature telling a tale that included many of concerns of our own planet, but she failed to see the connection. She inquired, "How is all this related to the nuclear detonations in India here on Earth?"

"It was on one of the extended expeditions," Nivla continued. "Three Treretumian spacecraft arrived on Earth. The environment was relatively hospitable, and the inhabitants appeared to be advancing as we had many millennia before. Well into our mission of assisting Earthlings with the advancement of their civilizations, the presence of a substantial Muimdac contingent was uncovered. The enemy that had been presumed to be vanquished was very much alive and in our midst. They seized control of one of our spacecraft to attack the Treretumians on the other two . . . and you can imagine the rest. In the end, the only way to ensure that the Muimdac posed no threat to the Treretumian mission or the inhabitants of Earth was to destroy the spacecraft and the Muimdac within it."

Ⅰ⅃ⅠⅣⅠⅣⅠⅣⅠⅣⅠⅣⅠⅣⅠⅣⅠⅣⅠⅣⅠⅣⅠⅣⅠⅣⅠⅣⅠⅣⅠⅣⅠⅣⅠⅣⅠⅣⅠⅣ

The fantastic story they had just heard was alarming, almost unbelievable, but plausible. Olga and Gavilán exchanged opinions in a private huddle. Everything the alien had divulged fit. Previously unanswered questions had been answered for Gavilán. Olga and Gavilán turned toward the alien.

"How can we possibly help you?" Olga inquired. "You appear to come from a far more technically advanced society than ours."

"My brother, Nomis, was in an accident that occurred on this planet several decades ago. The wreckage and the remains of the accident victims were removed from the crash site and transported to an unknown location. I have come to collect my brother's remains and those of the other two victims. They died in the service of their planet. They deserve to be treated with honor and their remains returned to Treretum where a place of honor is reserved as their final place of rest.

"You have just returned from Area 51, the place that is most likely the location of the spacecraft wreckage and my brother's remains. Please share with me the information about this heavily guarded site that I will need to recover our dead. That is all I seek."

"Again, how can we possibly help you?" Olga repeated.

The alien continued, "Once we find the remains, we could seize them by force, but that is not our desire. We prefer to remove our honored dead silently, undetected. Our best information indicates that Hangar 18 is the most likely location."

"I have extensive photographs of Hangar 18," Olga volunteered. There was something about this being that Olga found honorable and admirable.

"Yeah, but that place is locked up tight as a drum," added Gavilán. He shared Olga's sympathetic views, but he was very concerned about how the conversation was going—he felt they were being drawn into an untenable situation. "Even the airspace is patrolled all around the area.

Security is probably tighter there than at Fort Knox." Gavilán paused. "Can't you do your wrinkled fabric routine and just slip in and take your brother's remains?"

"Another detail that I must mention—this recovery is not sanctioned by the authorities in charge of our spacecraft. This mission—"

Gavilán interrupted, "You mean this is your own personal mission, in the name of family honor."

Nivla raised his head, paused for a few seconds and softly responded with a single word, "Yes."

"You've got to be kidding!" Gavilán exclaimed as he began to wave his hands up and down. He turned to Olga, continuing with his dismay, "He's got to be kidding."

Olga continued to look straight at the alien as she reached to capture Gavilán's arms in calming gestures. "Maybe we can help."

CADMIUM POISONING

FACTS

- Sirius, also known as the Dog Star, is the star system containing Nivla's beloved Treretum. Dogs and cats in our solar system, much like their owners, are being exposed to high levels of cadmium in their diets, and just like humans, dogs and cats get diabetes, and they die of kidney failure, liver failure, and cancer.

- You may have heard your vet say that the first organs to go out on a dog are the kidneys—"They start passing protein in their urine, so make sure you keep them on a low protein diet." Well, that's hogwash. They start passing protein in their urine because their kidneys are starting to fail, and that is likely due to their high-cadmium diet. The grain and animal by-products that are likely the mainstay of their diet are low in zinc and high in cadmium, respectively.

- Animal by-products, whether it's beef, chicken, or otherwise, are the parts of a slaughtered animal that are left over after the parts considered suitable for human consumption have been removed. They can include, for example, the pancreas, liver, lungs, kidneys, stomach, feet, backs, heads (including brains), ovaries, testicles, spleen, and intestines.

- Many of the same organs are sold for human consumption (e.g., chicken giblets, which contain hearts, livers, and other organs; hot dogs, bologna, and sausage, which can contain the same organs that go into dog food. The deciding factor as to whether these organs go into dog food versus hot dogs is how they are handled after slaughter. For example, giblets for human consumption must be refrigerated immediately after slaughter, but meats that go into dog food can be stored for up to 24 hours without refrigeration. Refrigerated or not, including the organs where cadmium tends

145

to accumulate results in both man and man's best friend being cadmium poisoned.

- Another cadmium-rich ingredient in many dog and cat foods is animal by-product meal, made from animal by-products that are rendered (i.e., made into a stew, with the fat skimmed off the top and cooked until the remaining water is eliminated) and then baked and ground into concentrated protein powder.

- The FDA Center for Veterinary Medicine (CVM) tested pet foods from major manufacturers and found trace amounts of sodium pentobarbital. This is the primary chemical used to euthanize animals. Generally, in addition to processing carcasses from slaughterhouses, rendering plants process dead zoo animals, euthanized dogs and cats, and even road kill. It all goes into the animal by-product vat to make meal.

- Animal by-products and animal by-product meal are high-cadmium products. Because of their high protein content and relatively low cost, they are a major component of pet foods. Phosphates are often added as well. Read the ingredients—not only the labels on the food products that go on your table but also on the labels on products that go into your dog's and cat's bowls.

Chapter Thirteen

The Powwow

It was like homecoming for both of them. The Bay Area was near and dear to their hearts, a haven that was so conducive for personal growth that neither could imagine having gone to school anywhere else. It was Olga's turn at the wheel, but Gavilán was wide awake, sitting at her side. Although he often worked in the Bay Area, Gavilán seldom found his way to the campus or the surrounding area. Both looked forward to visiting their old stomping grounds: Stanford Stadium and Maples Pavilion, Mem Chu, the Quad, the Rodin sculpture garden, Lagunita, the bookstore with the nearby fountain, Mem Claw. This was what they had been looking forward to before destiny, the DHS, and a large alien had changed their plans for them.

The night drive had placed them in Palo Alto shortly after sunrise, and without thinking, Olga elected to enter the campus by driving in on the scenic route—Palm Drive. The palm trees on either side of the road with the Quad visible off in the distance brought back many memories. They passed the turnoff for the Stanford Museum and the Old Chemistry Building and approached the Oval, a dedicated grassy area surrounded by flowerbeds and paved pathways—a perfect place for Frisbee enthusiasts. But Olga kept looking to the right, peering in the direction of the Old Chemistry Building.

Gavilán noticed her preoccupation and remembered hearing Olga talk about her experiences there. He held his fist up to his mouth as though he were holding a microphone, saying in a faint voice, "Dr. Olga Ramos returns to campus as a lead research engineer at the NASA Jet Propulsion Laboratory in Los Angeles. She received her PhD from Stanford University and fondly remembers seeing the elderly Nobel Prize winner, Linus Pauling, answering questions after his advanced organic chemistry class as she and the rest of her quantum mechanics class shuffled into the classroom that they shared."

"How is it that you remember things I said in passing years ago?" she asked. Gavilán made a funny "I don't know" face and shrugged his shoulders.

They drove up the right side of the Oval and approached the Quad where Memorial Church—affectionately referred to as Mem Chu— could be seen on the far side of the Quad through a set of arches near them. Olga brought the car to a stop and looked beyond Gavilán to her right as the engine idled. Gavilán could see a million things going through her mind by looking at her eyes.

"¿Muchos recuerdos, preciosa?" [Many memories, precious?]

She responded with a faint, "Sí." [Yes.]

෴෴෴෴෴෴෴෴෴෴෴෴෴෴෴෴෴෴෴෴෴෴෴෴෴෴෴෴෴

They made their way back to Campus Drive and over toward Stanford Stadium. The unmistakable smell of eucalyptus was everywhere as were the towering giants that were perpetually shedding the thin outer layer of their bark. Suddenly, Olga turned to Gavilán and said, "You know, Leland Stanford brought the first eucalyptus trees to California from Australia." She glanced forward to make sure she kept the car on the curved road.

"Yes, I know," Gavilán responded calmly. He saw new buildings encroaching on the open spaces that he remembered as they drove. Gavilán commented, "The campus continues to grow, filling in open spaces."

"Yeah, you're right," Olga said with a big smile on her face. "I remember climbing this gigantic loquat tree in an open area—I think it was out toward Mayfield Drive. I used to pick the loquats, eat half of them while I was in the tree, spitting out the big brown seeds. I'd have my pockets full before climbing down from the tree . . . and they were sooooo good." This was obviously one of her fond memories, but then the smile went away as she continued in near disgust, "Now, there's a dorm in that space."

"I know," chimed in Gavilán. "You know, we had to worry about where we were going to live after freshman year, and it was no fun. Some were lucky to find dorm slots, others found on-campus housing by going the Greek route, and some of us wound up off campus, but it was part of growing up."

"Yeah!" interjected Olga jokingly.

Gavilán's tone changed as he mimicked Olga with "Yeah!"

Olga, knowing that another one was coming, paused, and took a deep breath. Then in unison they exclaimed with another "Yeah!" They laughed briefly, but then it was time to get back to matters at hand. Olga asked, "When are you supposed to meet your friend?"

"Oh yeah, Puma!" answered Gavilán, as though he had almost forgotten about his scheduled meeting. "We're supposed to meet this afternoon at three by the fountain in front of the bookstore. That's always been one of my favorite meeting places on campus—I guess because that fountain reminds me of the talons of an eagle."

Olga nodded in agreement. "You're not alone. Why else would it have been dubbed Mem Claw?"

"Anyway, we're supposed to meet after he finishes with his part of the tribal presentation," continued Gavilán. "He is with the contingent from the Shoshone-Bannock tribes right now." Gavilán glanced at Olga and added, "I also met Puma at a Stanford Powwow, many years ago."

"Interesting name," Olga commented.

"Yep, and it suited him well—sleek and graceful yet powerful and demanding of respect. He was one of the Shoshone dancers—quite impressive, decked out in his native dress.

"I spoke with him last week. He was telling me that two of the elder members had to cancel on the Powwow because they were diagnosed with cancer and needed to be with their families."

"Oh no!" exclaimed Olga, sympathetically.

Gavilán added, "It seems they've been having more than their share up in Idaho."

ℿℿℿℿℿℿℿℿℿℿℿℿℿℿℿℿℿℿℿℿℿℿℿℿℿℿℿℿ

Gavilán saw Puma approaching. He rose from his concrete seat at the edge of the fountain and began walking toward Puma with his hand extended to greet his friend. Gavilán's upbeat "Hello, my brother" rang out in the open-air plaza. The two men embraced, and after several pats on the back, they separated.

"Cuauhtémoc Gavilán, it's been a long time," Puma said in a low voice. There was sadness in his voice.

Gavilán lowered his head slightly and looked up into his brother's tired and troubled eyes. "Too long," he responded. His concern showed on his face. "Brother, what is wrong?"

Puma turned his head to the left, away from Gavilán in an effort to hide the tears that wanted to flow. "Nothing." He paused and then continued in a mumble, "And everything."

Gavilán put his hand on Puma's left shoulder. "I know much has happened in my life since we last met, but your demeanor tells me that you are troubled. The young man that I remember was invincible. But now, before me, I see a warrior who has been beaten—someone who is ready to give up."

"You read me well," Puma replied. The two men turned and walked back where Gavilán had been waiting. "My people are in distress. We are plagued by disease, and no one seems to be able to do anything about it or even know why." They sat down at the edge of the fountain.

Gavilán's natural curiosity and environmental background were already kicking in. Knowing that two of the tribal elders had been diagnosed with cancer and dreading the possible answer, he asked, "How is your family?"

Puma replied as tears again began to collect in his eyes, "In the seven years that have passed since our last meeting, my mother developed diabetes, and my father's coronary arteries became clogged. They were both treated, but then my mother was diagnosed with kidney cancer. My father remained strong despite his inoperable heart condition. The chemotherapy was very hard on my mother. I felt so impotent, so helpless. There was nothing I could do—just watch her die. When she passed, I was unsure as to whether it had been the cancer or the treatment that did her in."

Gavilán offered his sympathy—"I'm so sorry, my brother." It was clear that recounting the recent past was stressful because of the clouds that formed in Puma's eyes. He knew that Shoshone men do not cry.

Puma continued, "It was shortly after that that my father was diagnosed with stomach cancer. After they removed half of his stomach, it was his turn to endure the ordeal of chemo. He would tell me that the days immediately after his chemo were absolutely miserable. After a brief remission, the cancer returned. In the end, his doctors were making bets as to whether it would be his heart or his stomach cancer that would get him, but the cancer won."

Gavilán interjected, "But your parents weren't that old."

"I know," responded Puma. "They both died in their mid-sixties. And then we lost an aunt to breast cancer and an uncle to pancreatic cancer, both diabetic. The list goes on. That generation is rapidly disappearing from my family."

"Cancer! Why so much cancer in your family?" inquired Gavilán.

"It's not just my family," Puma explained. "The health concerns of the tribe are on display on the Shoshone-Bannock website—diabetes and cancer."

The scene was somber, and Gavilán hated to see his friend in a state of depression. He changed his tone and exclaimed jokingly, "I know I probably shouldn't do this, but how about we go over to Tressider Union and have a couple of beers—so we can cry in 'em?"

Puma reacted sternly. "I assume you mean that figuratively."

Gavilán responded instantaneously, "Of course."

Puma smiled, nodded, and whispered, "Yeah."

ꙮꙮꙮꙮꙮꙮꙮꙮꙮꙮꙮꙮꙮꙮꙮꙮꙮꙮꙮꙮꙮꙮꙮꙮꙮꙮꙮꙮ

Gavilán's phone rang, and he quickly answered, noting that Olga was the caller.

"Hola, mi amor," [*Hello, my love.* This is a common greeting.] came rolling off Gavilán's tongue.

Olga responded with "Hola-a-a-a. Are we still going to connect at Chef Chu's for supper?"

"Sounds right to me," he replied.

Inquisitive, Olga then inquired, "How was your visit with Puma?"

Gavilán described what had happened and conveyed the story Puma had shared. He then commented, "I wonder if it's a genetic issue."

"Mmmm, maybe, but I doubt it," she responded incredulously. "You know, this reminds me a little of something I read about that happened in a village in Japan, where everyone was suffering from bone pain, diabetes, and cancer. They gave it a special name—*itai-itai* disease. That's 'ouch-ouch' in Japanese. It didn't matter how old they were—it affected everyone. Eventually they traced it back to contaminated rice that everyone was eating because they had built their rice paddies on cadmium-contaminated soil. In other words, it was cadmium poisoning."

"Like what you said we were getting from the phosphate fertilizers the farmers use to grow their crops, right?" interjected Gavilán.

"Yeah, but more so," she responded. "I'll bet there's something going on in their food or their water—something that results in chronic, low-level cadmium exposure. You know cadmium accumulates in the body over time, so a little goes a long way. Do you know if the CDC or EPA has done an epidemiological study on this, Eagle Man?"

Gavilán was sensitive to the plight of his brother's tribe. "I don't think so. Somebody from the tribe needs to look into this—get whatever help they need from the outside—but it needs to be someone who has direct involvement, a vested interest." He continued more slowly and in a lower tone, "Phosphate fertilizers . . . hmmm. I'll pass it on."

"You know, I feel bad for Puma and his people. After all they have endured at our hand—and I say 'our' only because I am a U.S. citizen—they certainly don't deserve this." Olga paused, and then she mumbled in a low voice, "Que lástima." [What a pity.]

"¡Que pecado!" [What a sin!] responded Gavilán in a much more resolute tone.

"¡Que verguensa!" [How shameful!] exclaimed Olga in a tone of utter disgust.

꘎꘎꘎꘎꘎꘎꘎꘎꘎꘎꘎꘎꘎꘎꘎꘎꘎꘎꘎꘎꘎꘎꘎꘎꘎꘎꘎꘎꘎

The hustle and bustle of Chef Chu's was always invigorating for both of them, and the food was a true delight that made the wait well worthwhile. The word about town was that the delicate battered prawns, the tasty sauces on the lettuce-wrapped Mushu pork, and, of course, old spicy standards like Kung Pao chicken all made every visit to Chef Chu's an evening to remember.

After being seated and placing their orders, Olga and Gavilán had a chance to relax and get caught up with Charlie, the maître d', and be updated on his family's achievements since the last visit. Charlie and his wife were proud Chinese Americans, and their three children—two sons and a daughter—had names that were as American as apple pie. After Charlie excused himself so that he could go do his job, Olga and Gavilán began to reminisce.

There was the standard chitchat about how much the area has changed, how many more people have moved into the area, the traffic, the weather, how wonderful it is to be back, etc. But then Olga made a departure in the conversation. "The good old days were good, but they are old . . . ancient history. Inquiring minds want to know—what's *new* in your life? Tell me more about Gavilán's current endeavors."

He responded, "Well, my current project is probably the most important undertaking of my life. If this works as effectively in the field as it does in the bench-scale studies, it will revolutionize the way that remediation of soils and groundwater contaminated with chlorinated solvents is carried out. Cost will no longer be prohibitive, and the low-income families that live near contaminated industrial sites will be less likely to be exposed to the chlorinated solvents or their partial degradation products, which in some cases are far more toxic and more mobile than the original contaminants. I just wish it had been available a few decades ago when the environmental restoration movement was in its heyday. Even so, we would be lightening what I think of as a *poverty tax* on people who live around contaminated sites. These people are subjected to injustices due to things that are beyond their control. And their ability to just pick up and leave is strictly a function of their economic status. Most just can't afford it."

"Sounds interesting," Olga responded. "I also feel strongly about the poverty tax, as you put it. I became aware of poverty issues back when I was a little girl." She paused and bowed her head in modesty for an instant. Then she said with a smile, "Knowing you, you'll keep working on your new technology until it is so affordable that anyone can set up a remediation system in his or her back yard."

Gavilán nodded his head as he continued, "I may not know all of the fundamental, underlying principles, but I know enough to be able to apply the science for the benefit of humanity and my Mother Earth."

"Hey, wait a minute, she's my Mother Earth," interjected Olga jokingly.

Gavilán looked her rather sternly and responded in a very somber tone, "She is the Mother of all living things . . . well, all things living of which the ancients were aware. She provides for all our needs, and we must protect her."

Olga could see she had touched a nerve. She reached across the table and took his hands in hers. "I know. I wasn't trying to make light of our environmental woes. I realize that our fathers' and our generations have adversely affected our environment more than any others in the history of the planet. We are the cause of global warming, destroyed habitats, and the spread of toxic contaminants beyond belief."

Olga hoped that her few sentences had restored her in Gavilán's esteem. She lowered her head slightly to be able to look up into Gavilán's eyes. When they made eye contact, she saw what she had interpreted as anger melt away. "I'm sorry," Olga said. "I didn't mean to offend you."

Gavilán smiled and said in a much calmer voice, "Ms. Cause and Effect."

Olga saw this as an opportunity to steer the conversation away from environmental remediation while staying with the "cause and effect" theme. She smiled back at Gavilán and commented, "You know, our society is too caught up in treating the symptom without knowing the cause. I remember in graduate school, one of the concerns regarding every line of investigation that was pursued in the department was that it had to have the goal of getting to a fundamental truth. Certainly, the application of the research results was of the utmost importance, and those that were interested in the application of those results were ultimately footing the bill. But we were never to lose sight of the fundamental research goal, and the distinction between fundamental and applied research was never in question.

"One day, my veterinarian told me that most dogs die of kidney failure, that they begin to pass protein, and that protein was a dog's worst enemy. For years, I sought out the dry dog food with the lowest advertised protein content. Today, I'm convinced that he was wrong, and my dogs get zinc supplements because the real enemy isn't protein. It's something else altogether—something that is causing the kidneys to be unable to filter out the proteins. Dogs are natural carnivores, and how many carnivores do you know of that are on a low-protein meat diet?"

"None in my family," he replied jokingly.

Olga continued, "My mother was the first diabetic I ever knew but certainly not the last. The dreaded disease struck others in the family, and my aunt repeatedly lectured me, 'Ya no comas tanta cosa dulce . . . te va dar diabetes.' [Don't eat so many sweets . . . you're going to get diabetes.] But like the story about my dog, it made no sense to me. My body was designed to make sugar, glucose to feed the cells of my muscles, my nerves, my brain—and the inevitable fluctuations are dealt with by the storage of the initial surge by my liver and the production of insulin by the beta cells of my pancreas.

"If my pancreas is functioning as designed, the insulin will be produced, circulate in my bloodstream, and attach to the cells of my body. It is the key that allows the glucose to be absorbed. The glucose can then be drawn out of my bloodstream to nourish the cells of my body. As the available glucose in my bloodstream is depleted, liver reserves are tapped, then fat is converted to glucose—if necessary—and the cycle continues until the next tasty morsel passes my lips. The high blood sugar is the symptom, not the cause of diabetes."

Gavilán felt the discussion was getting too technical, but he decided to go with the flow. "But how can you be so sure?" he asked.

"I'm an engineer and a damn good one. I have studied design, and the body is a marvelous and miraculous design, far more complex and interrelated that any man-made chemical plant or refinery could ever be. The liver alone is capable of performing thousands of different reactions to detoxify the organic poisons that are contained in our food. As an engineer, methinks that the designer of the human body would not have overlooked this little detail regarding sugar. Besides, why would we have been given taste buds that can appreciate *sweet* if we were never to indulge in *la cosa dulce* [the sweet stuff]? Of course, if something has gone awry, and the body no longer processes sugar as it should, eating sweets is just adding fuel to the fire. No, Gavilán, I'm a firm believer in *cause and effect*, and with regard to diabetes, sugar in the blood is the latter rather than the former."

Just then, the food arrived and was served with the grace and elegance that both Gavilán and Olga had become accustomed to expect at Chef Chu's. They decided to share their generous and aromatic servings to add variety to their delight. Olga reached forward with her fork to sample the Kung Pao chicken while Gavilán picked up a piece of broccoli from Olga's beef and broccoli plate with his chopsticks. They looked at each other, and then both glanced to the table next to them where platters of butterflied prawns and Mushu pork were being set down.

Gavilán said, "Maybe I should have ordered the prawns."

Olga reached across the table and touched Gavilán's hand. "No, you made the right choice," she reassured him. "But I don't want to spoil it for them. I'll tell you later."

"Is it hot?" he asked.

With her mouth half full, Olga responded, "Thermally hot or spicy hot?'

Gavilán chuckled as he responded, "Ah, spoken like a true engineer."

After glancing at the platter of prawns on the next table, Gavilán leaned forward and lowered his voice, saying, "But we all have roughly the same cadmium exposure, don't we?"

"Nope," she said defiantly.

"Okay, give me an example," he insisted.

"Eskimos," she declared. "Lots of protein and fat in their diets from seal and whale blubber, no industry, no crops, no fertilizer, no cadmium, no cancer, and no heart disease. The body does what it's supposed to and breaks down the fat to make glucose for the cells of their bodies."

"Hmmm . . ." muttered Gavilán. His opportunity to lighten the conversation had arrived. "Strange. But funny that you should mention Eskimos. Just the other day, I read about a disease that has become very serious among the Eskimo population. It is very contagious, and it is transmitted when Eskimos kiss."

"Really? I hadn't heard anything about that. What is the disease?" Olga asked inquisitively.

"*Sniffilus*," said Gavilán, trying to keep a straight face.

"¡Pendejo!" [Dummy!] she exclaimed as she reached across the table and punched him in the arm. They both laughed for a long time, with tears coming to Olga's eyes. During the laughter, their waitress dropped off the bill for their meal. Slowly, the laughter subsided. Gavilán picked up the bill and began to examine it.

Olga looked at Gavilán, knowing he was so right for her. She was very fortunate to have crossed paths with him so many years ago. She said softly, "Thank you."

Gavilán briefly took his eyes off the bill and glanced at Olga, gently smiling as he said, "Sure. But what's that for?"

"For being you," she said.

Gavilán looked at Olga. There was a brief pause, and then Gavilán took a deep breath before saying, "Let me pay the tab, and let's get outta here."

"All right, Eagle Man," Olga said in a voice filled with self-determination. "That was very sweet of you, but I'll pick up the next one."

"Deal!" he responded.

ꂚꂚꂚꂚꂚꂚꂚꂚꂚꂚꂚꂚꂚꂚꂚꂚꂚꂚꂚꂚꂚꂚꂚꂚꂚꂚꂚ

Olga and Gavilán arrived at their suite, and as usual, they had their separate rooms awaiting them. The suites they booked when traveling together always had a common area that allowed them to discuss things and explore ideas in a comfortable, relaxed setting.

The meal had been the usual treat for all the senses. The first things they did upon entering the suite were to set down their bags, kick off their shoes, and plop down on the comfortable easy chair and sofa.

With her arms draped over the arms of the easy chair, Olga chuckled and said, "Sniffilus."

Gavilán chuckled with her, but his thoughts returned to the stories about cadmium. "You know, you seem to know a lot about this cadmium issue, and I can see that you want to share the information with others, but I also see that you tend to hold back."

"There's a time and place for everything, and people generally don't want to hear it. I learned my lesson one time at the Little Red Barn in San Antonio. One of the Texas cowgirl waitresses—dressed up in her tight-fitting red blouse, short skirt, string-pull cowboy hat, boots, and a gun belt and holster holding a toy six-shooter at her hip—came up to the table next to mine to take the order of the couple sitting at that table. When the man asked for a steak and shrimp platter with a baked potato instead of plain ol' French fries, I cringed. After the waitress finished taking the order, he leaned forward and said to the lady sitting across the table from him, 'Baked potatoes—you know, I just love the potato skins because not only do they have more flavor than the rest of the potato, that's where all the vitamins and minerals are.'" Olga paused, moved her head back, made a face, and shook her head slightly from side to side—como si tuviera asco [as if she had been grossed out].

Gavilán squinted slightly, nodding his head, affirming he could envision exactly what she was describing.

Olga continued, "I couldn't contain myself. I blurted out in a voice of near-desperation, 'But one of the minerals is cadmium . . . DON'T DO IT!'"

Gavilán began to laugh, and Olga continued, speaking over his laughter, "The normal high-noise level of people enjoying themselves dropped to zilch. You could have heard a pin drop, and everyone was looking at me. And the man at the next table gave me the dirtiest look with the ugliest scowl on his face you can imagine. I felt like melting and oozing under the table. Once people started talking again, and the noise level went back up, I tried to discretely excuse myself from the restaurant."

꙰꙰꙰꙰꙰꙰꙰꙰꙰꙰꙰꙰꙰꙰꙰꙰꙰꙰꙰꙰꙰꙰꙰꙰꙰꙰꙰꙰꙰꙰꙰꙰

Before retiring, Olga wanted to check her e-mail, so she pulled out her computer. This reminded Gavilán that he had not heard a word on the results from their grand balloon adventure. Olga announced that she would be going to bed.

"Okay, but before you do, what did your super-duper camera and computer collect at Area 51?" inquired Gavilán.

Olga got up from the sofa where she was sitting and walked over to the table by the window. She set the computer down next to the computer case that was already on the table and replied, "Well, let's take a look and see." She quickly began typing. The rapid "tick-click" of the laptop keyboard dominated the sound waves in the room. "I just have to run the data analysis program, upload the collected data, and then we're in business." Within minutes, Olga had produced an amazingly detailed image of Hangar 18, complete with guards standing at the fence and hangar doors. She motioned to Gavilán, who stepped behind her to look over her shoulder.

"That's nice," he said in a tone that clearly indicated disappointed expectations.

Olga raised her right hand with her forefinger extended. With the touch of a key, the image began to zoom in closer and closer. Gavilán began to show interest as the center of the image became larger and larger. With another keystroke, the images began to move—armed guards paced back and forth in front of the compound gates. Olga selected the head of one of the guards with the touchpad, and soon, the face of the guard began to dominate the screen. Closer . . . closer . . .

"Ooo, a bad shave day!" Olga exclaimed sarcastically. She continued to zoom in until a single hair from the guard's inadequately shaved face occupied the entire screen. "Should I continue?"

"No! I'm very impressed," Gavilán said as he took a step back and shook his head.

"Oh, but I must," she replied playfully. With another keystroke, the view zoomed out to include the guard's entire face. Olga continued slowly in a low comical voice as she lifted her right hand, again with forefinger extended, "Observe."

With the click of another key, the head of the guard rotated 180 degrees, exposing the back of his head. "Uh oh!—a bald spot!" Olga announced. "Time for some Rogaine . . . or better yet, some zinc and sulfur."

"Huh?" exclaimed Gavilán. "How can you get the back side of his head? We were in the balloon. How could you have gotten a shot from this angle?"

"Calm down, my little eaglet," she said in a calming voice as she motioned with both hands, palms down. "The footage we took wasn't individual photographs but, rather, scans, capturing any and all movement in the field of vision. The software I just used to analyze the scans keys in on moving objects, compiling data to develop three-dimensional images, if possible. If the object rotates 360 degrees during a scan, we have a pretty good idea of what it looks like from all angles and how the object moves. The guard was a piece of cake since he was constantly moving. The building, on the other hand, is a different matter, and we have to depend on the different angles from the balloon for resolution and definition of the building's features."

"Wow! Now I'm really impressed," responded Gavilán enthusiastically.

ꙨꙨꙨꙨꙨꙨꙨꙨꙨꙨꙨꙨꙨꙨꙨꙨꙨꙨꙨꙨꙨꙨꙨꙨꙨꙨꙨꙨꙨ

Olga had just retired, and Gavilán still sat on the sofa in the common area, enjoying the moment. There was a knock at the door. Gavilán stood up, walked to the door, and cracked it open, but no one was there. Gavilán locked the door, turned, and much to his surprise, Nivla and two companions had appeared out of nowhere and stood before him.

"Nivla!" he exclaimed. "How did you get in here?" Gavilán caught himself and, with a change of expression on his face, said, "Never mind . . . I remember—we have wrinkled dimensions in my neighborhood."

Olga heard Gavilán talking and reentered the room but was taken aback when she saw the three aliens standing in front of Gavilán.

"Oh good," Nivla said. "I'm glad I will be able to speak to both of you."

"Wait a minute," interrupted Cuauhtémoc Gavilán, feeling a little overwhelmed and threatened by the presence of the two additional Treretumians. "Show us a little courtesy. Why don't you introduce your friends?"

"These are my two drones, Cinz and Reppoc," replied Nivla.

Cinz, a tall, muscular Treretumian, was clearly of the same clan as Nivla. Reppoc, on the other hand, was short and strong, but more delicate with piercing green eyes. All were dressed in dark-gray hooded robes that extended to their feet, and all wore a pale-blue sash around the waist.

Gavilán was immediately captivated by Reppoc's eyes and caught himself staring as the conversation ensued. He interrupted, apologetically, "Reppoc (re' pok), I'm sorry for staring . . . it's just that you have such amazing green eyes.

Before Reppoc could respond, Nivla interjected, "Yes, but they change color—to blue, depending on his state." Everyone's attention was now focused on the smallest of the Treretumians.

Reppoc uttered his first words, starting in a low, almost-growl, accelerating as he progressed, and ending in a crescendo, "And my name is not Reppoc (re' pok) —my name is Reppoc (re pôk)!" Cinz placed his hand on Reppoc's shoulder in a calming gesture.

Gavilán turned with his head down slightly, raised his right eyebrow as he looked at Olga, and muttered, "Space cholos." [Homeboys.]

In response, Olga tilted her head to the left, raised both eyebrows, stretched the corners of her mouth downward, and halfway shrugged her shoulders—all at the same time.

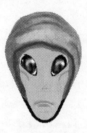

ꗃꗃꗃꗃꗃꗃꗃꗃꗃꗃꗃꗃꗃꗃꗃꗃꗃꗃꗃꗃꗃꗃꗃꗃꗃꗃ

Nivla uttered several seconds of unintelligible sounds that were apparently completely understood by Cinz and Reppoc because they responded with a glance to the ground and an immediate change in their demeanor.

He then continued by addressing the Earthlings, "I apologize to both of you. My drones have not visited Earth before, and they need to make a few adjustments. Cinz and Reppoc are my trusted companions. I trust them with my life. Should I need to get a message to you at some point in the future and not be able to contact you directly, I will send one of my drones."

Olga and Gavilán looked at each other in puzzlement.

Nivla continued, "And from what I can detect, you may need protection from Muimdac—and perhaps from a few members of your own species. My drones have been directed to provide assistance in my absence as necessary without being detected."

Olga appeared a little irritated. "Members of my own species? I can imagine to whom you are referring, but Muimdac? What the hell are you talking about? I think we can take care of ourselves, thank you. Right, Gavilán?"

Before Gavilán had a chance to respond, Cinz took a step forward speaking rapidly in a low, deep voice, "The tiny airborne Muimdac invade the bodies of their victims. These insidious creatures congregate in vital organs, waiting for more of their kind to arrive until they have amassed enough of their kind to launch an attack on the target organ, rendering it incapable of performing its life function. By incapacitating vital organs, the impact is felt throughout the body. Believe me, you are not currently equipped to defend yourselves from the Muimdac."

The Earthlings exchanged puzzled, disbelieving looks. Then Cuauhtémoc spoke sarcastically, "I get my flu shots every year. But you seem to think that what you tell us should have us terrified."

"Wait up, Gavilán," Olga interjected in a less agitated voice. "Maybe these guys aren't entirely off base. I remember hearing about an event that took place shortly before I was born, the return of United States Apollo astronauts from the moon. Federal government and NASA officials responsible for the safety of the public and the personnel in the space program, as well as scientists interested in obtaining accurate analytical results from collected samples, agreed unanimously that the astronauts and lunar samples would require *special handling.*"

A strange look of vindication came over the faces of the Treretumians as Olga continued, "A facility especially built for the occasion, the Lunar Receiving Laboratory, was constructed at the Johnson Space Center in Houston so that returning astronauts could be observed under quarantine. They collected biological samples that could be analyzed in a *glove-box* environment, free of terrestrial contamination." She paused briefly, reaching for Gavilán's arm. "On the health and safety side of things, concerns were raised regarding the potential for alien life being introduced into our world, the potential for that life to propagate in its new environment, and the potential for adverse consequences for the human race. Perhaps because our nation had just experienced mass vaccinations the previous decade to bring polio—a dreaded microscopic but formidable adversary—under control, it was deemed better to err on the side of caution."

Gavilán probed, "Why are you so afraid of the Muimdac?"

Cinz responded defiantly, "I am not afraid of the Muimdac." Nivla placed his hand on Cinz's shoulder, and Cinz continued in a calmer tone, "I have studied their ways. You must know your enemy to defeat him. Learn where he goes and what he does. I do not fear him, but I respect him, and I try to frustrate his efforts at every opportunity."

Nivla took his hand from Cinz's shoulder and took a step forward, saying, "The Muimdac have infected our planet, our society, and they threaten our very existence, with most of the inhabitants of Treretum being unaware of their being manipulated and consumed by their enemy." The massive alien continued, "This is perhaps not the proper time to discuss the details, but know that before you stand three Treretumians that are aware of their presence and are not afraid . . . simply determined to do what they can to protect their families and preserve their society."

Cinz stepped forward to Nivla's side and again took the spotlight. "We are but different levels of the same family. I know how they think. But by the same token, they know how I think. They can have a presence within a target organ for decades undetected, waiting for the right moment when their numbers have reached the threshold needed to launch a successful attack. This is why I never let my guard down. The Muimdac I do not fear, for I know the Muimdac. Those who fear, fear the unknown. Knowledge of my enemy gives me valor . . . and valor conquers fear."

Nivla spoke in a low, somber tone, "If the Muimdac are present in this sector as we suspect, you will need help." He gestured toward Cinz as he looked directly at Olga. "Cinz sometimes instills fear in those he is trying to help, but you will need him." He then placed his hand on Reppoc's shoulder as he continued, "And Reppoc may be small in comparison, but you will need him as well. I have discussed the situation with my drones. If the Muimdac are confirmed to be present in this sector, my drones will remain behind when our spacecraft departs for Treretum. They know the enemy . . . and you *will* need them.

〔〕

It was agreed that Nivla's drones would provide assistance in Nivla's absence, if necessary, and then Olga's curiosity got the best of her. Here she was having conversations with aliens. She needed to know about their world—the part of the universe from which they came. She took the floor as Gavilán looked on. "So, Nivla, tell us a little bit about Sirius, the Dog Star. Is it as it appears—two suns that circle each other? How did this situation come about? It seems unusual, and inquiring minds want to know."

Nivla, *the teacher*, was happy to oblige. "Our planet, as with Earth in your solar system, is an extinguished ember, a sloughed-off bit from the primary star around which it rotates. These second-generation stars are the consequence of the disintegration of first-generation stars that originated from the initial 'explosion' of sorts, what we call the Explosion of Conception. However, they were unstable, stemming from the relatively high content of heavy material that was formed by fusion under intense heat and pressure.

"In spiral galaxies, like ours that emerged at the beginning of the current universal cycle, just over half a bin-bak'tun (over thirteen billion years) ago, a central spinning mass sloughed off spinning droplets that emerged to form entire star systems. Imagine these droplets, the primary stars in a new galaxy like our Milky Way, are like the droplets of water that were slung away due to centrifugal force."—he paused for a moment to think of an example and then continued—"like . . . from the spinning inside tub of one of those machine you use to wash clothes, but there was no outside tub to capture the droplets.

"The heavier masses were ejected along with vast amounts of hydrogen to reform into first-generation stars, but as these stars aged with gravity holding each of these turbulent masses together—still spinning, spinning, spinning—centrifugal force pushed the heavier materials formed by the fusion process and other nuclear processes to the outside of a spherical inferno. In the course of a few billion years, more heavy material migrated to the outside of the sphere, impeding the release of energy, destabilizing the central mass until the instability was too great, causing the first-generation star to fragment into smaller stars. The heavier parts that were not recaptured into the daughter stars emerged as molten pieces of slag from the inferno that still raged with a renewed intensity."

Olga and Gavilán were fascinated with what Nivla was saying and in terms that were understandable and appeared plausible. "You mentioned other 'nuclear processes.' So then, what else is going on if fusion isn't the only nuclear reaction involved in the formation of the heavier materials?" asked Olga. She already knew part of the answer, and wasted no time . . . time to test *the teacher.*

It was a fair question, and Nivla was happy to see that the brain cells were working. "Many things are occurring, but I'll give you an example. In the intense environment of a star, subatomic particles are plentiful and flow freely in the 'stellar soup.' The heavier materials tend to result from neutron capture by nuclei of atoms that are already multiprotonic. It is interesting because depending on the energy of the neutron and the point at which the neutron strikes the nucleus, it may be absorbed to form a heavier nucleus, or it may split the nucleus that it strikes into two or more fragments. In other words, in terms of building atoms of higher mass, there is a lot of 'one steps forward, one step back' activity in the stellar environment."

Gavilán just nodded his head and said, "Interesting."

"Getting back to the general discussion of star formation and how it applies to the situation in my solar system," continued Nivla, "some large daughter stars sloughed off additional heavy matter along with substantial amounts of hydrogen, as in the case of Sirius B. The mass of Sirius B is approximately half of its much larger sister due to the heavy material it contains. The higher associated gravitational forces were sufficient to capture the hydrogen, and lighter materials that had been sloughed off so that a new stellar furnace, rich in heavy material, was formed. Eventually, the fuel will run out, and Sirius B will become a large planet that influences the movement of the surviving sister star, Sirius A.

"But what about the formation of other planets?" inquired Olga, "The ones that revolved around both Sirius A and B? They would be much older planets, wouldn't they?"

"Yes, they would," replied Nivla. "At the disintegration of a first-generation star, many of the relatively small bits of heavier material, rich in elements substantially heavier than hydrogen and helium, much like the planet on which we stand, were slung into space. Their momentum was great because of the heavier nuclei of the atoms that comprise them. If they were not captured directly by the daughter star, they were captured by gravity and became planets that revolve around a star made primarily of hydrogen, the fuel for the fusion reaction that keeps the star alive. This would be a more common mechanism. Daughter stars that contain higher concentrations of lithium, the next element after hydrogen and helium, are more likely to be associated with these heavier-element satellites that were sloughed off originally . . . and may have turned into habitable environments for life-forms like yours and mine."

"From what you have described," commented Gavilán, "I can see that every star and its planetary system is likely to be unique, and any life-form that evolves is obliged to adapt to that particular environment. Give us more details regarding your star system, Sirius A and B, which in turn will give us a little insight into the nature of your species."

"The trajectory of the center of mass of every star system is relatively straight but influenced by gravity. The gravitational pull of every satellite that orbits the primary star in the system, including your own solar system, impacts the trajectory of every other mass in the star system to some extent. In my home star system, because the minor star, Sirius B, contains a substantial fraction of the total mass, its motion moves the principal star, Sirius A, and all planets in the system. To distant observers, the trajectory of Sirius appears to be wobbling, and the intensity of its energy emissions appears to be variable—as does its apparent diameter. But all these are due to the interaction between Sirius A, B, and C . . . yes, a third small star. The existence of major sources of secondary and tertiary energy is why Treretum's climate is so variable and so severe."

Olga interjected, "But I thought Sirius was a binary star system."

"From a distance Sirius C is difficult to detect. Sirius C is much smaller, its emissions are very faint, and it is nearly extinguished. Sirius C revolves solely around Sirius A, within the elliptical orbit of Sirius B, which also orbits the much larger Sirius A. Not far into the future, Sirius C will be the largest planet in the Sirius system, but it will require more than a billion years to cool sufficiently for exploration and habitation. Sirius B will eventually suffer the same fate."

Olga and Gavilán found Nivla's discussion captivating. Gavilán glanced at Olga's hands and caught her pinching herself. He understood why—he too could barely keep from pinching himself to make sure he wasn't dreaming.

"On a larger scale, the trajectory of the center of mass of each galaxy is relatively straight but, again, influenced by gravity. When the gravitational fields of adjacent galaxies pull them toward each other, the galaxies collide, as is the destiny of our Milky Way with our neighbor, Andromeda, in about five billion years."

Gavilán interjected sarcastically, "And all this time I had thought our planet was to see its doom in 2012."

Nivla responded quickly, "The myth of 2012 is not a myth. Your Earth and my Treretum and our entire galaxy await the same fate, but that is far beyond your lifetime or mine. Information included in an ancient Mayan scripture regarding 2012 was simply misunderstood. The scripture marked the end of the thirteenth bak'tun in 2012. Each bak'tun is a period of about four hundred years, and it was during our first expedition to your planet more than five thousand years ago that the Mayan astronomers began to keep track of the four-hundred-year bak'tun cycles. The astronomers and those who wrote the scriptures felt that it was sufficient to look thirteen bak'tuns into the future. Scholars at places like your University of Texas understood the true meaning of the scriptures, but sensationalists continued to derive personal gain from the misinterpretation and the concerns that it raised among many Earthlings."

"In any case, 2012 has come and gone," said Olga with a sigh, "and our lives are influenced by events of much smaller time scale and dimension.

"Like a visit from *a teacher,* an extraterrestrial from a neighboring star . . . a mere 8.6 light-years away," added Gavilán.

꒱꒱꒱꒱꒱꒱꒱꒱꒱꒱꒱꒱꒱꒱꒱꒱꒱꒱꒱꒱꒱꒱꒱꒱꒱꒱꒱꒱꒱꒱꒱꒱

Later, after the extraterrestrials had left, Olga approached Gavilán with a question. "Do you think that Nivla's comment about the 'explosion at the beginning of the current universal cycle' was a reference to the Big Bang?"

"Reference?" exclaimed Gavilán. "I don't know how much clearer he could have been."

"Do you think that from what Nivla said, Earth was once a tiny star fragment that sloughed off the sun?" she asked.

Gavilán raised his hands to his cheeks, stroking upward past his temples as he offered his opinion. "It seems plausible that all of the stars in the galaxy, and all their planets, and all their moons . . . that they all came from the same original glob of mass that was slung out into space at the time of the Big Bang. Therefore, all of them could potentially have the same basic elemental building blocks. And depending on the size, mass, and distance of each from other large, heat-emitting masses, the planets and moons all cooled down at different rates. With the discovery of water on the moon . . . that just supports this perspective. All of the history of Earth could have also occurred on the moon, only in 'fast forward' due to the relative size of the moon and much faster cooling rate. Similarly, all the apparent dry river beds that are observable on the surface of Mars suggests that what we see on Mars may be just a preview of what will occur on Earth during the course of a couple of billion years."

"Just more to think about," uttered Olga as she went into a big yawn and stretch of the arms. "I guess we'd better get some rest before tomorrow's activities at the Powwow."

Gavilán agreed. "Good night, my good doctor," bade Gavilán as he rose to his feet to retire to his room.

"Good night, sweetie. See you in the morning."

നനനനനനനനനനനനനനനനനനനനനനനനനനനനനനന

Booths were set up near the stadium, on both sides of a long, broad promenade that widened into an arena where performers could share their talents. The booths housed small stands where food vendors prepared traditional and not-so-traditional culinary delights, which, of course, included tacos and barbecue. Artisans were busy in their booths demonstrating how some of their wares were made, adding to the handicrafts that were already on display—everything from dolls to fine silver and turquoise jewelry. Several temporary poles had been set along the perimeter, and loud speakers mounted to disseminate information regarding events, displays, races, and tribal dance performances that were about to begin.

The promenade was filled with people in all types of attire— everything from jeans and T-shirts to beaded buckskin dresses, loincloths, and ornate feathered headdresses. There was the hustle and bustle of people of all ages interacting—exchanging currency for food and goods, exchanging ideas, exchanging contact information. It was an opportunity to introduce the very young to different cultures or to parts of their heritage that were not part of the day-to-day routine. Although it was a diverse crowd, bringing together an international audience from the Stanford campus, there was a sense of unification in the air, a coalescing members of the many Native American tribes with Eskimo and Polynesian representatives into a cohesive group of people, assembled to celebrate their commonalities and diversity.

A group of men and women carrying drums of all sizes—some decorated elaborately and others very plain—formed a semicircle in the arena as the announcement came over the loud speakers, piercing through the dull roar of the crowd. It was a continuation of the tribal dance competition. Gavilán took Olga's hand, and the pair made a beeline to the arena to see the presentation.

The featured dancer had an envious physique and was dressed in a loincloth of buckskin. He displayed the muscle tone of his legs and upper body proudly. In his right hand he held a rattle of some sort that appeared to be made of bone, and in his left hand he held a single arrow. His feet were covered with beaded moccasins. The colorful part of his attire was his headdress—an assembly of colorful feathers that clung to his head like an extended Mohawk haircut, extending from his eyes, over the top of his head, and halfway down his back.

The assembly of drummers began to pound out a fairly fast and rock-steady beat as the elder members of the group began to chant—single-beat notes interspersed among longer pulsing tones, focusing on one or two pitches. In rhythm to the drums, the dancer pranced around, high stepping with his headdress leaning first to the right, circling until he had made a full 360, and then to the left, again making a full 360-degree circle—always in perfect sync with the drum beats.

"This guy is really good," proclaimed Olga.

"Yep," affirmed Gavilán. "He reminds me a little of the dancer at the Powwow years ago when we met."

She turned, grabbed his hand, and gave it squeeze, with a "Yeah."

At the end of the performance, the loud speaker sounded in the midst of the applause, giving credit to the tribe and dancer, and announcing the time of the next performance in the competition.

The crowd in the arena area began to disperse, and Olga and Gavilán headed up the promenade once again. About twenty yards into their walk, Olga announced, "You know, sheep skin moccasins are just the best in the winter time. I saw that one of the vendors up ahead is selling them, and I think we need to stop in so I can get a pair."

Gavilán responded playfully, "As you wish, mademoiselle."

They proceeded a few more yards when Olga stopped suddenly and reached into her purse, explaining she had put her phone on vibrate before the performance. She had just received a text message from Sam at the conference in San Francisco. Sam indicated that Dr. Welch wanted to contact her but thought it best that he send a text message because it would be less likely to be intercepted. She read the message aloud to Gavilán, commenting at the end, "Sounds a little paranoid, to me."

Gavilán just frowned.

"Where do you want to have dinner tonight?" she asked.

In an instant, Gavilán responded, "How about Frankie, Johnnie, and Luigi's?"

"Great! Hold on." Olga began typing out a text response with her thumbs. After hitting *Send*, she looked up at Gavilán and said, "Something's up."

They took a few steps, and Olga began to put her phone back in her purse when she received another message from Sam. She read the message and said in a slow, concerned voice, "They'll drop in if their conference session adjourns early enough, and they can find their way down there in their rental vehicle."

In a Bogart voice, Gavilán mimicked, "Just go with the flow, sweetheart."

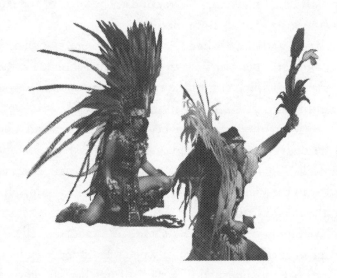

Olga tightened her lips and, after a few small nods of the head said, "Let's go find those moccasins."

"He really is a teacher," Gavilán declared as he raised a slice of pizza to his mouth. The smell of fresh pizza filled the hole-in-the-wall establishment, known throughout the Bay Area for their hand-tossed pizza and delectable Stromboli, made with only the freshest of ingredients. Gavilán continued, "I was truly impressed with Nivla and his patience in explaining things when we went to the Big Apple."

"He's been pretty awesome with us too, if you think about it," responded Olga as she scraped the toppings from a slice of pizza onto a plate. She stopped what she was doing, reached into her purse, and pulled out a small bottle. Olga shook the bottle, which sounded like a deep-toned baby rattle. "You'll need one of these."

"*What?*" exclaimed Gavilán.

"I know that we picked ingredients that were low in cadmium," answered Olga. "No mushrooms, no sausage . . . but if you're going to eat the crust, you should at least take a zinc tab to minimize your assimilation of the stuff. It works for rats, and no offense, but you're not that different."

Gavilán raised his hand to scratch his head, looking a little bewildered.

"Trust me. Just pop one of these," she insisted as she extended her hand with the container of zinc toward Gavilán.

Doing as directed, Gavilán took a tablet from the jar, popped it into his mouth, and quickly chased it with another bite of pizza. With a full mouth, he spoke in muddled English, "Mmmm . . . Frankie, Johnny, and Luigi's . . . I remember thinking their Stromboli pizza was the best pizza in the Bay Area back when I was at Stanford, and I have to say that nothing has changed. Their pizza is out of this world."

"Yeah, I know. I remember," Olga uttered as she raised another forkful of melted cheeses and other toppings to her mouth.

"Oh come on, you've got to try just a little piece of this," Gavilán declared as he took a slice and waved it gently in front of her nose.

"Gavilán, I can't do it," she said sternly. But Gavilán continued to entice her, waving the pizza in front of her and blowing gently over it, sending the aroma in her direction. "Well . . . maybe one bite . . . with an extra zinc tab." She dropped her fork, popped a zinc tablet, and washed it down with water. Then she took a bite of the pizza that Gavilán held before her. "Mmmmm, just as good as I remembered it. But you know I have a good memory, so that I can still appreciate this wonderful concoction with just one bite and without ingesting all the cadmium. I'll just go back to my scraped-off toppings."

The meal was amazing, and the conversation was enlightening. Olga explained what she knew about cadmium and zinc and the essential role that zinc plays in human health. It all made sense to Gavilán, and he promised that after doing a little investigating on his own, he would likely become one of Olga's converts. Once the zinc formalities were out of the way, they were able to relax and talk—just enjoy the conversation. They talked about the Powwow, the dancers they had watched earlier in the day, and the great deal she had gotten on the sheepskin moccasins.

And then Olga recalled the text messages she had received from Sam. Gavilán commented, "I guess they got tied up and couldn't make it down here."

"Yeah, I guess you're right," she responded. They were both puzzled.

They started to plan their departure from the area, and Gavilán mentioned, "Don't forget, I need to drop in on one of my old professors. He lives just off Mayfield, so it won't really be out of the way."

"Sounds great," she said wearily. It was clear that Olga was getting fatigued. But then out of nowhere, she got a jolt of renewed energy as the sound of Tchaikovsky's *Romeo and Juliet* interrupted the conversation. She reached into her purse, pulled out her cell phone, and flipped it open like a switchblade. It was a reflex. "Hello, Sam. What did you guys decide?" Olga paused. "Oh, I'm sorry, 'cause you're really going to miss out on some world-class pizza. We were starving, so we didn't wait for you. We'll just have to survive without you this time, but maybe we can meet later at the suite where we're staying." She again paused. "Okay, call or text us later for directions when you're getting ready to head out."

After closing her flip phone, Olga began to explain, but Gavilán nodded to indicate he understood what had just transpired in the conversation, and Olga's explanation slowed to a complete stop. "It's going to be a late night," he said.

"I know," she agreed. Neither seemed too happy about the pending visit.

With a change in demeanor, Gavilán suggested, "Then let's enjoy the rest of our visit to FJ&L's, and not mention Sam or Dr. Welch until we get back to our suite."

With an extended hand and a smile on her face, Olga agrees enthusiastically, "Deal."

They sipped on their ice water with lemon, and there was silence between them for a minute. Then Gavilán spoke. "You know, I've never asked, but it struck me the very first time I heard your phone ring and again just now. Why did you pick that music for your ringtone?"

"Well . . . it reminds me of someone I really admire," she replied solemnly.

This was Gavilán's cue. He enthusiastically started with, "Yes, I know. I too admire Pyotr Ilyich Tchaikovsky and the countless beautiful masterpieces that he left us in his music." He continued, "His genius . . ." but he immediately lowered his tone and slowed the pace of his discussion to a halt when Olga raised her hand, palm facing outward. He gazed at her with a puzzled look.

"Well . . . I was referring to Miss Piggy," she interjected. "She's always so cool and collected . . . and so loyal. She's a one-frog pig, and she's not afraid to use her karate on anyone that threatens her Kermy. I often find myself asking, 'What would Miss Piggy do if she were in my situation?'" She looked at Gavilán, lowered her head slightly, and muttered, "Oops, TMI."

Gavilán tried to hold back his chuckles at first, then he giggled, and then they both began to laugh out loud.

Olga continued, "Well, since my secret is out, what *would* Miss Piggy do in a situation like ours? On one hand, we have an alien . . . *acquaintance*, apparently friendly, who says he just wants to recover his deceased brother's remains. On the other hand, we have a government that—after sixty years—has released very little documentation regarding the spacecraft crash and, to this day, is still trying to convince the public that the fallen object was just a weather balloon. This is the same government that dismisses valid sightings of what turned out to be an approaching alien spacecraft from a neighboring star system but insists that the technology used to make the sightings is needed for national security."

"Well, I tend to agree with what you're saying," Gavilán responded, "but I think it's a little more complicated than that. How well do you know the alien acquaintance, and can you trust him?"

With a pouting, frustrated look on her face, Olga responded, "I can ask the same questions about our government."

CADMIUM POISONING

FACTS

- The South Pacific island nation of Nauru, home of the "fattest population on earth," is an example (heads-up Michelle Obama and others!). It has a land area of only 8.1 miles. Do the math. If it were in the shape of a circle, the diameter would be just over 3.2 miles. The island had a limited era of prosperity when phosphate deposits were discovered and then strip-mined, leaving open pits of the remaining phosphates exposed to the atmosphere. The native inhabitants' diet changed from mostly fish to burgers, hot dogs, and fried foods. The change in diet is blamed for the change in accumulated fat on their bodies and the skyrocketing diabetes rate. Now, the life expectancy of the average male citizen of Nauru has dropped to between 48 and 49 years. With the small area of the tiny nation, the sea breezes that are always present, and the open pits of what is left of the phosphate mines, all the citizens of this country inhale airborne cadmium when the wind is blowing from the right direction. Also, rain that falls into the abandoned strip mines provides a transport mechanism for cadmium into the groundwater. While about 10% of the cadmium they ingest is assimilated, nearly 50% of the inhaled cadmium is assimilated. The impact of cadmium on the thyroid gland and pancreas results in a reduced metabolic rate, accumulation of fat, reduced capacity to generate insulin, reduced capacity for cells to extract insulin from the bloodstream, and greatly improved conditions for developing Type 2 diabetes and various types of cancer.

- Similarly, in a report aired on Univision, Salvador Castañon described an "epidemic" of kidney failures among farm workers in agricultural communities in Mexico, Guatemala, and El Salvador. Footage in the report showed workers with no shoes walking in rows of tilled soil, spreading seeds and fertilizer. It was speculated that pesticides were responsible for the epidemic, while the more likely cause, cadmium in the phosphate fertilizers, was not mentioned.

- It is possible that the Shoshone-Bannock tribes of Idaho included in the storyline suffer from diabetes and cancer due to chronic exposure to cadmium associated with phosphates—potato farming using phosphate fertilizers and nearby phosphate mining, processing, and waste disposal.

- Cadmium in phosphate rock mined and processed in the western United States (eastern Idaho and most of Utah) contains 30-300 parts per million (ppm) of the heavy metal, compared with 5-15 ppm in phosphate deposits in Florida and the Carolinas.

Chapter Fourteen

The Many Balances

It had been a long and interesting couple of days, and as was customary for at least one night of the Powwow, both Olga and Gavilán were exhausted from a day in the sun followed by a grand meal—on this occasion at Frankie, Johnnie, and Luigi's.

Gavilán unlocked the door to their suite and opened the door. As both looked into the room to step in, they heard, "You've heard the saying 'Use it or lose it'?"

"Nivla!" Olga exclaimed. "How did you get in?"

Nivla's head cocked back slightly, a bit surprised by her question. "Remember wrinkles in the fabric and straight lines?" He resumed his previous relaxed stance and continued, "Anyway, you've heard the saying 'Use it or lose it'? Well, it's true."

"Wait!" Gavilán interjected as Olga and he walked into their suite, closing the door behind him. "You mean that Treretumians have that saying too, and you just wanted to share that with us?"

"No, it was just one of those quaint sayings that caught my eye when I scanned the data stream for archiving in our ship's data banks," responded Nivla. The inquisitive Treretumian was a sponge for colloquialisms, and the more time he spent among humans, the more comfortable and uninhibited in using them he became.

"Caught my *eye?*" exclaimed Gavilán, surprised at Nivla's use of slang.

"Yours too?" responded Nivla almost instantly.

And just as quickly, ending the rapid volley, Gavilán said, "No, no, I mean . . . never mind," shaking his head and waving his arms as he turned and walked away.

Nivla was a tall, massive creature. He looked like he might have been a linebacker on the All-Treretumian football team. The skin of his face was a pale green, while the scaly skin on the back of his hands was tan. His dark-brown, almond-shaped eyes were larger than most, even by Treretumian standards. The contrast between the espresso-coffee brown and his pale skin made his expressive eyes the most prominent feature on his face.

Olga gestured for Nivla to sit at the table where Gavilán was already sitting. Nivla sat directly across the table from Gavilán, and Olga sat at his side.

"Anyway, I think that saying is talking about a balance . . ." Nivla paused but then continued to clarify, "between use and non-use and the consequent loss of functionality."

"My sign is Libra, and I'm really big on balance," said Gavilán after a brief pause. Realizing he was directing his statement at Nivla, *the teacher*, he continued, "And I think the implication is that we need to maintain that natural equilibrium that is reached in every living creature in the course of carrying out its normal activities. No, not equilibrium . . . make that steady state."

"I am not familiar with that term," Nivla responded.

Olga jumped into the conversation, saying, "It's sort of like equilibrium but not quite, because there is something going in and something coming out, all at the same time. But the amount going in equals the amount coming out so that the amount inside stays the same. So, it's like the old *water-in-the-bucket-with-holes-in-the-side* analogy."

Gavilán picked up the explanation, getting Nivla's undivided attention, saying, "When you use your muscles, you are adding oxygen and nutrients by way of the bloodstream, and you build muscle tissue. But if you don't use the muscles, the adding of a few nutrients may not be enough, and your muscles shrivel up. You know, they atrophy—the water in the bucket eventually runs out."

Nivla, impressed and grateful for vivid illustration, said, "You explained that very well."

"We did?" responded the two instructors in unison, looking at each other in surprise.

Gavilán continued, "Isn't that what you were talking about when we came in the door?"

"Not quite," replied Nivla. "You see, I was thinking of the conditions on my planet. Although we have struggled for many thousands of your years to remove the impurities from our environment, there are still trace amounts that enter our world through the food that we bring in. Once each solar cycle, every Treretumian over the age of one bak'tun goes in to the health and detoxification centers for a cleansing and replacement of his or her toxic element filter. The filters remove toxic elements from the bloodstream—things that internal organs cannot break down and detoxify—by trapping them and retaining them until the next cleansing.

"It's like your mobile combustion units on Earth . . . the ones with the catalytic reactors mounted on the belly side of the units, approximately at the center of the rectangle formed by the four circular rubber friction dissipaters. Heavy metals, like lead, and other poisons gradually build up within the catalyst units until they cease to function. We are the same way. As our organs get poisoned with impurities from the environment . . . they cease to function. We have an organ similar to your liver that can detoxify many complex compounds, but it cannot detoxify a toxic element, because an element cannot be broken down further. It will always be toxic as long as it remains in our bodies. Thus, we have inserted toxic element filters to keep these elements that cause harm to our organs from circulating in our bodies, and periodically change the filters to remove the accumulated poisons. Actually, it is also similar to your *bucket-with-holes-in-the-side* example, but the amount removed is in discrete amounts, and our goal is to keep the bucket from overflowing with toxic elements that would kill us. Use the filter or lose your life."

"Ooo," whimpered Olga as she and Gavilán glanced at each other.

Nivla continued, "As with your bodies, our bodies require certain key elements to function properly, but they can be toxic when their concentrations get too high. For those elements, the trick is to keep the bucket from overflowing and, at the same time, keep it from running dry—a balance. A deficiency of essential elements is just as bad or worse than too much of those same elements in our diets because our bodies have mechanisms for maintaining certain elements in balance. I think your bodies have similar control mechanisms to maintain balance—what you call homeostasis."

"I feel like I'm in a class at a Treretumian med school," murmured Gavilán. Olga reacted by giving him an elbow jab.

Nivla continued, "The big problem is that things don't always stay in balance, and it is when too many systems become out of balance, that even with the removal of toxic elements with our filter units, we expire."

"Wow," uttered Gavilán in a low trancelike tone, thinking of their extended life span. "Thousands of years of knowledge, experience, and wisdom, suddenly cease to exist."

"Not quite. We have studied the chemical and physical changes in the brain that result from different experiences," elaborated Nivla, "but even today, the best we can do is to document the physical and chemical makeup of each brain before death and archive it for future reference. We have had some success in interpreting the data thus obtained, but we still have much to learn in this field."

"Cowabonga!" exclaimed Olga.

"Cowabonga?" reiterated Gavilán as he looked at her in surprise.

"Something I guess I picked up from my dad," she defended in passing, as she tried to get back to the original topic of the conversation. "So the bucket analogy applies to many situations. There are many things that we need to keep in balance."

"Yes, well, I have been challenged in distinguishing between some similar and some dissimilar terms," admitted Nivla. "In some instances the terms seem to mean almost the same thing with subtle differences, and in others they appear to have meanings that are diametrically opposed. I was hoping that you could help me understand some of these balances that I am having difficulty understanding."

"Sure." "Of course." Olga and Gavilán agreed enthusiastically and simultaneously. "What exactly are you having problems with?" continued Olga.

Nivla elaborated, "Well, to start with, I see individual balances and societal balances, and they sometimes appear to be in conflict." He proceeded to rattle off a long series of balances. "In the individual balances, I need help with

- the balance between pride and arrogance,
- the balance between trust and naiveté,
- the balance between caution and paranoia,
- the balance between patriotism and xenophobia,
- the balance between skepticism and cynicism, and
- the balance between ambition and obsession."

Nivla took a deep breath and then continued with additional comparisons involving phrases. "And then there's

- the balance between 'living for the moment' and 'striving to achieve long-term goals,'
- the balance between 'blindly accepting what we are told' and 'rational, individualistic thinking,' and
- the balance between 'hoarding wealth' and 'sharing one's good fortune.'"

Olga and Gavilán looked at each other silently in disbelief. It appeared that Nivla's list was well prepared and that perhaps the "balances" were simply Nivla's cues for orchestrating the conversation.

"Is that it?" asked Gavilán.

"Well, then there are the societal balances," continued Nivla, "which include

- the balance between environmental and economic considerations,
- the balance between what is expedient and what is right, and

- then there is the apparent imbalance between government bureaucracy and governmental actions that are for the good of the people."

Nivla ended with a question. "How do you control some of these things that appear to be in direct conflict, especially in the societal balances I just mentioned?"

Olga responded, "That is a problem. I suppose that each of us must focus on things that he or she can control—focus on our personal, individual balances, and encourage others to do the same. In that way, if everyone in the society is an active participant, the societal balances will take care of themselves."

"But, Nivla . . . you didn't just drop in so we could discuss different balances," declared Gavilán. "Help me out here. My impression is that you're already familiar with all those terms, and right now I'm having a little trouble with my skepticism-cynicism balance."

"Actually, I did, but with ulterior motives. I came to evaluate—assess the viability of Treretumian survival here on Earth."

Gavilán immediately leaned back in his chair as he mumbled, "Shit. Invasion."

Olga looked at Gavilán and quickly turned to Nivla.

"No," Nivla responded as he also leaned back and raised one hand in front of his chest, palm out. "I assure you that Treretum never had and never will have an interest in invading Earth. On the contrary, my interest is in assessing the feasibility of forming a team—the beginning of a Treretum-Earth alliance. And you are the ones I would choose to spearhead that team."

"This all sounds very interesting," remarked Gavilán, "but you will be returning to Treretum very soon, and we will remain here. So where is the connection—the interaction?"

"That is why I am evaluating the balances—trade-offs, if you will," Nivla explained. Leaving a Treretumian on Earth without the benefit of a periodic filter change would surely shorten his life expectancy drastically, especially since the Earth environment is so contaminated. I do not take the lives of my subordinates or the Earthlings with whom they interact lightly. Survival would certainly depend on support from interested Earthlings like you. If I were to leave someone here on Earth, I would be condemning him to a certain premature death. Earthlings potentially could reap overwhelming benefits, for example, in technological advancement . . . and in the future, there could be tremendous benefits for both our worlds.

"Why us?" questioned Olga. "We don't have political power. We aren't among the wealthy who wield influence. Why us?"

Nivla replied, "You are young, you are intelligent, you are open-minded, you are compassionate, you think logically and pay attention to detail, you have not been corrupted by forces in your society, you are dedicated, you are passionate about your work, you are concerned about your planet . . . shall I go on?"

"Gee, you're making my head swell," commented Olga sarcastically.

"Oh yes," interjected Nivla, "and you have the capacity to enlist the help of others who are of like mind. What lies ahead will require more than a handful of dedicated individuals if your planet is going to survive."

Olga and Gavilán turned toward each other with puzzled looks on their faces.

"Returning to your original question—why am I here, the reason for my visit this evening . . ." Nivla took a deep breath and continued, "Well, many lives are in the balance, but how can I assess whether a balance is practicable when I don't understand the true nature of both sides I'm weighing? I need your perspective." He tilted his head slightly, alternated looks between Olga and Gavilán, and continued, "That is why I am here."

CADMIUM POISONING

FACTS

- Cadmium solubility and mobility are pH dependent. The pH of the blood is well buffered, and the body is equipped with two additional balancing mechanisms to control pH: excretion of acids in the urine and exhalation of carbon dioxide.

- The pH in muscle cells drops slightly and temporarily during periods of exercise due to the formation of lactic acid and carbon dioxide. The increase in the partial pressure of carbon dioxide results in favorable conditions for the formation of carbonic acid. As the hemoglobin carries carbon dioxide away to the lungs for exhalation, steady state conditions are gradually regained and the pH returns to normal. Under conditions of extreme physical exertion, the oxygen supply cannot keep up with the demand for energy aerobically, and anaerobic energy production from glucose through the process of glycolysis is accompanied by the formation of pyruvate, followed by lactate, and a corresponding drop in cellular pH.

- The body maintains a mean blood pH of approximately 7.4; however, certain parts of the body maintain localized pH values that are less than the mean. The brain, for example, has a pH that generally decreases with age. (Should it? Or is that a symptom that something is changing [e.g., depletion of zinc and/or as a response to the accumulation of other heavy metals]?)

- Cadmium has been documented to increase localized pH (alkalinization), which improves its chances for retention, and it generally does not accumulate in the brain.

- In the range of normal blood pH, the solubilities of metal-containing compounds (e.g., compounds of aluminum, lead, mercury, iron, and manganese) generally increase with decreasing pH. Conversely, precipitates of metal compounds are most likely to form where the pH is highest.

- Metallothioneins provide a balancing mechanism to prevent excessive heavy metals in the bloodstream through excretion in bile discharged to the intestinal tract. The problems with cadmium are that (1) it doesn't remain in the bloodstream—it accumulates in bone and tissues, and (2) it tends to stay there (30-year biological half-life), showing no sign of a problem for decades until enough has accumulated to impede organ function and later cause cancer. Hence, you need to flush cadmium out into the bloodstream (with zinc and niacin) so that the extra metallothioneins generated in response to the zinc supplementation can sequester cadmium.

- Note that niacin is often prescribed to minimize arterial plaque accumulation and heart disease. For maximum effect, take niacin that is not "flush free" ("flush free" is typically in the nicotinate form). However, be forewarned that the "flush" may be accompanied by red skin and itching. For a stronger "flush," which will likely be accompanied by the red skin and itching, take the niacin shortly before or after eating a grapefruit, which contains a compound that enhances the effect of niacin.

- Ultimately, the cadmium issue will likely have to be addressed through legislation, addressing all potential sources (and recycle loops) of cadmium into the food chain. Without control of all sources, legislation to control one or a few sources (e.g., California's Public Health Goal for cadmium in drinking water) will likely be ineffective. That is not to say it is inappropriate; it is simply ahead of its time. The balance between overregulation in one area and underregulation in another is a problem (sneezing at gnats and swallowing camels).

- How and where do you strike the right balance between relying on a physician to be responsible for your health and taking responsibility for your own health? Relying blindly on anyone reduces your chances of survival. You need to be well informed so that you can make the right choices, getting information from reliable sources yet not necessarily waiting for the overwhelming evidence from human studies to be published in the *Journal of the American Medical Association*—we may not live that long. Besides, when it comes to mammalian response to cadmium exposure, are we really qualitatively that different from rats or rabbits?

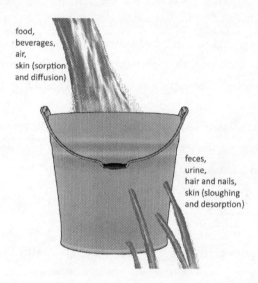

food,
beverages,
air,
skin (sorption
and diffusion)

feces,
urine,
hair and nails,
skin (sloughing
and desorption)

- The trick is to keep the bucket from overflowing (e.g., cadmium or zinc or copper poisoning) because when it does, it means organ malfunctions, cancer, pain, suffering, and death. At the other extreme, you want to run the bucket dry for cadmium while keeping it from running dry for zinc and copper (i.e., zinc or copper deficiency) by minimizing cadmium in the diet with concurrent supplementation of zinc and copper.

- Changes in diet can cause unexpected imbalances to develop. For example, when I changed my diet to try to avoid cadmium, I began eating large quantities of almonds. What I didn't realize was that almonds contain oxalates and are categorized not as a high-oxalate food but as an "extremely high-oxalate" food. Because of the low solubility of calcium oxalate, I developed kidney stones. Approximately 75% to 80% of all kidney stones are caused by this black precipitate that forms inside the kidneys when the calcium and/or oxalate concentrations get too high, so be careful. Also, be cautious about the form of vitamin C that you take since large doses of sodium ascorbate (as opposed to ascorbic acid) can cause localized elevation of the pH in the kidneys, enhancing the precipitation of calcium oxalate (i.e., formation of kidney stones). The majority of the remaining 20% to 25% of kidney stones are caused by the precipitation of uric acid (as in the cause of gout), with a few percent of kidney stones resulting from the precipitation of phosphate compounds.

- Homeopathic/semihomeopathic treatments for kidney stones include the following:
  o Glycerin, antibiotics, beer, and lots of water—facilitates passing of the stones
  o Te de pelo de elote [tea from the hair of corn (on and including the corn on the cob)]—helps dissolve calcium oxalate kidney stones
  o Te de palo azul [tea from the bush "palo azul" (blue tree)]—helps dissolve uric acid kidney stones

- Some individuals may have problems swallowing all the supplements. Pills can be crushed and capsules emptied into a favorite low-cadmium beverage (e.g., orange juice, water with a wedge of lemon and honey) to make the process easier. I have told my daughter on many occasions since I began my cadmium detoxification program that I feel like I am getting younger. Thus, in honor of Ponce de Leon, Florida orange growers, and the fountain of youth, I call the mixture of the following supplements in orange juice *Agua Ponce*: zinc, vitamin A, vitamin B complex, vitamin B_1, vitamin B_3, vitamin B_6, vitamin B_{12}, vitamin C, vitamin D, gamma vitamin E, magnesium, copper, selenium, and one or two glugs of apple cider vinegar. (I guess we could add a little lithium to make it more authentic.) To provide extra liver support and boost glutathione levels, consider adding N-acetyl cysteine, lipoic acid, and silymarin. To provide extra thyroid support, consider adding iodine. To provide extra joint support, add Boswellia and/or a little sulfur in the form of methyl sulfonyl methane (MSM).

- Although countless formulations intended to provide joint pain relief contain glucosamine and chondroitin, these supplements are almost universally derived from the shells of crab or other shellfish and, therefore, are *not* recommended due to potential (likely) cadmium contamination.

Chapter Fifteen

Alien Observations (Part II)

Egroeg summoned Suturb to his quarters to continue the presentation of findings regarding the Earthlings and their characteristics. He felt that the information in Suturb's report should be analyzed back on Treretum. It would influence future missions to Earth and interactions with its inhabitants. *I wonder if the second half of his presentation will be as informative,* Egroeg thought to himself. *I suppose I shouldn't expect much from a Kcalb Clansman . . . but who knows? We shall see.*

Suturb arrived at Egroeg's door and raised his hand to knock on the door announcing his arrival. The sleeve of his uniform slid down his arm exposing the watch Egroeg had given him. He glanced at the watch, paused, and then turned his hand to knock with the knuckles of the three fingers at the end of his hand.

The door evaporated as "Come in, Sucram Suturb" rang out from within the officer's quarters. Suturb entered and approached Egroeg. "Good to see you, Sucram." Egroeg appeared much more relaxed than during Suturb's first briefing. As before, Suturb set up for the presentation placing his holographic cube on an end table. He was preparing to pick up where he had left off, but he was interrupted by Egroeg. "I notice you are wearing the present I gave you."

The muscular Treretumian smiled and responded, "Yes, sir," as he raised his right hand to look at the digital watch strapped to his wrist.

"It helps me be more in tune with Earth's shorter daily cycle. It is quite helpful. Thank you again."

The pale, beady-eyed Treretumian appeared to smile as he said, "Good. So what do you have for me today?"

Suturb passed his hand over the cube, and the holographic displays began. "In my presentation today, I will further describe some characteristics of the human Earthlings of the country we are currently canvassing, and then I will touch on ways in which special groups they call corporations and their government interact with them. I will finish with a preliminary assessment of how their peculiar characteristics will likely affect future Treretumian contact."

"Good ... excellent, please proceed," Egroeg said as he motioned with his hand and nodded his head.

"Human Earthlings make rules to try to incorporate some semblance of order in their lives. Most obey them, but some relish in performing acts that break those rules. Consequently, they enlist the assistance of hired officials to serve as enforcers. Examples of these enforcers include proctors on exams, umpires at baseball games, referees at boxing and wrestling events, football games, basketball games, and other sporting events, truant officers, marriage counselors, policemen and women, sheriffs, deputies, and other law enforcement officials, school crossing guards, and judges. And then they have these people called lawyers who get paid to try to convince everyone that their clients didn't break the rules even when they know that they did. Everyone accepts it as being correct and appropriate behavior, but they also make light of it. For example, 'What's the difference between a lawyer and a catfish?' The answer is, 'One is a scum-sucking bottom dweller, and the other's a fish.'"

This drew a snicker from Egroeg's small mouth. Suturb began to explain the joke, but Egroeg raised his hand in front of his chest, palm out. "I'm familiar with that species. I understand. Please go on."

"Human Earthlings are creatures of habit," continued Suturb. "To their own detriment, they don't seem to care about their health, taking part in habitual chemical abuse of their bodies. They build 'comfort zones' around themselves that appear to be sacred, even when the elements of their own demise are built in as integral parts of the polluted environment of their comfort zones. Then, when they start having symptoms of their own making, they get into another routine of going to their doctors so they can shed the responsibility of taking care of their own health. They are too busy seeking financial gain . . . looking for something they call the American dream, the next free meal, members of the opposite sex, and, of course, the next party. They are so wrapped up in the chase that they lose sight of where the path is leading them."

"Yes, well, very interesting and sad at the same time," commented Egroeg. He had been looking forward to the presentation and was already engaged, asking for more detail. "Could you elaborate on the 'comfort zones' you mentioned? I am not familiar with that term."

Suturb elaborated, "Earthlings, in general, don't want anyone or anything to disturb their comfort zones. These zones can be physical surroundings, or they can be behavioral patterns that they refuse to alter. They can be made aware that these zones have problems—even to the point that they will eventually lead to their deaths—but their comfort zones are sacred, and no one need try to disturb them. Examples of stubborn Earthlings that try to preserve the physical attributes of their comfort zones are humans who remain during floods that inundate their homes, while humans who refuse to modify the habitual behavior associated with their comfort zones include those who smoke cigarettes and humans who eat things that they know will harm them, as do many referred to as diabetics."

"Tell me more about these health-related issues," urged Egroeg. "Of course, you are aware that this is very relevant to our mission."

"Yes, sir, I know," answered Suturb in a low voice. He then continued, "The illness, pain, and suffering of the masses and the accepted institutional response—treating the symptom rather than the cause—comprise a substantial part of their economy. A large segment of the earnings of the individual family units is spent on supporting the doomed health of the elder members of the society. But the elderly are doomed because nothing is done to correct the causes of their failing health. They have a system that pays those who have vested interests in seeing that cures are not found for the health maladies.

These Earthlings have so many quaint sayings. The one that seems particularly appropriate right now relates to *leaving the fox to guard the hen house*. In this case, the *fox* is the group of individuals and corporations that benefit from maintaining the status quo—continued illnesses among the masses, the *hens* being guarded, and their continued dependence on services, drugs, and associated paraphernalia sold by the *fox*. Instead of looking for the cures, the *fox* focuses on ameliorating symptoms. In some cases, the *fox* develops destructive treatments that do more damage than good and then subject the *hens* to these inhumane treatments that render their bodies' natural defenses—what they call their immune systems—incapable of responding to the insults inflicted on their bodies."

"Are you saying," Egroeg interrupted, "that different factions within their society do not act in the best interest of the sick and disabled because they have potential personal gain in just treating symptoms and promoting ineffective and potentially harmful—even life-threatening—treatments?"

"Yes, sir . . . well put," praised Suturb. "They do little or nothing to keep the same maladies from developing in others in the future because the money is in the treatment, not the cure. And the exploitation of the ill goes beyond prescribing expensive drugs or injecting toxic chemicals into their veins. They exploit those who are in poor health to maximize the financial impact of their illnesses. For example, it is not uncommon for a person with diabetes being treated to control blood sugar levels to be subjected to multiple amputations and then treated for other related problems, like kidney failure or stroke, independently, without treating the common underlying cause.

"After the partial dismemberment of a patient with a disease like diabetes or cancer and without addressing the root cause that is likely impacting the entire body, they say that the disease has 'spread' to other organs or has impacted other organs as a result of 'complications,' when in many cases, the cause of one diseased organ is likely to be an accumulating poison such as a toxic heavy metal that has concurrently reached critical concentrations in many organs. With the repression of the immune system that usually accompanies the prescribed treatments, maladies in other organs often manifest themselves as new and aggressive diseases such as cancer. But by addressing all the ailments individually, profits are maximized."

There was a pause in the presentation. Suturb wanted to give the information presented time to soak in. Egroeg just raised his left hand to his forehead and slowly shook his head.

Suturb decided to continue, "Another quaint expression that is very apropos in describing the protective function of the government is *penny-wise, pound-foolish.* They impose strict standards on the concentration of cadmium, for example, in the wastewater discharged to streams and rivers, but they apply it liberally on their farmlands in the form of phosphate fertilizers and sewage sludge for products labeled 'organic' to grow the tainted food that they distribute for consumption, leaving a deep imprint of death, pain, and suffering on the populace. Furthermore, the rivers that they say they are trying to protect get contaminated with cadmium by the highly contaminated agricultural runoff. Little or no attempt is made to control the spreading of this poison on the soils or the runoff from the contaminated fields that are becoming more contaminated each growing season."

"Is there no outcry from the masses because of the introduction of lethal contaminants into the food chain?" Egroeg asked.

"Most don't understand the nature or extent of the problem," explained Suturb. "But the vast majority of Earthlings don't want to know. They don't want to take responsibility for their own health and safety, and they don't take the necessary precautions to protect themselves or the people around them from the hazards in their immediate environment. For example, they drive two-wheeled motor vehicles with no helmets to protect their heads in case of an accident. They inhale smoke from paper rolls filled with shredded cadmium-laden leaves of a plant they call tobacco, exposing everyone around them to the toxic gases and aerosols particles. They attempt to drive vehicles when they know that their senses have been dulled by alcohol-containing beverages. They spread cadmium and other toxic materials on the agricultural fields and directly on the crops that are going to be consumed by others in their society. They prepare food for friends, family members, and themselves using ingredients that they know are contaminated with toxins like cadmium. And they go to events where foods made of marine creatures like oysters and shrimp—creatures that are especially high in cadmium content—are the featured delicacy on the menu. And the worst part is that if someone tries to bring the presence of the hazards to their attention, they are, for the most part, ignored or even ridiculed for pointing out the hazards and sharing their concern."

"It sounds like a masochistic society, intent on inflicting and perpetuating pain on themselves and those around them," Egroeg observed.

"As it relates to the food chain," Suturb continued, "the behavior is almost understandable, because those who are vocal about the hazards are few in number, while powerful entities with substantial financial resources and influence have vested interests in maintaining the status quo of continued pain, suffering, and illness. They don't want to tell the public—starting with the producers of phosphate fertilizers. The series of culpable parties continuing with agribusiness that uses the phosphate fertilizers, manufacturers that use the tainted agricultural output in products such as cereals, pastas, coffee, breads, baked goods, and chocolate, to produce foods that are consumed by the public—which, as a result, falls victim to cadmium poisoning—members of the medical community and operators of hospitals and clinics that treat the inflicted, the pharmaceutical companies that sell drugs to ameliorate the symptoms and treat the many diseases associated with cadmium poisoning, and the insurance companies that feed off the public's fear of developing cancer and other dreaded illnesses."

"What is the problem here? Don't they have the technology to be able to separate cadmium from phosphate that they mine?" asked Egroeg.

"Yes, sir, the technology exists," Suturb explained, "but it would add cost to the final products, and it is not used in this country. In fact, it is rarely used at all. Science and technology are used differently here than on Treretum. On Earth, rather than using the advances in basic understanding that come with scientific breakthroughs to benefit the masses, technological development and new scientific information is usually promoted only if there is substantial financial gain for the promoter. Sometimes the new information is 'bought,' and new and superior products are withheld from public offering by interested parties that would potentially suffer financial losses on other well-established and, in many cases, inferior products. And if the technological breakthrough is promoted, it is controlled by a select few who exploit it, hoarding information that could save lives and diminish levels of suffering in the general populace.

"In their medical community, for example, they sell some of the potentially beneficial products that evolve for exorbitant sums of money with little regard for the masses that cannot benefit from them because of their financial constraints. Other products that could cure substantial numbers of the ill are often withheld or their use prohibited, promoting the use of other, more expensive remedies. The focus is on advancing the financial status of the few who, in fact, view the masses, along with their maladies and diseases, as an essential part of their society, necessary for their own financial gain. They amass huge fortunes and isolate themselves through their extravagant lifestyles, losing touch with the reality of the hundreds of millions they exploit. Quite curious—this image they have of individual success—when the world they leave behind on the day they expire is no better off for their having lived."

"You mean they attempt to achieve individual success by amassing financial resources?" queried Egroeg in disbelief.

"Indeed, sir. The values of Earthlings appear to be very different from those of Treretumians," responded Suturb. The tone of his response clearly indicated that Suturb was idealistic and proud of his planet's moral code.

Egroeg leaned forward. "You know, Sucram," he said in a low voice—as though he were taking the presenter into his confidence. "That has been the downfall of many Treretumians." Egroeg resumed his former posture. "When individuals place their own interests above the good of the masses . . ."

"But it is not just individuals," interjected Suturb. Egroeg raised his head abruptly in surprise at being interrupted by his subordinate.

"Corporations and health-related organizations, for example, continually try to take advantage of their governments and government programs that were intended to benefit the sick and poor."

Egroeg was amused. He resumed his relaxed stance and smiled at Suturb's almost emotional outburst. "Well," he responded in an encouraging tone, "at least the government is looking out for the best interest of it citizens."

"Sir, before you draw any conclusions, you must realize that things are not always as they appear," cautioned Suturb. "At times, the Earthlings are abused by their own governments. The government of the country over which we are currently hovering, for example, clearly feels that it has the right to perform large-scale experiments on its citizens—to use them as guinea pigs. It is commonplace to test reactions to different drugs and chemicals on the young members of their armed forces, but they also do large-scale biological testing on the general public. It has been going on for many years. For example, there is a now-famous incident where they were studying a curable social disease in a place called Tuskegee but refused to administer treatment so that they could document the progression of disease, leading to the suffering and deaths of the subjects of the study. And when that was done, they traveled to a nearby country to infect mental patients with the disease to perform further study, all without the knowledge or consent of any of the victims or their loved ones."

"This is disturbing," interjected Egroeg. "The intentional spread of disease among the masses is completely contrary to our goals for this planet."

"I know, sir," responded Suturb. After a brief pause he continued. "In another example, in years past, they released cadmium powder over cities in the middle of their country, from a state they call Minnesota in the north to the state we will be visiting next, Texas, in the south. They released the powder over heavily populated cities like Saint Louis and Corpus Christi, to study *atmospheric dispersion*."

"Why a carcinogenic metal and why over heavily populated areas?" muttered Egroeg.

"Perhaps the real interest was in gleaning information about atmospheric dispersion over heavily populated areas," responded Suturb, "for possible use in the future with their biological warfare program. There is no rational answer." Suturb paused due to the puzzled look on Egroeg's face.

"They do this to their own kind—not an enemy?" asked Egroeg incredulously.

Suturb continued, "Now they are again dispersing cadmium across the skies, along with other metals including aluminum, a major contributor to memory loss and the dreaded Alzheimer's disease. Reportedly, this is to shield the surface of the Earth and its inhabitants from exposure to the sun's radiation and reduce what they call *global warming*. It has recently become more widespread and has been dubbed *chemtrails* by the few that know about the program. It goes virtually unnoticed by the public because the appearance of the chemtrails in the sky is much like that of the condensate trails, or *contrails*, that normally forms behind the high-altitude internal combustion engines of their aircraft. It is amusing the way they treat one of their self-imposed maladies, specifically global warming, by creating another, namely the poisoning of the atmosphere with toxic metals that will eventually settle to the surface to be inhaled by the same people they are supposedly trying to protect."

"Disturbing . . . very disturbing. They don't appear to understand the function of government, or they are so corrupt that they have completely lost touch with what government is supposed to be about," Egroeg commented. He then queried his massive associate as he leaned back in his lounge chair, "Now, what can you tell me about the corporations you mentioned earlier in the session?"

"That was my next topic, sir," responded Suturb rather casually. It was clear that both Suturb and Egroeg were becoming comfortable with each other. "Corporations are groups of individuals that behave as a single body, and they are intimately associated with the prevailing economic systems of the planet. In the world of commerce on planet Earth, nothing is more important than maximizing the profitability of an enterprise that individuals or a group of individuals undertake. The basic premise is that those that are profitable are better equipped to deliver products and services, and they should be rewarded accordingly, reaping the benefits of their labors. But oftentimes things go awry, especially in large organizations where a few control the actions of many. In this situation, buyers must beware, simply to improve their chances of survival.

"When one or more scientific investigations identify toxic materials contained in a product, for instance, the ensuing actions proceed in several phases." Suturb's hand motions brought up a holographic image describing three phases of corporate actions. "The phases generally occur sequentially, and there is often overlap between activities related to two or more phases."

Egroeg interrupted, "Are these corporate actions related to our mission goals? I'm not sure I follow where you are going with this."

"Yes, sir," responded Suturb. "The three phases of corporate actions described here explain to some degree why toxic materials in the Earthlings' environment persist. We will need to understand the mindset before we can effectively deal with it."

Egroeg nodded his head as he said, "Alright, Sucram. I trust your judgment. Please proceed."

"First comes the *denial phase*. The fathers of the product use direct advertising and general announcements, stating that the results of the scientific investigations are incorrect. This is usually accompanied by claims of financial damages, along with threats of lawsuits. Sometimes, subject matter experts are hired to try to discredit the scientific investigations, and invariably, other sponsored investigations are conducted that are said to show no adverse impact despite known flaws in the experimental design or analysis of the experimental results. Standards that are accepted as being protective of human health and safety are often cited, as in the case of toxic materials leaching out of plastics that come in contact with food products. What is not mentioned is that the standards may have been established without the benefit of critical experimental data, resulting in the setting of norms that are too lax to protect the masses. In light of new data, regulatory authorities have the right and responsibility to modify the prevailing standards. But in general, the organizations that are supposed to protect the public are too busy approving new drugs to treat symptoms and fail to address basic causes of the problems."

Egroeg changed his position, leaning forward, right elbow on his knee. "It sounds as though this could go on for some time. And how long does this phase typically last?" he inquired.

"Sometimes decades," answered Suturb. Egroeg motioned for Suturb to continue.

"Yes, sir. Then comes the *lobbying phase*, where influential people are sought to put their names and support behind the cause, regardless of whether they understand the related issues or possible consequences. It oftentimes includes the transfer of large sums of money to the influential individuals.

"And finally, the *cut-your-losses phase*, which comes about only if the previous phases to maintain status quo are ineffective. This phase includes placing the tainted product in other markets so that production can continue. And the health and safety officials within the country do nothing to keep this from happening. At no time does the ethical issue of doing the right thing arise. The moral issue is never considered when it comes to reducing or stopping production. Instead, terms like 'demanding stockholders' and 'meeting stockholders' expectations' are used as excuses to continue behavior that is ultimately destructive for the masses of the planet. Another peculiar thing is that those responsible don't lose a bit of sleep over their actions, nor do the bribed government officials that allow it to happen. In fact, more often than not, they are paid handsomely for their deeds."

Egroeg sat up, openly expressing his disgust. "So what we have is a situation where those with financial resources, power, and influence are allowed to harm others . . . in mass. And it sounds as though enormous sums of money are exchanged to treat countless diseases and to allow the highly toxic heavy metals and other substances that are responsible into the food chain. Did I understand that correctly?"

"Yes, sir. As I have already mentioned," stated Suturb, "the planet is populated by societies that treat the symptoms without addressing the causes of their problems. This propensity is widespread and includes health problems, of course, such as the treatment of diabetes and kidney failure without addressing the root cause of the illnesses. But it also includes issues that are not recognized as health issues—for example, the incarceration of the mentally ill. Earthlings with abnormally high manganese and other heavy metals in their brain tissues are more prone to violent behavior in situations that are not to their liking. They incarcerate the mentally ill with true criminals, not questioning the *why* of their actions and not realizing that their behavior may be due to mineral imbalances and accumulation of heavy metals. Research has shown this to be the case, but the solution that their society has chosen to respond to violent behavior is incarceration, again treating the symptom rather than investigating and treating the underlying cause."

"Separation of portions of the society is never a good thing," declared Egroeg. "In fact, it is counterproductive. Even on our planet, history has shown that complete isolation of different groups creates distrust—to the point of paranoia—so that when members of the different groups do interact, the result is often violent out of ignorance and lack of understanding."

Suturb simply nodded. He was seeing a side of Egroeg he had not seen before—a side that possessed wisdom and understanding. Ironically, the talk among Kcalb crew members included Egroeg's paranoia. Having found common ground with the mission commander made it more difficult for Suturb to see Egroeg as one of the Drutsab he had been taught to distrust.

Egroeg continued, "The we-versus-them mentality has its place but only when dealing with an aggressive enemy that is beyond reason. But enough of personal philosophy. Please go on."

"Yes, sir." Suturb looked at the holographic display to reorient himself and continued, "In some areas of the planet, they segregate themselves into groups with similar physical characteristics. In other areas they are segregated by force. And almost everywhere, they are segregated by financial status. The wealthy are generally reluctant to share, and the poor are often unable to better their own situations, although in some instances, they are satisfied to remain poor, taking advantage of charities from the rest of their society.

"Another strange yet accepted behavior is the exploitation of those who are less fortunate and have fewer financial resources. They are typically penalized for their financial status, as shown here." Suturb spoke authoritatively as he motioned to the cube and then paused, allowing Egroeg sufficient time to read the list that was on display.

- *They pay more for products that cost less to produce and are often of inferior quality.*
- *Financial considerations lead them to live on a diet high in starchy foods such as breads, noodles, and rice . . . eating things that are not very nutritious and some things that are actually harmful, resulting in pervasive illness and premature death.*
- *They are criticized by others for not protecting their own health, and they are criticized by their own for taking measures to protect their health and the health of their loved ones.*
- *They live in slums because they cannot afford to leave them.*
- *They are preyed upon by "investors"--vultures that come in from the outside—and are charged outrageous interest rates because they are less "credit worthy."*
- *Poor diets cause internal conditions that promote violent, antisocial behavior.*
- *They are forced to endure higher crime rates in and around their homes.*
- *Because of the conditions, they often seek escape through drugs that ultimately add to the crime rate, to support the resulting drug habits and addictions.*
- *It leads to an atmosphere of resentment, animosity, and mistrust.*
- *Life is cheap; death is expected, even welcomed (ergo, some members of this sector are happy to do the dirty deeds of death for others who maintain clean hands and a safe distance from the violence).*

When Egroeg looked up from the display, Suturb continued, "One of the things that is beyond my capability to reason is why there is a tax of sorts, imposed on those who are least capable of paying it."

Egroeg's reaction was somewhat compassionate and sympathetic. "It sounds rather hopeless from what you are reporting. Is there no way that the downtrodden can better themselves and their condition?"

"Some escape by excelling at sports, others by excelling at illicit activities," responded Suturb. "And then there are the young males from this pool that serve as the primary instruments for increasing the power and wealth of those responsible for the munitions and weapon systems of war. It is in the schools of the poor neighborhoods that the military actively recruit. It is on what they call the Hispanic television networks that the advertising is so intense that they present the same recruiting ad two or even three times during a single advertising break in the main programming, and the message is one of helping to pay for educational expenses." Suturb continued with a Treretumian Spanish accent, "Eso es parte del plan. El army me va ayudar."

Egroeg straightened up his posture and asked, "What does that mean?"

"That's part of the plan. The army is going to help me," Suturb replied. "Of course, there is no mention of the war and the killing that awaits them should they enlist. These young males supply the muscle behind the war machine, a self-perpetuating wholesale distributor of death. In a sense, those young males are helping perpetuate the conditions that so many of them wish to leave behind. Those who enlist join the ranks of those who are told what to do and what not to do. But that is not entirely foreign to them since they are coming from a society where independent thinking is discouraged. They take the easy way out so they don't have to struggle, even if it means compromising principles.

"For many young Earthlings, it means financial security and includes pumping up their own egos in the process of fighting, attacking, and even destroying other societies that they are told are 'the enemy.' It appears that—depending on which area of the planet you focus—they may fight among themselves for reasons of 'religious, racial, or ideological differences,' invade neighboring territories to gain access to additional lands and resources, or attack others half a world away because their leaders tell them that weapons of mass destruction are threatening their way of life. And after it is all said and done, some profit from perpetuating the war machine, while countless innocent victims are killed or maimed in the process."

"Is there no legitimate reason for organizing and maintaining these armed forces? Is it all related to financial gain?" asked Egroeg.

Suturb responded, "Indeed there are reasons—for example, to ward off aggressive behavior of another country or to combat the insanity of groups they call *terrorists*. But the bulk of the resources expended and lives lost are wasted unnecessarily with the accumulation of big profits for those supplying the war machine."

Egroeg shook his head as he commented, "For our purposes, this is very nonproductive behavior. It does not help with the overall progress of the planet. In fact, it undermines progress, diverting attentions from the true challenge of controlling the quality of their environment." Again, Egroeg shook his head.

Suturb continued, "And when they return from combat, many of them will have suffered loss of limb or other permanent injuries. Others return with mental and emotional disorders."

"What a waste of human potential," muttered Egroeg as he slumped into his seat.

"Yes, there is great waste of young human resources," answered Suturb instinctively, "but the biggest waste among humans is their willingness as a race to accept death for all individuals, saying that they are going to a 'better place,' when in fact, something precious that has taken a lifetime to acquire is lost—knowledge, experience, acquired and innate talent—and no attempt is made to capture it before it is truly lost."

Suturb concluded, "In summary, the current condition on Earth and the societal maladies around this world can be distilled into a single phrase—*the domination of greed over ethics*. It manifests itself in a few powerful individuals taking advantage of the uneducated and uniformed without regard for their plight. Information is withheld or misrepresented, resulting in a race of beings that have great potential but still lack the understanding and focus to control its own environment or destiny. Consequently, the many suffer, while the few prosper. And our goals for them remain frustrated."

"Your report paints a gloomy picture of the conditions on Earth," commented Egroeg. "Are there no saving attributes of these Earthlings?"

"On the contrary, sir," answered Suturb enthusiastically. "Overall, these human Earthlings are resilient, resourceful, compassionate, courageous, diligent, enthusiastic, loyal, generous, friendly, kind, forgiving . . . I could go on. But they are also very trusting, which makes them vulnerable. It is the few that assume control and take advantage of the masses who are thwarting our efforts to foster good health and a clean environment for all Earthlings."

Egroeg rose to his feet slowly. "Yes, well . . . Sucram, you continue to amaze me, and I am certain that the examiners of your report back on Treretum will be equally impressed," as he walked over to Suturb to pat him on the back. "We will probably have additional special assignments for you on this mission. I see good things in your future, Sucram Suturb. Well done."

Suturb stood erect, saying, "Thank you, sir. I simply try to do my best—not just for myself but for all of Treretum."

CADMIUM POISONING

FACTS

- Numerous reports on caloric reduction have been published recently. Some support the idea of periodic fasting as an essential means of reducing caloric intake, but all link reduced caloric intake to an increase in life expectancy. In part, this is likely due to reduced cadmium intake. The process of life is self-perpetuating until the buildup of poisons in the body reaches a level that keeps organs from functioning properly. Cadmium's long biological half-life in the body, approximately 30 years, results in its accumulation in the pancreas, kidneys, and liver, causing problems with assimilation of nutrients and removal of toxins, both ingested and generated in the body. Bottom line: Don't overeat—not because of the calories but because of the cadmium.

- As for cancer treatment, "avezes el remedio es peor que la enfermedad" [sometimes the cure is worse than the disease]. Consider taking phosphate-free zinc supplements as a preventive measure. Many people are afraid of taking zinc supplements. All Earthlings need zinc and copper, especially in later years, when cadmium has had a chance to accumulate, pushing both zinc and copper out of the body. Both metals can be toxic at high concentrations, but the body has a regulating mechanism that keeps the available concentrations in the bloodstream fairly stable. Metallothioneins are sulfur-containing proteins that attach to metals in the bloodstream. The body makes these proteins of varying molecular weights, primarily in the liver and kidneys, in response to high concentrations of zinc and other heavy metals in the blood. Some of this zinc is made available for rerelease into the bloodstream should concentrations of this essential metal begin to fall. High concentrations of zinc in the bloodstream trigger the synthesis of additional metallothioneins, and an associated benefit of generating additional metallothioneins is the chelation of cadmium. Metallothioneins preferentially attach to divalent metals in the following order: copper>cadmium>zinc. Thus, zinc supplementation not only improves conditions for mobilizing cadmium, but it also stimulates the production of additional metallothioneins for sequestration of cadmium and its removal from the body. However, since copper is removed preferentially, individuals taking zinc supplements should consider concurrent copper supplementation based on the copper in their diet (a little copper goes a long way).

- Changes in color are not confined to eyes. Embarking on a regimen of zinc and other supplements results in the gradual flushing of cadmium from the body. Removal of accumulated cadmium is accomplished primarily through the excretion in feces and urine to a lesser degree. The color of the urine may become more yellow due to the vitamin B complex that is part of the routine supplements to be taken, and the color of the stool may become lighter due to the zinc, even if no other supplements are taken. Increased fruit consumption (at least five pieces per day) will ensure plenty of roughage in the diet, regularity of the system, and softer, lighter colored stools.

- One might suspect that metal workers and welders might be at higher risk of cadmium poisoning (welders should *never* weld on galvanized pipe due to the formation of breathable cadmium-laden aerosols), but bakers run the same risk (high risk of lung cancer) by breathing air containing cadmium-laden flour.

Chapter Sixteen

Organization

Gavilán answered the door then opened it wide as he stepped back, motioning for the two men to enter.

Olga scurried over and greeted Dr. Welch. "Billy Ruben, nice to see you again," she said as she leaned forward to give him a kiss on the cheek. She then took Sam's hand and leaned forward to touch cheeks. Sam's eyes widened, and a glow of anticipation came over his face, but that look quickly turned to a look of disappointment when instead of a kiss, he heard in a semiwhisper, "Good to see you too, Sam."

Gavilán shook hands with both men and mumbled, "Hello. How ya' doin'?"

Dr. Welch took Olga by the arm and pulled her several steps away from the others, and concurrent conversations ensued.

Dr. Welch spoke in a low, concerned voice, "Your life is in danger. So is your friend's. I don't know if it's because of your Area 51 preoccupation or my cadmium investigation, but we have been linked by the powers at be, and now we're in this together.

"Gavilán, you have an interesting last name that I recognize to mean 'eagle,' and I know that you have a traditional Mexican first name, but what exactly does Cuauhtémoc mean in plain English?" inquired Sam.

We've been followed by multiple Homeland Security teams since the Houston conference. When we got back to Atlanta, both Sam and I returned to houses that had been broken into and ransacked. Somebody turned them inside out, but nothing seemed to be missing from either Sam's home or mine. Olga was noticeably shaken. "Well, we'd better get Gavilán in on this conversation." She broke loose of Dr. Welch's grip and took a step toward Gavilán.

"Wait!" exclaimed Dr. Welch. Olga stopped cold. "We're being watched right now. There have already been attempts on our lives, both made to look like accidents. With as much money as is at stake, I wouldn't be surprised if the pharmaceuticals haven't bought some very influential government officials, including Homeland Security agents."

"I really think Gavilán needs to be part of this conversation," reiterated Olga as she turned and took a step toward Gavilán.

"Well," responded Gavilán, "the name actually has an Aztec origin. I was named after an Aztec chieftain who was in power very briefly when Hernán Cortez and his Spanish conquistadores invaded Mexico. However, I have no plans of sharing his fate. To answer your question, Cuauhtémoc translates as 'descending eagle' in *plain* English." "Descending eagle," Sam repeated slowly with a puzzled look on his face.

Gavilán extended his arms as he elaborated, "You know . . . like a diving eagle that swoops down to snatch up its unsuspecting prey."

"Oh," reacted Sam with a look of semidisgust on his face.

"Simón, esé. I'm all eagle," continued Gavilán in his cholo accent as he abruptly turned and took a step toward Olga.

Olga and Gavilán bumped into each other as he gave her an abrupt one-armed hug that put her slightly off balance. "Dats why chee calls me her Eagle Man."

They sat around a table in the common area of the suite where Olga and Gavilán were staying. All but the low-hanging light over the table were off, giving the scene the air of an illicit poker game—Olga, Gavilán, Dr. Welch, and Sam, each at an edge of the square table with a pitcher of water, four glasses, and napkins placed at its center.

Olga began the conversation with, "Billy Ruben thinks that because of our experience at the NASA conference . . . our lives are in danger. Billy Ruben, would you elaborate so we are all on the same page?"

"My feel is that Olga and I are the prime targets, and I'm speculating that it's related to the research we reported on, but I can't tell for sure. I can only address the issues associated with my project . . . and it's all about money—big money." Dr. Welch stretched his arms, exposing the cuffs of his white shirt, brought his hands together on the table top, leaned forward, placing some of his weight on his elbows and forearms, and began to tell the group about some of the background on his project.

"You see, officials at the CDC knew about the problem with cadmium in phosphate fertilizers decades ago, but nothing has been done about it because the right people and the right political campaigns have received millions of dollars to do exactly that—nothing. The combined forces of agribusiness and the pharmaceutical companies, with the paid assistance of key personnel in government and the insurance and medical fields, have been able to keep the truth about the carcinogenic heavy metal cadmium under wraps and out of the public eye . . . and for that matter, off the radar screen of the medical community.

"There are rumors that Frank Boudreaux at the CDC, a diabetic who lost his wife to kidney cancer thirty years ago, had mysterious circumstances surrounding his own death shortly after he began investigating the cause of his wife's demise. He had come to the conclusion that it was related to cadmium poisoning from the food that they had eaten all their married lives. Mr. Boudreaux's untimely death due to injection of tainted insulin came as a great shock to his friends and coworkers at the CDC, but with him died the investigation regarding the impact of cadmium on the health of the general population.

"There were rumors that the unfortunate accidental contamination of his insulin was not an accident at all and that some very influential individuals with substantial financial backing had decided the cadmium issue should remain a secret. The word was that they had 'binding agreements' with people in high places to conceal the issue using whatever clandestine methods were deemed necessary, and they had the tacit approval of individuals at all levels of our nation's political spectrum, all the way to the highest office in the land. Politics at the CDC too often interfere with the important task of protecting the public, but when Frank died, no one was foolish enough to risk his or her life by picking up the Boudreaux cadmium project. It was just something that no one talked about. But that was then, and this is now, and I'm not just anyone at the CDC."

The story was incredible, and Olga and Gavilán were full of questions they alternated firing at Dr. Welch: How could Mr. Boudreaux's insulin have been contaminated? Were pharmaceutical interests involved? Was it a well-planned conspiracy? Do doctors really not know about what's going on? How is the medical profession involved? What other kinds of cancer does it cause? How is agribusiness involved? What about the staggering financial implications? Do small family farmers know about cadmium in phosphate fertilizers? How can the insurance companies that pay for all the diagnoses and health care let this continue, or are they okay with it because much of it is being subsidized by Medicare and the federal government? Are they part of the possible conspiracy?

Dr. Welch leaned back in his chair and said, "I don't have all the answers, but did you know that nearly 20 percent of the gross domestic product of this country is tied up in health care?"

All this was news to Sam. He summed it all up in one question. "Dr. Welch, are you saying that there is collusion between the pharmaceutical, agricultural, and insurance industries, along with the medical profession, to perpetuate the spread of a carcinogenic contaminant in our food supply?"

Olga, Gavilán, and Dr. Welch exchanged looks of surprise to hear Sam pose the question.

Sam was a little uncomfortable with the pause and glances. He continued with an additional question. "You mean that farmers sacrifice quality in exchange for quantity?"

Again there were glances exchanged, almost in relief, because this was more like what they expected to come from Sam's lips.

"No," Dr. Welch replied. "I mean they sacrifice you, me, all of us"— he motioned with the index of his right hand in a horizontal circle—"for a buck." He paused and continued in an almost apologetic tone, "I shouldn't be so harsh on the farmers. Most of the small farmers and farm workers probably don't know a thing about cadmium in the phosphate fertilizers they are using. That's why cancer rates in the farming community are up—it's not just the pesticides."

Again, glances were exchanged by all. Billy Ruben knew he was on a roll. He could see the wheels turning in all their heads. He continued, "You see, there's nothing wrong with using phosphate fertilizers. The problem is when people who know about them are too greedy to bother to take out the cadmium—the lethal contaminant in the phosphate rock that they grind up to make the products that are spread on the fields."

Dr. Welch paused, poured himself a glass of water, and took a sip. He appeared dismayed as he bowed his head, shaking it to the left and right as he muttered, "It's all about greed." He stopped shaking his head and stared at the floor for a few seconds before raising his head and continuing in full speaking voice, "And as for the first question you so eloquently posed . . . Son, agriculture is big business in this country, and so is the prescription drug trade.

"The selling of health insurance and cancer insurance and handling of related claims employs a lot of people in this country. And the prestige that goes with being the healers of the sick, constantly searching for the cure for one dreaded disease or another just wouldn't be the same. What would happen if most of the diseases that strike fear into the hearts of the masses were to virtually disappear, resulting in a glut of qualified medical personnel vying for a much smaller number of potential clients? How would that impact the medical 'brotherhood' that currently reigns supreme, by and large unwilling to expose the incompetent and unscrupulous within their own profession?"

Dr. Welch paused, took another sip from his drink, and then continued, "As for the staggering financial implications, the numbers are truly staggering, and that's why there's room for so many to belly-up to the trough. For example, when drugs that cost pennies to produce are sold for many dollars a pill to millions of desperately sick people, there's plenty of room in the budget for 'staying connected' with the right people at the FDA—making personal contributions to the people who not only help them introduce their new products to the public but also place stumbling blocks before those who would introduce products that would threaten to change the status quo."

Sam, Olga, and Gavilán sat silently, listening to their elder like apprehensive school children, uncertain as to whether they were supposed to be hearing their teacher venting his frustration with the world.

Dr. Welch again paused, looked at each of them, and then continued, "You see, to feed the masses, we need high-volume agricultural production. But in our country, there has been a dramatic shift away from an agrarian society and a concentration of the population to the big cities. We have allowed the production of our food supply to fall into the hands of too few. And when decisions about production become strictly business with a focused eye on the bottom line, there is too often a sacrifice in quality for the sake of quantity production and reduction in production costs. The nation's agribusiness, the pharmaceutical industry, hospitals and the medical profession, insurance . . . each of these is a multibillion dollar industry, and each would be impacted dramatically. It's too easy to turn a deaf ear to all the warnings when it perpetuates lucrative conditions for the right people."

Everyone sat silent for a moment. Then, Gavilán muttered in a low voice, "I guess it would take someone with pretty big cojones [pronounced *ko-ho-nes*, defined as testicles but slang for courage and boldness] to try to change the momentum of the big machine."

Olga interjected, "Or an FDA that really protects the public from potentially toxic foods and drugs that could hurt us all."

It was as though she had struck a nerve. Dr. Welch straightened up and again took the floor, except this time, it was almost in an angry tone, "Don't get me started on the FDA and other federal agencies that are supposed to protect us. You see, I'm a government employee, and I pride myself in doing something that I feel is in the public interest. That is the only legitimate justification for the existence of any governmental organization. But not all of us think that way. As in any governmental agency, you have some dedicated people at the FDA, and then you have some bad apples . . . you know . . . the ones that are cronies of the pharmaceutical and agribusiness executives and insurance industry lobbyists. They tend to be so busy with all the to-do from these special interest groups that they lose sight of their real responsibility—to protect the public."

Dr. Welch rose from his chair, and he continued. "*Food* and Drug Administration—*food*—how basic can you get? They're letting our food supply get increasingly contaminated with cadmium not just by letting contaminated phosphate fertilizers be used to grow fruits and vegetables that we consume but also by allowing highly contaminated animal products onto our grocery store shelves and into our restaurants. And then to top it off, they're permitting the use of cadmium-laden phosphate food additives in everything from pudding and evaporated milk to bacon."

Dr. Welch unbuttoned his suit coat and raised his right hand to his hip, exposing more of his white shirt in the process. He began to pace up and down as everyone watched in silence. Then he resumed his rant.

"They know about cadmium . . . they have to! They must have someone in their organization that realizes that the cadmium goes with the phosphate when they are making the sodium, calcium, and potassium phosphate food additives. But if you look at the ingredients listed on the food products you buy at the store, those phosphate additives are showing up more and more, adding more and more cadmium to the burden our bodies have to bear and getting us that much closer to cancer and the grave. Who are we kidding? The FDA isn't protecting us!"

It was clear that Billy Ruben was passionate about his role in society and the government, and his frustration was evident. When he stopped, he appeared almost exhausted, having worked himself into a tizzy. In a disappointed, low voice, Dr. Welch continued, "If only our governmental agencies functioned in concert, with a common goal of promoting in every sense a healthy nation, like our organs work to promote healthy bodies . . . . But greed is ultimately the poison that keeps our organs from functioning and eventually ends in our bodies' demise."

Olga raised her right hand even with her face, with her index finger extended to address Dr. Welch. "It's funny that you mention organs in the discussion. It's not just the cadmium issue where government agencies are dropping the ball. I don't understand why federal agencies seem to be putting stumbling blocks in front of things like stem cell research and treatment, when there are so many people who could benefit from current stem cell technology and when there is the potential in the future of generating entire organs to replace ones that are failing. Some say it's a moral issue, but they don't need stem cells from fetuses—they can take our own stem cells to do treatments and virtually perform miracles. But currently, insurance companies won't cover stem cell procedures because they say they're experimental. I wasn't trained in the medical field, but I can recognize a potential solution to many of our health problems when I see it—and it's been demonstrated to be effective countless times on humans. You don't have to be a rocket scientist . . . ."

Dr. Welch placed his right elbow on the table and leaned forward slightly to rest his chin and half his mouth in the palm of his hand. "You're absolutely right," he muttered into his hand. "There is no moral issue associated with placing the right cells in the right location in your body so they can do their job of repairing failing tissues. It's just a matter of logistics." He straightened up and continued, "You see, treatments that are accepted elsewhere in the world are frowned upon or banned in this country because there is little financial incentive. For many, the answer to their health issues is in cells within their own bodies and not in some expensive miracle drug. Since the stem cell treatments are relatively inexpensive and involve almost no drugs, lobbying by 'friends' of the FDA and other agencies is strong and consistent. The money spent by the pharmaceuticals not just at the FDA, but also in the form of financial contributions to certain religious organizations that raise the moral issue about extracting stem cells from fetuses, as well as the political campaign coffers of key individuals, is considered money well spent. You see, that clouds the real issue and paralyzes our system's ability to react rationally." He slumped his shoulders forward slightly as he mumbled, "At least that's my two cents' worth on how things work."

Everyone paused. Some showed expressions of surprise, others of concern, but all were grateful for being present to hear the insights Dr. Welch had shared.

ᘁᘁᘁᘁᘁᘁᘁᘁᘁᘁᘁᘁᘁᘁᘁᘁᘁᘁᘁᘁᘁᘁᘁᘁᘁᘁᘁᘁᘁᘁ

After a few minutes of almost compete silence, a faint voice came out of an unlit corner of the room. "We couldn't help but overhear the conversation regarding the logistics issue for having the right cells in the right place at the right time within the body."

In a startled fashion, everyone turned to see who was in the corner as three creatures stepped into the light. Sam reacted by clumsily getting out of his chair, arms waving to maintain his balance, pushing back, knocking the chair over, and almost falling down.

"Please forgive us. We didn't mean to alarm you," apologized Nivla, accompanied by his two drones. They were dressed in dark hooded garments, and the characteristic light-colored sashes that would normally appear at the waist could instead be seen partially hanging out of their loose sleeves. Nivla raised his sash, saying, "I thought it might be best to remove these to avoid being seen." He pulled back his hood, and his drones followed suit.

Sam's jaw dropped as he took another step back, bumping into the overturned chair, while Dr. Welch's eyes widened as he grabbed the table and pushed his chair away from the visitors. A curious smile came over Gavilán's face as he just sat and watched the spectacle. Finally, he rose from his chair and swung his right arm over his head as he turned ninety degrees, saying in a loud, boisterous voice, "Nivlaaaaa, so good of you to rejoin us."

Olga cleared her throat. "Hmm, hmm. I think that introductions might be in order."

ꆆꆆꆆꆆꆆꆆꆆꆆꆆꆆꆆꆆꆆꆆꆆꆆꆆꆆꆆꆆꆆꆆꆆꆆꆆꆆꆆꆆ

After all the introductions had been made and the initial shock wore off of being introduced to not just an extraterrestrial but one who spoke perfect English, Dr. Welch asked Nivla a few initial questions. Nivla's responses were clear and concise. Dr. Welch was attentive but appeared skeptical and cautious. Then Sam asked in a somewhat demanding tone, "I still don't quite understand. How did you get in here without being noticed?"

Nivla responded calmly, "By redirecting ourselves into incongruities in the time-space continuum."

Gavilán interjected, "It's sort of like going in a straight line when the space we perceive is the surface of a wrinkled tablecloth."

Sam looked at Gavilán, then at Nivla, and then he leaned back in his chair as to distance himself from both. The look on his face turned into one of concern that he was listening to two strange creatures, both quite insane.

Olga reassured Sam by touching his sleeve as she said, "Don't worry. We'll explain later."

"The conversation that we overheard regarding your anatomy was very interesting. Like your species, Treretumians are *organized* in the design of our bodies and in our society. Certain groups have specific functions, and the proper function of all groups is essential for the survival of the whole."

"You mean you have organs like a heart and lungs?" blurted out Sam.

"Yes," responded Nivla, "and our society has a group that serves as the head to guide the masses. From the little we heard, it appears that in your society, you have a few who are trying to control the masses . . . or should I say *exploit* the masses?"

Olga and Gavilán looked at each other, amazed at Nivla's perceptive comment. Dr. Welch lowered his chin, looked over the top rim of his glasses, and squinted his eyes in a show of skepticism. Sam just sat there, nodding his head affirmatively.

"In the early days of my world," Nivla shared, "a group of Treretumians banded together to try to control the masses . . . to try to change the destructive path on which the planet was headed. The group had many good intentions, but eventually, their relationship with the masses became exploitative."

Sam leaned forward abruptly, moving his hands forward on the table, and blurted out, "But why?"

Nivla's two drones immediately took a step toward Nivla in a protective stance. Nivla looked at them and motioned for them to exercise restraint. He then focused his attention on Sam, responding, "Simply put . . . greed. I suspect that the same is true of the situation you were discussing when we entered."

Still looking over the top of his glasses, Dr. Welch asked, "So what do you suggest we do about it?"

Nivla shrugged his shoulders and said, "As individuals, you can do very little. But if you work together in a coordinated effort, you can bring about change. The individuals who exploit the masses must be exposed, and there must be a public outcry of rage so that your governmental leaders take action to correct the situation, possibly through legislation. Achieving this can be very difficult, depending on how close the ties are between those who are exploiting the masses and your governmental officials."

Everyone mumbled simultaneously with "Tell me about it," "Yeah," and "No kidding."

"And do not think that the exploiters are above making threats on your lives," continued Nivla, "for there is a lot at stake."

Olga, Gavilán, Sam, and Dr. Welch began to huddle to discuss their problem and Nivla's suggestion when Nivla raised his voice, "Now that I have solved your problem, perhaps you can offer suggestions as to how I can solve mine."

Everyone looked up in surprise. After a moment, Gavilán spoke out in a tone of amazement, "You are asking us to help resolve *your* problem?"

"Yes, of course," responded Nivla. "My planet has been struggling with this problem for a long time with no lasting resolution to date. Involving others with a fresh perspective can only help."

All the Earthlings resumed their seats at the table as Nivla proceeded. "My world has experienced exploitation, both internal and external. By that I mean that the internal exploitation was by Treretumians, as I described before . . ." Nivla paused for a moment, "and the external exploitation was by invading beings of unknown extra-Treretumian origin, the Muimdac."

The group was mesmerized as Nivla continued, "The internal exploitation problem is difficult, but we were, and still are, dealing with a situation involving Treretumians seeking to expand their wealth and power. The external exploitation problem, on the other hand, becomes a matter of life and death for every Treretumian that is involved, and it threatens our very existence. You see, the Muimdac are masses of microscopic beings that *cooperate* to take any shape and appearance that suits their needs—they are, one might say, 'Borganized.'"

This term drew a snicker from Gavilán. Olga's eyes squinted, and her head pulled back as she muttered slowly, "As in the Borg?"

Nivla nodded his head, causing Gavilán to add, "Nivla, you've been watching too many old episodes of *Star Trek*." Gavilán was getting uneasy and began to pace around the room.

Nivla could sense that his credibility was in question and that tension was rising. He continued in a slightly louder tone. "One of the Muimdac characteristics is that groups of them take the form of the organ or body part of their host as they devour it. At some point the impacted organs cease to function. Affected body parts can be detached without major functional impairment to the rest of the body. For example, a Muimdac-transform warrior—that is, a warrior that has been completely assimilated with no outward change in the victim's appearance—can lose an arm in battle and continue to be a threat. In fact, he can regain full functionality by attaching additional Muimdac to the location of the lost limb. The warrior who lost his arm could go to an incapacitated companion Muimdac transform, cut off a leg or some other body part, place it on his shoulder, and it would turn into a fully-functional arm to replace the one he lost."

Nivla's audience sat silently, dumbfounded by what they were hearing.

"Transformations occur rapidly," continued Nivla, "because their skin is a sheath that confines light signals transmitted continuously to all cells within the body. Information travels at the speed of light beneath the sheath. This nearly instantaneous transfer of information allows the entire Muimdac assembly to act and react in a coordinated manner."

Sam appeared fidgety and finally stood up exclaiming, "This is freaking me out! You're saying that what I saw in an old Arnold Schwarzenegger *Terminator* movie is really happening on your planet? Never in my wildest dream did I imagine that anything like that *mercury* guy could be real."

Dr. Welch also stood up, placing his left hand on Sam's right shoulder. "Calm down, son. I don't think that in your wildest dream you ever saw yourself sitting at a table, talking to a being who came from a planet located many light-years away either." The two men sat down slowly.

Nivla reveled in the reactions and watching everyone exchanging glances, with looks of astonishment on their faces. He continued, "When a limb is physically severed from the rest of the body, this light-speed mode of communication ceases between the disconnected parts. The sheath covering each part quickly heals itself, closing the wound to keep the light within the individual Muimdac assemblies. Until the severed part is physically reconnected or additional Muimdac are available to assume the role of the severed part, the rest of the 'body' continues to function normally."

Intrigued, Gavilán inquired, "So how do you deal with something like that?"

"With great difficulty," responded Nivla. "Part of the problem is simply identifying the hosts that have been or are in the process of being transformed. Once a Muimdac transform is identified, it is taken to a confined area where we can be certain that all of the microorganisms that make up the transform can be destroyed. Incineration is one of the preferred methods, but special care is taken to ensure that there is no escape in the exhaust gases."

"Nivla," Olga interjected, "I am sorry to say this, but I don't see how you're going to cleanse your society and an entire planet of an insidious enemy such as the one you just described. But you're right, it reminds me a little of the Borg in that they are very well organized, and—"

Gavilán chimed in, "And communication among all the invading party members is constant. Each one knows what all the others are doing, what is happening to all the others."

Nivla was entertained by the way that Olga and Gavilán complemented each other. It was as though each knew what the other was thinking and where their thoughts were leading them—together. He also found it interesting that Dr. Welch, Sam, and his two drones all took a back seat to the conversation led by Olga and Gavilán.

"There's got to be a way," mumbled Gavilán.

Then Olga suggested, "Since the Muimdac appear to be something like the Borg . . . how did the Federation manage to defeat the Borg?"

For a moment, Nivla thought the conversation seemed to be going astray. But he decided to remain silent and see what the two Earthlings came up with.

Olga and Gavilán discussed the elements of the strategy used to defeat the Borg. "You know, it wasn't so much strategy as it was sheer luck," contended Olga.

Gavilán agreed, "What was really key was that Captain Riker had inside information from Captain Picard."

"Yeah," continued Olga. "If he hadn't been transformed into the Borg, Locutus, and then been in the process of being 'un-Borged,' they would never have stumbled on the Borg's Achilles' heel."

Nivla, anxious in listening to the ping-pong match between Olga and Gavilán regarding the weakness of the Borg, blurted out, "What was their vulnerability?"

Olga and Gavilán looked at each other, turned and looked at Nivla, and in unison said, "Sleep."

They were like two children telling a story. Olga went on, "Well, actually, that's only part of it because they had to sleep to replenish their energy supply."

Gavilán continued, "And because their channels of communication with Captain Picard hadn't been severed, they were able to send the message to the mother ship—this giant cube—that it was time to sleep."

Olga: "Yeah, so everyone 'powered down' and went to sleep."

Gavilán: "But their *real* weakness was that they followed instructions blindly—"

Olga: "—without considering the consequences. They were obviously not of a 'cause and effect' mentality."

Gavilán: "And since no one was minding the store, systems started to go astray."

Olga: "Yeah, so much so, that the giant cube eventually self-destructed—boom."

Nivla was visibly upset with the back-and-forth presentation and the contents of the "strategy," or lack of one, that had been described. He tilted his head forward slightly, oscillating left and right, like a fan set at minimum angle. His eyes emitted tiny flashes of light, almost like sparks, with each frequent blink. "I appreciate your good intentions, but this will not be effective against the Muimdac. Unlike your fictitious Borg, Muimdac do not sleep—they simply accumulate, going unnoticed until they are in numbers sufficiently large to cause problems. Also, unlike your Borg, which, by the way, appears to be modeled after another species on your planet—the honey bee—the Muimdac do not have a hive and a queen around which their society is focused and for which each member would fight to the death to protect.

"They don't even need a spacecraft. They travel in the cosmic winds until they find a promising host or group of hosts, and each infected host becomes its own Muimdac colony. The Muimdac concentrate in certain areas within each body they invade until they are again dispersed. They find and infect new prey, waiting patiently for reinforcements to arrive. They accumulate until they have sufficient numbers to cause problems within. But they never have to report to a central figure outside the host prey. Not until the host is vanquished does one victorious Muimdac colony communicate with another."

"Nivla paused for a few seconds, took a deep breath, and continued, "Each victim is a unique case with specific strengths and weaknesses, and each victim presents different challenges for the Muimdac invaders. Consequently, due to the differences in vulnerabilities and the distribution of Muimdac within, victims may display different or multiple symptoms. But it's all the same underlying Muimdac infestation that is responsible for their ultimate demise. The process may be slow, but the outcome is always the same."

Dr. Welch, Sam, Cinz, and Reppoc joined Nivla, Olga, and Gavilán in the discussion. They analyzed, conjectured, and exchanged ideas until they finally forged a plan on how they could battle the Muimdac on their own terms. As with the Borg, it required an understanding of how the enemy functioned, recognizing their vulnerabilities, and crafting a plan of action to capitalize on those weaknesses.

The strategy hinged on introducing an antagonistic element that would initially have similar behavior so that areas of localized Muimdac colonies could be identified and their locations invaded by overwhelming numbers of the antagonists. Successful recovery of Treretum was possible only by dealing with the invaders on their own level—beating them at their own game. Whenever possible, supporting factions would be enlisted that would surround, sequester, and expel individual Muimdac, one at a time.

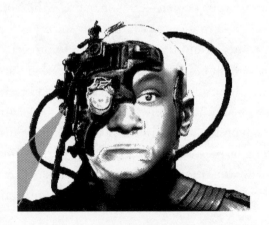

They all agreed this was the beginning strategy for addressing the problem of the Muimdac on Treretum. It was understood that the struggle would be long and painful, both physically and emotionally, and that only by persevering, always focusing on the end goal and keeping an open mind to make adjustments as new information was obtained would victory be attainable.

ꡌꡌꡌꡌꡌꡌꡌꡌꡌꡌꡌꡌꡌꡌꡌꡌꡌꡌꡌꡌꡌꡌꡌꡌꡌꡌꡌꡌꡌ

After resolving the issue of an initial strategy for combating the Muimdac on Treretum, the conversation turned to more basic questions, led by Sam. "Where have you been hiding that you go undetected by our national security sensors and equipment? Why was your arrival unnoticed?"

Olga interjected, "Wait! Their approach didn't really go undetected." Her tone and volume went down as Nivla raised his hand to speak.

"Phobos, I think you have named it, the hollow inner moon orbiting Mars, has served and continues to serve as a staging area for the our work done on Earth. The monolith that inspired the film *2001, Space Odyssey* was, in fact, a homing device to guide our supply ships to the vicinity of the mission—a staging area. The cavernous interior of the moon resulted from the collision in the distant past of a large, cold asteroid with a moon that was in the process of cooling. The asteroid penetrated the outer crust and was absorbed into the molten center. The odd-shaped result was ideal for storing supplies and assembling equipment. The caverns were sufficiently large to accommodate dozens of ships within the orbiting satellite, shielding them from detection."

Dr. Welch, a man who believed in everything being aboveboard and transparent, voiced a concern, saying, "No disrespect intended, but why should we believe anything you say? If you always have to go sneaking around, hiding, why shouldn't we think you are trying to deceive us . . . to trick us into doing something strictly to suit your purposes? Why did you have to hide your ships within Phobos?" It was just Billy Ruben's way—he had to play devil's advocate, whether he believed what he was saying or not. "You probably have other motives . . . other things you are hiding . . . things we know nothing about. What else are you concealing?"

At first, Nivla was offended, but he didn't reveal this to his audience. Instead, he decided to provide examples of concealment and deceit in the context of Earth history that might strike a chord. "Don't be so quick to judge. It is simply a convenient staging area. I have not deceived you, unlike many of your elected officials. I have much information to share but each bit in its own time. I have openly sought your help and unselfishly offered mine and that of my drones." He paused for a moment. "You have so many quaint phrases that are so appropriate at this time, like 'People who live in glass houses shouldn't throw stones.'" The crowd exchanged glances once again, wondering where Nivla was going with the statement. "I recall seeing documentation about your president Dwight D. Eisenhower boarding a UFO in 1955, and in his farewell address, he warned the people of your nation to beware of the powerful 'military-industrial complex.'"

"Nivla, what are you talking about?" interrupted Olga in a whiny voice of incredulity.

Gavilán followed with, "Yeah. Even if it were true, what would that have to do with anything?"

Calmly, Nivla continued in a low but deliberate tone of voice, "There was no active Treretumian mission on Earth at that time. With the crash of the spacecraft in which my brother died, all activities were suspended, and all of my planet's representatives returned to Treretum. However, it is impressive that the engineers and scientists of your military-industrial complex were able to reverse-engineer enough of the control and propulsion systems found in the wreckage to produce several prototypes in a few short years. By 1955, they were ready to demonstrate them to the president at what today you call Holloman Air Force Base."

"What?" exclaimed Olga and Gavilán simultaneously. Sam's jaw dropped, as did Dr. Welch's, but to a lesser degree.

"Yes, Eisenhower was his name . . . at Holloman, in New Mexico, not far from the site of my brother's crash," elaborated Nivla. "The desert southwest is remote, sparsely populated, isolated, and perfect for conducting aircraft and spacecraft research and development. It is no coincidence that nearby Kirtland Air Force Base was the original location of the Air Force Space Technology Center and Weapons Laboratory and is the current home of the Air Force Space Vehicle Directorate and Directed Energy Directorate—also in New Mexico . . . Albuquerque to be more precise."

Dr. Welch, with composure regained and now more pensive, interjected, "Kirtland AFB played a key role in ending the conflict with Japan at the end of World War II. The base provided logistical support for key components and delivery of the final products of the Manhattan Project in nearby Los Alamos. No doubt Kirtland had areas where access was restricted, accessible only to those with secret or top-secret clearances. The secure environment at Kirtland would have made it the ideal initial location to store and examine a large object that no one was to know existed."

Nivla continued, "Yes, well, you may have heard about the Kirtland Air Force Base UFO sightings two years later. Two veteran air traffic controllers at the base tower spotted an approaching aircraft on their radar, and then viewed it with binoculars, hovering just off the ground and then leaving the scene at a high rate of speed, higher than any aircraft with which they were familiar."

Everyone sat in silence. Nivla was on a roll. He thought he had gotten their attention, but he wasn't sure if they were convinced their government officials might be less than honest about the occurrence of events, so he continued, "And what about your president Lyndon B. Johnson who deceived your entire nation about an attack in the Gulf of Tonkin, just to keep the war machine going? Was he misinformed or simply influenced by the military-industrial complex that your president Eisenhower had warned against just a few years earlier?"

"What are you talking about? You've got your wires crossed," proclaimed Gavilán.

"Wait up, Gavilán," said Olga in a much-subdued tone.

Dr. Welch picked up the explanation, saying, "He's pretty much on the mark on that last one. Of the two attacks on a U.S. warship in the Gulf of Tonkin during the Viet Nam War, the second one never happened. But that was what was used to justify *retaliatory* air strikes in North Viet Nam."

There was a pause. Gavilán looked at Dr. Welch in disbelief, and then he turned to Olga. She looked at Gavilán sympathetically and then at Nivla. Being a Texan herself, Olga had mixed feelings about LBJ when she found out about the Gulf of Tonkin incident. Olga interrupted the silence. "I guess we'll never know for sure what caused LBJ to make that speech to the American people. He took that one with him to the grave." She paused for a moment then continued, "Let's give Nivla a chance and listen to what he has to say."

The spotlight was definitely on Nivla. His audience was primed for the punch line, so he continued, "I wasn't here during those years, but neither were any of my fellow Treretumians. To an unbiased third party, it appears that your president Eisenhower's concerns were well founded and, in part, it is likely that it is related with how work had advanced on making Air Force UFOs and the purpose for which those spacecraft were intended. UFO sightings since that time have occurred all over the world, and by and large, reports have been dismissed as mistaken sightings of weather balloons, or so the government would have you believe."

Dr. Welch verbalized the question that everyone shared. "Are you suggesting that all the UFO sighted around the world since the time of the Roswell incident are U.S. reconnaissance aircraft?"

"You can draw your own conclusions, but I think . . ." Nivla paused briefly, raising his right hand, palm forward, as though he was asking for everyone to pause, and then he continued, "not all . . . just most." He then lowered all but two fingers of his extended hand as he finished the thought, "There must have been at least one or two weather balloons in the mix."

Where did he pick up this sarcasm? Olga thought to herself.

௫௫௫௫௫௫௫௫௫௫௫௫௫௫௫௫௫௫௫௫௫௫௫௫௫௫௫௫௫௫௫௫

Included in the early morning discussions was Olga's presentation of scans from the hot-air balloon, hovering over the boundary of Area

51. Everyone was involved in the inspection of the scans, looking for something . . . anything that would indicate the presence of wreckage and/or recovered bodies from the crash near Roswell. Because nothing was uncovered, the consensus was that an airborne visual inspection of Kirtland Air Force Base facilities was in order.

"Now let's get organized," said Dr. Welch as he took the bull by the horns. Tactfully, he had made it clear that he wanted to be more directly involved. "I'll phone in to Atlanta to let the folks at the CDC know that Sam and I will be taking vacation to be able to drive back and enjoy the scenery."

Sam's jaw dropped in surprise, hearing Dr. Welch dictate how his accrued vacation hours would be spent. "But . . ." he uttered. He cut his sentence short because he realized there was no better use of his vacation time. "Never mind."

Dr. Welch continued, "It's a long trip to Albuquerque, and we're all tired, so I suggest that once we get to Los Angeles, we stop at a motel near the Interstate and get some rest. That way, we can be fresh for the long haul across the desert." Everyone agreed.

He placed his hand on Sam's shoulder and said in a lower voice, "Son, can you find us a place that would be suitable? I know you have a fancy phone with GIS/GPS on it. Maybe you can even give us the exit number off the highway so we don't waste time searching for the place."

"Yes, sir. You got it!" Sam replied enthusiastically; he also was eager to be more involved. He immediately pulled out his cell phone and began work on his task while Dr. Welch continued. Dr. Welch made suggestions that were solid and with which everyone agreed. Meanwhile, Sam proceeded with his task. After getting a list of LA motels that advertised locations close to IH 10, he used his GPS to identify the motel closest to the highway.

"Piece of cake," Sam whispered to himself. "All right, everyone listen up," he said.

Olga and Gavilán exchanged glances, and Olga commented in a whisper, "That's a little weird." Gavilán raised his eyebrows and nodded yes. It appeared that Sam thirsted for recognition and authority. They took note as Sam announced where they would rendezvous in Los Angeles.

ꙨꙨꙨꙨꙨꙨꙨꙨꙨꙨꙨꙨꙨꙨꙨꙨꙨꙨꙨꙨꙨꙨꙨꙨꙨꙨꙨꙨꙨꙨꙨ

The discussions in Olga and Gavilán's suite continued into the wee hours. The topics were varied, and they tended to wander, but they were either directly or tangentially related to what had brought them all to the Houston conference. Cinz and Reppoc remained relatively calm and quiet during the discussions, and even Nivla took a back seat in the conversation.

Olga commented that she didn't understand why scientists and engineers with such different backgrounds and research interests had all been invited to the same conference in Houston, and the majority did not appear to have anything to do with national security.

"Olga, I think that my cadmium issue and your space observations are ultimately linked," stated Dr. Welch energetically. "And I can think of three ways right off the top of my head.

"First, they are both related to the future of the human race. We're getting too big for our breeches. We need more space if we want to continue to grow as a species. Space exploration and colonization will be a big part of our future. The heavens await us. However, protecting our current environment here on Earth so that we live long enough to achieve our destiny is paramount. Meeting the increasing global demand for food production means that fertilizers are here to stay, and we need to cope with it here on Earth.

"Second, they are both potentially related to big bucks. We need less expensive resources to support our increasing demand for goods without destroying our planet. We will need to reach to the heavens, for example, by mining asteroids or other planets on which certain raw materials are more plentiful to supply increasing demand on Earth. Those who are successful in this endeavor will reap the rewards.

"And third, they are both related to control. Your field will be an essential tool for gaining and maintaining control of the heavens, while mine is linked to food production. And with today's and the future's exponential growth in our population . . . whoever controls food production will control the Earth."

"Hmmm . . . interesting analysis, Billy Ruben," said Olga. "I guess I never looked at it that way. And I guess they see the 'control of heaven and Earth' to be synonymous with 'maintaining national security.'"

"I'd say so," responded Dr. Welch.

"But the big bucks you spoke of—the rewards to be reaped," interjected Gavilán, "they're earmarked for the wealthy. You won't find too many entrepreneurs from the barrio scraping up the funds to send miners into space to retrieve those valuable resources. In fact, that's the way it is with all of this. The poor will spend the little they have just to survive, but there are so many of them that it'll be more of . . . like that old song says 'the rich get richer, and the poor get poorer.'"

"Uh, I think we struck a nerve," remarked Sam. "It is what it is, Gavilán. The poor don't have the vision . . . and they just let time pass them by."

"Nah, you're right . . . they just don't have the vision," retorted Gavilán. "They don't have the vision 'cause they're too busy trying to put food on the table for their families."

It was evident that poverty was a sensitive issue for Gavilán. "And yeah, I guess time flies . . . whether you're having fun or not," Gavilán muttered.

Nivla found the interaction interesting and entertaining. It demonstrated the disparity in points of view among the Earthlings. He stepped away from the table for a moment. Just then, Olga received a text message on her phone. "Who could be sending a message at this hour?" she asked.

Nivla responded, "I did. I thought that the document I just sent you might be of interest in light of the current discussion."

"Adding fuel to the fire," said Dr. Welch as he shook his head.

Olga began to read the lengthy text message aloud:

Poverty exists for a number of reasons, and there are a number of reasons why it continues to grow. Many people are born into a life of poverty.

Olga stopped and looked up at Nivla, astonished and slightly disturbed, her eyes narrowed and her jaw dropped. "Wait a minute!"

she exclaimed. "How did you get this? I must have written this when I was twelve years old."

Nivla looked at her calmly, tilted his head slightly to the left, and said, "Google knows all."

Olga squinted her eyes in disbelief and muttered, "Wait a minute . . . that's my line."

Nivla continued, "A quick Google search on Olga Ramos left a trail a mile wide. It was a simple matter to investigate your past, something that was a vital part of our assessment. I had to know whether you were the right person to approach. Please continue."

Olga gave Nivla a dirty look, and reluctantly, she slowly picked up where she had left off.

Most of these people end up making the same mistakes that their parents did because it's the only way of life that they know. Lack of education also adds to the problem. Different circumstances cause people to have to discontinue their educations. For example if a family needs another income in order to make ends meet, one of the children may have to quit school in order to get a job. This puts the child at a great disadvantage in the future. Then the cycle begins all over again.

Overpopulation also adds to the problem of poverty. If there are too many people, there is not enough food, clothing, or proper shelter to go around. And again, the problem of employment. Often times, there will not be enough jobs to go around. One reason why overpopulation is a growing problem is because of the lack of birth control, or rather the lack of knowledge of birth control.

The government also has a lot to do with the poverty situation. Many countries spend their money on defense, and artillery, when that money could be spent on food or shelter for the poor. This is evident even in our own city. We spend hundreds of thousands of dollars on rebuilding roads, and laying bricks down on our downtown streets for that "cobblestone" effect, when that money could be going to a much better cause.

Although there are many problems that add to the problem of poverty, there are also many solutions. The lack of education can be overcome by people simply staying in school. This gives the person a greater chance of getting a better job with higher wages. This could eventually pull their family out of poverty, in which case their children would not be born into a family of poverty. This right here eliminates two causes of poverty: lack of education and being born into a life of poverty.

The government could redistribute the budget and put more money to use in feeding the poor, and giving them shelter. This would put the people back on their feet. The government could also contribute to projects to educate the poor. In other words, the government would help people to help themselves.

Lastly, the people who do have money could donate a portion of their money to worthy causes.

Of all of the solutions, education is the most evident. Actually, all of the solutions eventually boil down to the need of an education. When someone is educated and willing to work, he can do what he puts his mind to. Through education, we, as a country, can pull ourselves out of poverty if we are willing to work together.

"Quite insightful for a twelve-year-old," commented Dr. Welch.

However, Sam was not impressed. "What is the problem here? People wind up where they are because of the choices they make. This is the land of opportunity—a place where anyone can make it because we're all on the same playing field . . . and y'all are making it out to be a place that oppresses the poor."

"We may be on the same playing field," rebutted Olga, "but the playing field isn't level. There are many ways that the poor are required to pay what has been called a 'poverty tax.'"

"What? I don't understand," said Sam. "Why should low-income families not have to pay taxes? In our country, everyone pays his or her fair share."

Olga responded, "Maybe on paper, but the tax to which I refer can take many forms, and the end result is that it stratifies the distribution of health, wealth, and well-being. Even in the formal sense, the wealthy hire others to help them evade paying taxes, while the poor have little recourse but to pay the amount they are told that they owe. But on top of that, they generally pay higher interest rates on credit cards and loans—"

Gavilán interrupted, "And if there is an environmental issue, they don't have the resources to move away, and in some instances, their neighborhoods may even be used as a dumping ground for heavy-metal-contaminated soils from a major construction site . . . sanctioned by high-ranking city officials . . . and not to mention any city in particular, let's just say I heard it from Olga."

Olga continued resolutely, "The implications of the poverty tax extend into the health of the community in many ways, and it takes its toll every day. In my hometown, San Antonio, the diabetes capital of the country and possibly the world, the poverty tax is in full swing. The basic diet for Hispanics—whether they are extremely poor or not so poor—who choose to cook at home includes substantial quantities of relatively inexpensive items like noodles and rice. Oh, and let's not forget the flour tortillas."

"Sopa de fideo y sopa de arroz [vermicelli soup and rice soup] . . . yum," mumbled Gavilán.

"See what I mean!" exclaimed Olga as she pointed at Gavilán. "It's a cultural thing."

"Ha! You just contradicted yourself!" exclaimed Sam. "Is it a 'cultural thing,' or is it a result of the 'poverty tax'? I say it's all about choices."

"You got me, Sam," conceded Olga. "It's actually a combination of both. But what about the woman at the grocery store, with several little ones in tow, who buys six loaves of white bread at a time, ramen noodles by the case, and rice and four tortilla mix by the twenty-five-pound bag so that she can stretch her dollars to feed her eight children? Does she really have a choice? The meat in her shopping cart, if there is any meat, is probably the cheapest sausage available, likely loaded with organ meats that are laden with cadmium. She thinks that the medical profession, the FDA, the EPA—the federal government—are all looking out for her and her children. Isn't that what they are supposed to be doing?"

Dr. Welch decided to contribute to the conversation. "Yes, federal agencies are chartered to look after the public interest. But whether it's related to cultural preferences, or it's being perpetuated by poverty, the long-term health impact of this cadmium issue is a society that is riddled with maladies like diabetes, kidney failure, kidney cancer, pancreatic cancer, liver cancer, osteoporosis, lung cancer, prostate cancer, breast cancer, stomach cancer, vascular disease and strokes, arthritis, and Alzheimer's disease. They are all linked. The long-term financial impact is that nearly one fifth of the nation's gross domestic product is diverted to health care issues."

Nivla approved by giving Dr. Welch a thumbs-up.

Olga added, "And for those who choose to eat away from home, those wonderful tortillas de harina [flour tortillas] that everyone loves and eats with their breakfast tacos every day are loaded with cadmium. But if you ask to have your tacos made with tortillas de maíz [corn tortillas] at a Mexican restaurant or taqería, the proprietors may want to charge you as much as 50 percent extra per taco, even though the corn tortillas are actually less expensive to produce, and the tacos that are produced typically contain less filling. Why? Because they have to stop and switch gears since their operation is not geared for making corn tortillas. The immediate result is that it discourages people from asking for corn tortillas. Even those who are aware of the consequences are much more likely to eat the high-cadmium alternative to avoid the minor but noticeable financial impact or the extra preparation time associated with the healthier option."

But Sam was stubborn, and he insisted, "There you go! You just admitted it. People have choices. Everyone has to take responsibility for his or her own health."

Olga shook her head, while Gavilán quickly responded, "How can people have a choice on this issue when they don't even know that there is a problem?" He was angry, not with Sam, but with all the greed, all the deception, and all the corruption that was responsible for the current conditions that were causing distress among countless millions. He could not contain himself and broke out in his first tongue. "¿Como pueden decidir cuando no saben lo que está pasando, cuando no saben cuales son las alternativas, cuando ni saben que el enemigo ya está adentro de ellos mismos?"

Sam squinted, not knowing what Gavilán had just said, while Olga leaned against Gavilán and placed her hand on his shoulder to calm him as she serenely translated, "How can they decide when they don't know what is happening, when they don't know the alternatives, when they don't even know that the enemy is already within them?"

Sam was on the defensive. "Y'all make it seem like a big conspiracy. This isn't anything new. There is no conspiracy. The information is on the Internet, right?"

"True," responded Olga, "but not everyone knows how to read, not everyone speaks English, not everyone has Internet access, and almost no one knows that the problem even exists, much less that they should be doing Google searches to find out about it on the Internet."

Gavilán picked up where Olga left off, saying "And don't forget that people need to be able to discern good information from bad . . . but you're right, Sam. People have choices, and when they are made aware, most people don't want to know. Once they know, they rationalize not doing anything about it by saying, 'Well, I'm going to die anyway,' or 'Something else will get me first,' or 'I've suffered emotional and psychological pain that is much worse than any physical pain could ever be,' or 'There are so many other things that are more immediate causes for concern, so why should I worry about this one?' or 'I can't afford to change the way I live.'

"The answer is that you don't have to worry about it. The cause-effect relationships are already well established. The real question is why—when you know that there is a problem that will likely cause you and your loved ones pain and suffering—why would you *not* make adjustments in your life and the lives of your children to try to avoid it? Any minor increased costs now—if any—are investments that will help you avoid the staggering costs and anguish associated with treatment later. Is it better to stick your head in the sand and pretend the problem doesn't exist?"

Sam shrugged his shoulders and said, "You can lead a horse to water, but you can't make him drink."

"True," acknowledged Gavilán, "but what if the horse drops dead of thirst because he was so dehydrated that he couldn't see the oasis directly in front of him? People need to know! They can't make a choice if they don't know!"

Nivla had second thoughts about what he was about to do, citing a rule that all *teachers* were to abide by. "I should not do this, but I feel that it is important to have all members of a team having the same vision so they can effectively work toward the same goal. We are not to take others on excursions through the wrinkles in the fabric unless it is to save their lives, but in this case, I shall make an exception."

Turning and directly addressing Sam, Nivla said, "Sam, you have successfully demonstrated your lack of compassion and lack of understanding of the plight of the poor. As a *teacher*, it appears to me that you have led a sheltered life, and you would benefit from seeing how the other half lives. I invite you to join me on a brief visit to the other side. Gavilán, I hope that you will agree to join us, and while we are gone, I hope that Olga and Dr. Welch will take advantage of the opportunity to become better acquainted with Cinz and Reppoc."

The evening of group discussion ended with Nivla, Gavilán, and Sam preparing to embark on a quick trip to New York City.

CADMIUM POISONING

FACTS

- The State of California has lowered the public health goal set for cadmium in drinking water from 0.07 parts per billion (ppb) to the even more stringent value of 0.04 ppb, based on a reexamination of literature on cadmium and its impact on renal function. But this is only one governmental body, and its impact on the general public is limited.

- Meanwhile, the FDA allows phosphate additives that contain cadmium to be added to more and more products that eventually enter our bodies. Why is the FDA allowing this? Stop the presses! Phosphates are even in our supplements! I was shocked when I realized that the zinc, vitamins B-6 and B complex, and other supplements I was taking contain phosphates. I have found phosphate-free substitutes, but *you have to look at the ingredients of every product you buy* to effectively minimize your cadmium intake.

- The strategy for removing cadmium from the body is analogous to the strategy for defeating the Muimdac and hinges on introducing an antagonistic element (zinc) that initially has similar behavior as cadmium (zinc is immediately above cadmium in the periodic table) so that areas of localized high-cadmium concentration (e.g., the kidneys, pancreas, liver, lungs, and bones), as with the Muimdac colonies, can be invaded by overwhelming numbers of the antagonists (daily dosages of zinc that are more than 10 times the RDA but still below the toxic dosage for zinc).

- Because members of the same families tend to eat the same foods, all are receiving relatively comparable cadmium dosages relative to the amount of food consumed. Older individuals generally will have eaten more food in their lifetimes and will have correspondingly higher quantities of cadmium accumulated in their bodies. The maladies exhibited will not necessarily be same in these individuals. In other words, two members of an adult couple living in the same household and consuming the same foods could develop different maladies—for example, arthritis and glaucoma, or diabetes and liver cancer, or breast cancer and gout. The possible combinations are countless, but all are related to the accumulation of cadmium, and the links between the different symptoms/illnesses continue to go unnoticed.

- Don't be complacent about your exposure to cadmium because its adverse impact is cumulative—it depends on how much and where cadmium has accumulated within the body. Don't accept others' complacency. Statements like "Así es la vida" [Such is life] and "Así son las cosas" [That's just the way things are] should be rejected—it is a matter of survival, and there is no room for complacency.

- Just as with the propagation of cellular malfunction and death in areas of high concentration of an antagonistic element, proper placement of the cells and essential nutrients that are expressly designed to maintain and protect can have a beneficial impact. There is power in numbers. That is why relatively high dosages of zinc, a metal that is needed throughout the body and is incorporated in every strand of DNA, are needed to inhibit and counteract the accumulation of cadmium. The objective is to raise zinc concentrations system-wide. However, localized repairs to damage caused by cadmium in specific organs and areas of the body can be enhanced by strategic placement of high concentrations of cells that are responsible for the body's own defenses and repair mechanisms. Stem cells, for example, are in each of our bodies. Work of pioneers like Dr. Roberto Fernandez Vina of Argentina have demonstrated repeatedly that by extracting blood already rich in células madres (stem cells), concentrating them further, and reinjecting them into ailing areas of the body can have miraculous results. (The treatment is available in Mexico, Germany, and elsewhere. While the treatment is also available in the US, it is not generally accepted, it is not government approved, and it is generally not covered by health insurance.) The same has been shown to be true when platelet-rich plasma (PRP) is reinjected into areas in need of repair. Given the right building blocks in the form of nutrients and the right vitamins and minerals, our bodies can heal themselves, but sometimes it is a matter of cellular logistics, and our assistance with those logistics can prove very beneficial.

- Autoimmune disorders (e.g., multiple sclerosis [MS], lupus, Hashimoto's disease) arise when the body's own defense mechanisms seem to turn on and attack the very organs they are supposed to protect.

Hypothesis: This occurs when the immune system becomes hypersensitive to a foreign substance that has invaded the cells of specific organs and, for example, the T helper cells, whose production has been documented to be stimulated by exposure to cadmium, then attack cells where cadmium has replaced zinc. (Recall that zinc is present in every strand of DNA and plays a key role in the function of every cell of the body, and cadmium tends to accumulate in specific organs.)

In other words, the invading cadmium not only triggers increased T helper cell production, but it also serves as the target that the T helper cells attack. Ample epidemiological evidence exists that suggests this may be what is happening in patients suffering from MS (see MS website that identifies MS "clusters" [areas of high incidence of MS] in the vicinity of zinc smelters). While it may appear that zinc is the problem, it is much more likely that the uncontrolled discharge of cadmium that is incorporated in the zinc ores being refined is responsible. (Cadmium is always present in zinc deposits, copper deposits, and phosphate deposits.)

- Stem cell therapy has been reported to repair damaged tissues that may be linked to cadmium poisoning (e.g., degenerative bone and disc disease, rheumatoid arthritis, osteoarthritis). It has been reported that stem cell production in the body, in general, can be enhanced by adopting a routine of fasting one day (24 hours) per week, restricting intake to grapefruit juice and water. This would also encourage maintaining a high metabolism rate and decrease the weekly caloric intake, which would decrease the likelihood of obesity.

• The zinc deficiency that usually accompanies cadmium poisoning results in a compromised immune system, but when it is coupled with iodine deficiency, the results can be devastating. Cadmium is a carcinogen, and iodine, in addition to being a key element for proper thyroid function, is responsible for signaling the normal process of scheduled cell death (cell apoptosis). Thus, the cancer caused by cadmium goes unchecked by the immune system due to zinc deficiency, and the normal programming of the death of the cells is disabled due to the iodine deficiency. It's "the perfect storm" (i.e., proliferation of cancer cells). Additional thyroid/cadmium/zinc comments are included in Appendix B.

Chapter Seventeen

The Environment Within

In the middle of the hustle and bustle of the emergency room of New York City's General Hospital, a woman is rushed in on a gurney with her husband in hot pursuit. The woman is in labor. The man, wearing a tattered, dark-blue overcoat, looks like someone from a World War II setting in Poland. His piercing eyes communicated his anguish as he pleads to the attending physician through his thick Eastern European accent, "Please, you have to save my wife and our little Bleema." The gurney, the patient, her husband, the hospital staff, and the drama continue to roll down the corridor.

Just then, the automatic doors open again, and a man is rushed into the ER. Medical technicians hover over the gurney to take the man's vital signs. Then a tall, slender dark-haired man dressed in green scrubs stands straight up and declares, "Too late—DOA." He pauses, lowers his voice, and continues, "Another dead on arrival—dead." The technician is clearly upset.

Another technician standing next to him turns and slaps him on the upper arm, saying, "Shake it off, dude. We just do what we can," as he starts to walk away.

The tall man in green pulls off his head garment and also starts walking away. He passes the two emergency technicians who had brought in the man on the gurney as they are being interviewed by an emergency room attendant. While the ER attendant writes on his clipboard, one of the ambulance techs says, "He'd been seen staggering in the streets by neighborhood residents earlier in the afternoon and evening. They said he had gotten 'totally polluted.'" Then the other ambulance tech mumbles, "It's a shame what people do to themselves."

Without regard for the ER attendant, the comments turn into a discussion between the two ambulance technicians. "Yeah, don't they know that they are killing themselves? With all the talk these days about the environment and environmental awareness, couldn't this dude feel that the environment inside of him was getting lethal?"

"No, man, he was so polluted that his senses were knocked out, and all he knew was that he wanted another drink. I've seen it with cocaine overdoses. It's like the frying egg commercial on TV . . . . Man, their brains are so fried that all they know is that they have to have more."

The other technician gestures toward the door, saying, "Yeah, but alcoholics develop cirrhosis of the liver. The scar tissue pinches off blood flow, and that destroys their bodies' major detoxifier, eventually killing them . . . like our boss is going to do to us if we don't get back on the road for the next call." The two men start toward the door of the emergency room, walking past three men in scrubs, complete with masks and headgear. One of the ambulance techs focuses on the trio as they walk past, turns to his companion, and mumbles, "Tall dude!"

Sam, Gavilán, and Nivla, disguised in scrubs, turn and walk down the hallway, looking for a more secluded spot where they can talk. The transient scenes had alarmed Sam. It was clear that this ER was a place where lives were in the balance.

Nivla places his latex-covered hand on Sam's shoulder, saying, "You just witnessed situations involving life-and-death decisions. In the first, the decisions of the medical team hopefully will save the lives of a woman and her child. It appears that the couple had little choice but to rush to the ER if they wanted to save their child's life. I wonder if they had proper prenatal care—care that would be considered even the bare minimum in your society—or if they knew what assistance might be available to a pregnant immigrant in a new country. Did they have any choices, and if they did, did they know what they were? Certainly, the couple must be aware that there are costs associated with their visit to the ER, but they chose life, knowing that the debt they would incurred would likely prolong their situation of living in poverty.

"In the other, the decisions were made long ago. The dead man was the result of abuse, both intentional and unintentional, and the damage caused by a toxic environment within. Sometimes, due to lack of information, people cause themselves harm. People living in poverty often choose to escape through drugs and alcohol, although drug and alcohol abuse is not restricted to the poor. They don't always understand the consequences of their actions . . . and sometimes they don't care."

"Yeah, like Olga says—cause and effect. It's all about choices," Gavilán mutters under his breath.

"And once your liver goes, your days are numbered," announces Sam authoritatively. "You don't have much time before the toxins in your body catch up with you." Then his tone changes—much more subdued. "I watched my father end his life at the bottom of a bottle." Sam's companions look at him in silence, and Sam continues, talking almost as though he were going into a trance, "You're right—it's all about choices. And no—we don't have much time."

In an attempt to change the tone of the conversation and get them back to home base, Gavilán declares, "We don't have time! We have to get back."

"No rush!" exclaimed Nivla, with a puzzled look on his face.

Sam snaps out of it, responding, "Oh, I forgot how you can control time and move about without our knowing of your presence. You can get us back in the blink of an eye because you can control time."

"Not in an absolute sense," Nivla, the teacher, responds. "Time is an attempt to measure the potential sequence of events. We use the ticking of a clock or the vibration of atoms. But these things are relative. Time, in its most absolute sense, is the tool we use to identify the instantaneous configuration of the universe."

"Do you always speak in such profound terms?" asks Gavilán.

Nivla replies calmly, "Remember that I am but *a teacher*."

Just then, a man in a wheelchair pushed himself past them. The man—an older Hispanic gentleman—appeared to have had his left leg amputated just below the knee.

"Pobre diabético," mumbled Gavilán.

"What?" asked Sam as he wrinkled his nose and squinted his eyes.

"Poor diabetic," responded Gavilán.

"How do you know he's diabetic?" asked Sam.

"Odds are pretty good that he is," responded Gavilán with great certainty in his voice. "So tell me, Nivla, do you have diseases like diabetes on your planet?"

"We had something like your diabetes, but it is an ancient disease that was eradicated tens of bak'tuns ago . . . when we took control of our environment and eliminated the unnecessary exposure to heavy metals. However, we do have members of our society that may lose a limb for one reason or another, if that's what you're asking. We deal with it very differently than you do here on Earth. You see, Treretumians have mastered what you are just beginning to explore—what you call brain-computer interface technology or BCI. On our planet, it was developed in four distinct stages. First, we developed robotics linked to the brain by electrodes and computers. Second, we included feedback to the brain from sensors on mechanical prostheses. Third, we developed a biological equivalent to replace the computer, and it was contained within the prostheses. And fourth, we stimulated development of relatively dormant portions of the brain—the ultimate controller—to be able to control additional prostheses."

"Additional prostheses?" queried Gavilán.

"Yes," exclaimed Nivla enthusiastically. "We have a class of drones that have two sets of prosthetic arms in addition to their own two arms and two legs—Spidermen, if you will. The availability of the two extra sets of limbs on a single drone eliminates two additional workers in some situations that require manual coordination. Your multi-armed Shiva is a very real possibility."

"Gee, it sounds surreal," commented Sam. "What's the name of that Indian goddess with all the arms? Or was she Cambodian?"

Gavilán responded to Sam's question in passing, saying, "Which one? Saraswati, Ganesh, Vishnu, Parvati, Lakshmi, Kali, or Durga . . . take your pick . . . and they're all Hindi," as he focused on Nivla and asked a question of his own as he gestured with his hands. "Did any of those drones—the ones with the extra arms—did any of them make it to Earth during one of your planet's previous expeditions? I'm just trying make sense of some pieces of a big puzzle."

"Yes," replied the alien in a very matter-of-fact manner. "They caused quite a stir among the Earthlings of that time, as I understand, so much so that they were declared gods by locals across the continent. From then on, those drones were kept on the spacecraft because their physical peculiarities detracted from the mission."

Gavilán raised his right hand to his chin and was pensive for a moment before continuing, "Do you foresee us—planet Earth—ever advancing to that point, where we could replace limbs and have prostheses or biological equivalents controlled by the brain of the individual who lost the limb?"

Nivla replied reassuringly, "I do, but to get there, you must continue the development of your current trajectory—that is, linking brain function to computers that can interpret the firing of synapses and respond by sending appropriate signals to robotic prosthetic limbs to perform specific mechanical tasks. The computers and associated power supplies should be sufficiently small to be contained within the prostheses.

"Then develop feedback loops that allow conditions detected by sensors within and on the outer surface of the prostheses—for example, heat, cold, the presence of wind, exposure to sun and moisture—to be converted into electrical signals that are channeled through and modified by the computer for that prosthesis and then sent to specific locations in the brain.

Once you have mastered that, the challenge will be to replace the computer hardware with a biological equivalent. Treretumians mastered this many bak'tuns ago, and you can as well."

Gavilán commented, "It all sounds so futuristic to me."

"Actually, this is ancient history on Treretum," Nivla responded. "Additional limbs will be, as you say, 'a piece of cake.' You graft additional limbs as desired and link them to appropriate 'unused' areas of the brain. As before, the biggest challenges are connecting the blood supply and nerves. Modern technology will help you to utilize more of the brain. On Treretum, we have individuals with two, three, and even four sets of arms that are specialized in performing tasks that require manual coordination. I shamefully confess, however, that some of these individuals have been adapted thusly solely for the task of giving pleasure to prominent members of the Drutsab Egral."

A faint "Oooh!" escaped Sam's lips, and everyone turned briefly to see if anything else would be forthcoming.

After a few seconds, Nivla continued, "As with any new appendage, the recipient has to learn how to use it. Unfortunately, the learning process is as it was with their original bodies—relatively slow and laborious. Despite this, drones often request to have appendages added because they feel it opens more doors for them—no pun intended."

Nivla's demeanor changed suddenly, and he appeared somewhat annoyed as he continued, "The Muimdac bypass all this development because there is no central processing station. Cells are multifunctional and signals travel at near the speed of light."

He continued, "At one point, we thought that victory belonged to Treretum. The Muimdac were vanquished. The battle was won, the violence ended, and a centuries-old quest of conquest foiled. At the time, it was perceived as the beginning of an era of rebuilding, of healing—an era for unifying a planet and preparing for the challenging future that lay ahead. The *perceived peace* was accompanied by an entire planet lowering its guard, and the potential recovery by the remains of a clandestine and relentless enemy was grossly underestimated. The victory was sweet . . . or so it seemed. But things are not always as they appear."

Gavilán refrained from mentioning that Nivla was straying off course with his conversation. It was clear he was a passionate patriot of Treretum, and the topic of the Muimdac invasion would always be a sensitive issue for him.

Nivla continued, "They were treating the symptom. They were monitoring declining concentrations of Muimdac in the bloodstreams of Treretumians who were known to be contaminated. However, the Muimdac shifted their focus, invading the bodies of those responsible for doing the monitoring. They then continued to have hosts that were unaware of their presence until it was too late . . . one Treretumian at a time.

"Their strategy was simple. They targeted key organs, amassing their forces in those organs while reducing concentrations elsewhere—for example, the bloodstream, which was routinely monitored. They lulled Treretum into a false sense of security, tricking us into thinking that we had won the struggle. Additional forces and needed resources were supplied during Treretumians' annual visits to the health and detoxification centers for replacement of their toxic element filters. This is also how the Muimdac inoculated additional unsuspecting Treretumians like my Oleub. With time, they amassed enough forces in the strategic locations to attack, disrupting the function of or taking over targeted organs. He did not last long. It was difficult to see his body incinerated, but it wasn't really his body anymore. It was only his image, and the reality is that we incinerated a colony of Muimdac in the body of a Muimdac transform . . . a very difficult time for my Aleub."

Gavilán and Sam were dumbfounded, and Nivla seemed to have drifted off to another world momentarily. But when he returned, he forcefully said, "Come, we must return," as he repositioned his green operating mask over the bottom half of his face and stepped out the door into the corridor with Gavilán and Sam following his lead.

CADMIUM POISONING

FACTS

- The liver is an essential organ that cleans and detoxifies the blood. It neutralizes oxygen free radicals to help the body cope with oxidative stresses that are placed upon it by our environment. The single most important and potent antioxidant in our bodies, glutathione, is present in all our cells, but it can be found in as high as a 5 millimolar (mM) concentration.

- The glutathione molecule is made from three basic amino acids: cysteine, glycine, and glutamine. The cysteine contains a thiol group (containing sulfur and hydrogen) that makes it versatile in the vital role it plays in every viable cell in the body. It is similar to hemoglobin in the sense that it functions by going back and forth between oxidized and reduced states. In a healthy individual, the majority of the glutathione is in the reduced state, ready to react with oxygen-free radicals and other oxidants that can damage cells. The oxidized molecule is then regenerated to its reduced state in an enzymatic reaction involving selenium. (Note that selenium, along with zinc, is also essential for a healthy prostate and found in high concentrations in foods like garlic.)

- Although the liver does an amazing job of detoxifying countless organic compounds, it cannot detoxify a toxic element like cadmium. It must be eliminated from the body. Together, two glutathione molecules can chelate heavy metals like cadmium for excretion through the digestive track. However, when this occurs, the glutathione molecules involved are lost and are no longer available for the oxidation-reduction interchange.

- Glutathione levels in humans tend to diminish with age, partly because as adults, we are more likely to be exposed to toxins that consume glutathione and because the production of glutathione is often limited by the availability of the amino acids that are required for its synthesis—cysteine in particular. In the aging process, the decrease in glutathione concentrations exposes the cells of our bodies to toxic compounds and oxidative attack. Because cadmium consumes precious, diminishing resources that are largely responsible for detoxifying ingested and inhaled toxins, cadmium takes its toll on the detoxification capacity of the liver.

- Since the carcinogen cadmium tends to accumulate in the liver, the liver becomes overburdened with glutathione production due to the continuing depletion via cadmium chelation. Therefore, anything that would help remove cadmium from the liver (e.g., zinc) and chelate it for removal from the body (e.g., vitamin A, vitamin B_1, vitamin C) would lighten the burden on the liver.

- As with reducing consumption of glutathione, anything that would increase glutathione concentrations in the body would also lighten the burden on the liver. Oral administration of glutathione has proved to be a slow and inefficient process because most of it does not survive the trip down the digestive track. Since it is a large molecule, absorption of glutathione through the skin also presents a challenge.

- It has been found that ingesting cysteine, its precursors, and/or compounds that break down to cysteine precursors (e.g., N-acetyl cysteine [NAC], lipoic acid, and silymarin) is a more effective way of boosting glutathione concentrations.

- Milk and eggs (especially the yoke) are both rich in cysteine, which is usually the limiting ingredient in the synthesis of glutathione. However, the high temperatures associated with pasteurization of milk and cooking of eggs destroy cysteine. Therefore, identify a nearby farm that is licensed to sell raw milk (ask Google—Google knows all) and consider adjusting the breakfast menu to include a ponche (a milkshake made with raw milk, a raw egg, and raw honey). Along the same lines, eat your eggs sunny side up and runny and explain to your friends why you prefer raw onions (on cheese enchiladas—yum).

Chapter Eighteen

So What's a Girl to Do?

It had been a very long night that had consumed most of the morning darkness. The dawn was nearly upon them, and Olga and Gavilán were finally alone in their suite. The activities of this trip's final night in the Bay Area had left them both exhausted.

Gavilán kicked off his shoes as he told Olga, "A visit with Sam and Dr. Welch, *two* visits with space aliens, and a quick jaunt to New York City while you get better acquainted with Cinz and Reppoc . . . I'd say that's 'bout enough for one night."

Olga was sitting on the sofa taking her shoes off as well, although she was taking them off quite slowly and seemed pensive. She looked up at Gavilán and said something that initially appeared completely unrelated as though she had been in her own world while he was talking. "You know, when I was fifteen years old, my dad took me on a trip in Mexico. We spent most of our time in and around Mexico City, and, of course, we spent a good while in the various mercados, shopping for loved ones back home. Dad had a grandaunt who had arthritis, and her wrists were always hurting. He got her a copper bracelet. And when she received the present, she immediately put it on. She swore that it helped relieve her pain. Billy Ruben and I were talking with Cinz and Reppoc, asking questions about their backgrounds and Treretum, and they were asking questions about Earth. They seemed very interested in metals, and in the conversation Dr. Welch mentioned that his mother wore a copper bracelet to help her arthritis. It turns out that Reppoc's grandmother did the same thing—she wore a copper bracelet too."

Gavilán squinted his eyes and said in a disbelieving tone, partly because the topic had come from nowhere, "Okay Ms. Cause and Effect—I'm having a hard time with that one. I know that copper has its place in the world of sanitation. I remember hearing in one of my environmental classes how the addition of just a few parts per million of copper sulfate to a reservoir is an effective way of controlling the microbial population of a water supply, specifically algae. Are you suggesting that arthritis is a manifestation of an algal or bacterial infection?"

"Calm down, my little eaglet," Olga teased affectionately. "Actually, Dad couldn't believe it either, but I guess that a little of my cause-and-effect mentality rubbed off on him . . . or maybe it was vice versa . . . so he did his homework. As it turns out, he concluded that it had nothing to do with microorganisms but instead with heavy metals, and specifically cadmium. According to Dad, copper has a high affinity for cadmium, and the presence of the copper bracelet next to the skin drew out minute quantities of cadmium from the skin. He said that the skin was an 'imperfect barrier' and that in the presence of perspiration, the skin allowed cadmium and other minerals to travel through it."

"My gosh, I feel like I'm back in school," interrupted Gavilán, "hearing a lecture on Fick's first law and the transport of a contaminant due to a concentration gradient across the transport medium."

Olga looked at him curiously. "He said that the removal of cadmium from the skin of his grandaunt's wrists," she continued resolutely, "resulted in a gradual removal of cadmium from the bones beneath the skin." She paused as though she'd been insulted and thought for a moment. She raised her head and stated indignantly, "And don't start making up profanities in the form of mass transport laws just because you don't agree."

Gavilán burst out laughing, uttering in a cackle, "I said Fick, with an *i*!" He looked at Olga and saw her look of consternation melt into a smile.

In an instant she was laughing with Gavilán, blurting out, "I guess you took more environmental classes at Stanford than I did." The laughter intensified, and Olga raised her left hand to cover her mouth as she repeatedly lifted and dropped her right hand like a puppy trying to balance itself on just its hind legs.

Gavilán hugged his petite friend. They hugged each other until the laughter subsided. They moved back a bit, gazed into each other's eyes, and again hugged. No words were needed to express their sincere and profound affection and respect for each other.

They separated, and there was silence. Then Gavilán spoke, softly and slowly, "I guess that might explain why our elders swore that soaking their aching feet in an Epsom salt bath helped relieve pain." He looked down at his hands like a shy adolescent and then continued as he looked up at Olga, "I always thought that it was just the warm water, but supposedly, even cold baths of the magnesium sulfate solution brought relief. It makes a lot of sense . . . right?"

Olga smiled sheepishly and said in a half-whisper, "Yeah."

〰〰〰〰〰〰〰〰〰〰〰〰〰〰〰〰〰〰〰〰〰〰〰〰〰

Gavilán started to swagger toward the door, saying, "Wow, it's been a really long day, and I guess we'd better get at least a couple of hours rest, because—"

Olga interrupted, "Wait, please, don't go. There's something else that's bothering me."

Gavilán turned and plopped himself in the nearest chair.

Olga began, "Cuauhtémoc, I am torn."

Gavilán thought to himself, *Cuauhtémoc? Uh-oh* . . . .

Olga continued, "My very patriotic fabric is being unraveled. I want to be a good citizen—a good citizen of this country that my parents fought and died for, a good citizen that still believes in the ideals that were instilled in me since my earliest childhood memories, a good citizen that does the right thing, doing things because they're right . . . living my life by the phrase 'do it because it's right,' and conversely, rejecting things because they are wrong.

"Gavilán, I grew up knowing the difference between right and wrong, but now the distinction is getting hazy. I see the government in control—my government— doing things that my conscience tells me are wrong. What I am being told is right seems very wrong. Gavilán, I see a being from another star system trying to preserve family honor, fighting for things that I once thought were the cornerstones of my country, my world . . . and now I am told that he is evil and that I must betray him. Gavilán, I am a citizen of the universe. If I don't turn Nivla in, they would have me believe that I am betraying my country. What do I do? What can I do?"

Gavilán saw the torment in her eyes. He reached out and held her hands in his, resting them in her lap. "Mi querida [my beloved] Olga, what would Miss Piggy do?" His interjection of comic relief was welcomed.

Gavilán went into his vato routine, reminiscent of Cheech Marin. "Joo [You] know, I am an ordained minister of the Shursh [Church] of Seester [Sister] Sonia the Flamingo [Flamenco] Dancer, registered in the State of California. Yeah, man, every Sunday I have to chine my choose [shine my shoes] to go dance during mass with the seesters [sisters] in their pink feathered outfits, and sometimes that's real hard for me to do 'cause I like to stay up Saturday nights talkin' on the shat [chat] line."

"Enough!" Olga exclaimed as she reached over to slap Gavilán on the knee. "I'm serious! Here I am struggling with issues that are making me examine my moral foundation—the cornerstones on which I have built my life—and you have the gall to make fun of me?"

"Mi querida, I'm sorry. How insensitive of me. Te suplico que me perdones [I beg you to forgive me]," he said softly as he lowered his head. "You know that I would never intentionally do anything to hurt you. I just thought that you were getting too serious and that we needed to change the mood." There was a pause, and then Gavilán continued, "No mas recuerda [just remember], EGBAR."

Olga looked at her friend. She felt bad for making him hurt as she knew she had. There was a long pause, and then to break the silence, Olga inquired, "Where do you come up with all that chit?"

Gavilán quickly raised his head to look at Olga. A big grin appeared on her face, and Gavilán knew he was forgiven. *I guess that's my cue to be a vato again,* Gavilán thought to himself. Then he boldly announced, "By the power *invested* [vested] in me, I now pronounce you mi hefita . . . or is that mi ruca [my woman]?" Olga giggled. Gavilán took Olga by the arms and looked her squarely in the eyes. His demeanor changed. He now spoke in a very serious, low tone, with great deliberation. "Olga, listen to me. I'm in love with you. I fell in love with you the day we met so many years ago. Olga, I love you. You have to have known that."

"Yeah," she responded sheepishly as she tilted her head to one side and momentarily looked downward. She raised her head slowly and continued, "I sort of thought that might be the case." She then focused on his dark eyes, looking straight into them. "When we first met, I was in awe." She paused. "But that has grown into much more. You are my best friend, my inspiration, the one that I know would never do anything to hurt me in any way." She paused again. "I just never wanted to jeopardize our relationship—"

Olga was interrupted by the forefinger of Gavilán's right hand touching her lips. She moved her head back slightly, initially in a state of surprise that quickly faded. She threw her arms around Gavilán's neck. They embraced, Olga standing on her toes. Gavilán straightened up, lifting Olga off the ground. Their kiss was long overdue; it was passionate and timeless.

CADMIUM POISONING

FACTS

- Adsorption and absorption are two important processes that influence the transport of cadmium in the environment and within our bodies. The former involves adhesion of a solute onto a solid surface, while the latter involves a fluid filling the void spaces in a porous medium (e.g., a sponge). Adsorption of both cadmium and copper on soil particles is enhanced by the presence of organic matter. Adsorption of cadmium is further enhanced in copper-enriched soils. The presence of nitrogen fertilizers enhances uptake of cadmium by plants (and probably animals as well).

- Copper bracelets are reported used to relieve aches and pains in the wrists and joints. Cadmium poisoning includes elevated concentrations in the skin, one of the body's methods of elimination of the heavy metal. In addition to enhancing cadmium removal, perspiration and skin contact with the copper, along with the concentration gradient across the skin, likely enhance migration of copper into the tissues and joints that are in pain. If cadmium was present in high quantities, it is likely that it had displaced zinc and copper (an essential component in connective tissues) from the tissues in that area.

- Moist skin absorbs cadmium and allows the heavy metal to migrate to areas of lower concentration and desorb into a fluid with which it comes in contact. In other words (*attention to gardeners, farmers, and anyone who handles fertilizers containing phosphates*), skin is an imperfect barrier that impedes but does not stop the transport of cadmium through it and into the tissues and bloodstream. Always wear gloves and at least a dust mask when handling phosphate fertilizers or products that may contain them (e.g., potting soil).

- The chemistries of vertical families of the periodic table are similar. Therefore, zinc, cadmium, and mercury are similar; sulfur and selenium are similar; and nitrogen and phosphorous are similar.

- As mentioned previously, in the periodic table, cadmium is located directly beneath zinc, and mercury is found directly beneath cadmium. The three metals are in the same family, and they have certain characteristics that are similar. However, while zinc has a biological half-life of approximately 78 days, cadmium's is about 30 years, and mercury's varies widely, depending on the form of the mercury and the location in the body where it accumulates. For example, ethyl mercury has a half-life of 7 to 10 days, whereas other forms typically have half-lives of 40 to 70 days. However, mercury can cross the blood-brain barrier, and in the brain, it has a biological half-life of 20 years and, in general, a reported half-life of 15 years in nerve cells. Like mercury, cadmium causes neurological problems and is linked to autism (see http://www.autismhelpforyou.com/Cadmium.htm). While the adverse impacts of mercury are widely recognized by our country's medical community and legislative bodies, the carcinogenic heavy metal cadmium is equally or more toxic than mercury and has a longer biological half-life but goes virtually unnoticed by the medical community, governmental agencies, and legislators.

- Mercury, like cadmium, causes neurological problems and, also like cadmium, is a contaminant in our food supply. High-fructose corn syrup (HFCS) is extracted from corn, using a process that involves caustic soda. Most of the caustic used is contaminated with mercury from the chemical process in which it is made. The quantity of mercury that winds up in the HFCS is small, but because the biological half-life of mercury is very high and because HFCS is found in so many products, mercury in HFCS is also a major health concern that remains unaddressed. (See http://www.washingtonpost.com/wp-dyn/content/article/2009/01/26/AR2009012601831.html).

- Contacting copper with mercury results in the formation of a relatively stable amalgam that is apparent from the resulting shiny, silver-colored surface.

- An amalgam of mercury is also used in dentistry. The relatively stable amalgam with silver is used in fillings that gradually leach mercury out of the fillings and into our bodies with the rate of leaching depending on the acidity of our saliva and the foods and beverages we consume. Since mercury is directly beneath zinc and cadmium in the periodic table, consider taking extra zinc for a day or two before having any dental work done that involves disturbing (i.e., removal) of silver/mercury amalgam fillings to minimize absorption of mercury that is likely to be introduced into your body during the procedure.

- Zinc and copper are the principal components of brass. Since cadmium and zinc have similar chemical characteristics, they are found in the same mineral deposits. In other words, most grades of brass contain mostly copper and zinc, but they also contain small quantities of cadmium.

- The rising cadmium concentrations in agricultural soil have an impact on the amount of cadmium being introduced into the food chain—the higher the cadmium concentration in the soil, the greater the plant uptake.

- This bullet, consistent with the title of the chapter, is intended to complement and provide a preview of Appendix A. So What's a Girl/Boy to Do?
  A. Take responsibility for her/his health and control of her/his life.
  B. Adjust her/his diet to minimize cadmium consumption— eliminate high-cadmium foods as much as possible.
  C. Eliminate contact with materials containing high concentrations of cadmium (e.g., soils containing phosphate fertilizers), using latex gloves, goggles, and dust masks as necessary.

D. Eliminate smoking, including exposure to secondhand smoke.

E. Eliminate ingestion of soft drinks and minimize consumption of alcoholic beverages.

F. Supplement with phosphate-free zinc. Take it without fail but *always with a meal*.

G. Drink purified water.
   1. Filtered with activated carbon
   2. Filtered by reverse osmosis
   3. Distilled
   4. Demineralized.

H. The Land of Agua Ponce. Spread the word—this is a bigger problem than the lead and mercury issues combined! The public needs to know!

I. *Read* the labels—inspect the product labels before you purchase.

J. Put on the pressure at/on
   1. Home
   2. Restaurants
   3. Public and private schools and institutions of higher education
   4. Doctors and pharmacists
   5. Legislators
   6. Health officials
   7. Media resources

Chapter Nineteen

Return to Albuquerque

The mild May morning was ideal for travel. Gavilán and Olga checked out of their suite on El Camino and loaded their gear into the car. It was time to depart the Bay Area and the site of the most memorable Powwow ever.

Gavilán tossed the last bag into the open trunk. As he closed the trunk, he turned to Olga saying, "I hope you don't mind my dropping off the thumb drive with my dissertation advisor. I had promised to let him see the initial results of the work we are doing at Moffett, and it was too much data to e-mail—or to put on a CD or even DVD, for that matter." Gavilán was proud of his work, and having validation from a nationally recognized authority would, if nothing else, gave him confidence and a bit of an ego boost.

"I already told you—no problemo," responded Olga.

The two hopped into the car, and Gavilán continued, "He's just off Middlefield, and it won't take but a few minutes." He started the car and turned out of the parking garage, and the two headed up El Camino Real.

About a mile up the road, Olga commented, "Things are not always as they appear."

"Were did that come from? What are you referring to?" queried Gavilán

"I don't know. I was just thinking about Agent Stevenson. From the first time I confronted him . . . he didn't seem like he was such a bad guy," she commented. "He was just doing what he was told to do."

Gavilán, el burlista [the tease], uttered, "Duh, use my brain? Duh . . . . I wussun tole to use my brain . . . dats not in my job description." Olga sensed a slight bit of jealousy mixed in with a healthy dose of sarcasm. Gavilán continued, "And as long as he think that way, that young man is dangerous. And you'd never think that from just looking at such a nice, clean-cut kid. Yeah, you're right—not everything is as it appears."

◻◻◻◻◻◻◻◻◻◻◻◻◻◻◻◻◻◻◻◻◻◻◻◻◻◻◻◻◻◻◻◻

Because one of Gavilán's advisor's neighbors, a Native American Stanford professor, was throwing a Powwow brunch for his friends and family, cars were parked up and down the street, and Gavilán had had to park the car a couple of blocks away. Neither Gavilán nor Olga minded because it was a beautiful day—the kind that makes you happy to be alive. Gavilán's elderly professor and his wife stood at the door of their home, saying their goodbyes to Gavilán and Olga.

"Adios, mi professor," hollered Gavilán as he waved his left arm over his head, and he and Olga made their way down the walkway to the street.

They reached the street and began their walk back to the car on the street side of what seemed an endless string of parked vehicles. Suddenly, a man who had appeared to be getting something out of his trunk slammed the trunk shut and stepped directly in front of them. It was Agent Stevenson.

"Oy vey, el tartamudo," [Oh my gosh, the stutterer] muttered Gavilán.

"So you came to see an Iranian," he began, "one we've had our eye on for quite some time now. Did you exchange information? Did you get instructions on what you're supposed to do next?"

"Gee, and all this time I though Dr. Mohammad was Irish. Actually, I only came to drop off data, and any direction that I receive will be after he has a chance to look over the thumb drive I left with him."

"Okay folks, I think I have enough to take you in for questioning," announced Stevenson.

Olga, in a burst of outrage, exclaimed, "What? We haven't done anything!" as she tried to maneuver around Stevenson.

Stevenson simply sidestepped, placing himself directly in her path.

"Listen," said Gavilán, in a tone of reconciliation. "Honestly, I just dropped off field data from some environmental work I'm doing at Moffett Field. He's going to give me his opinion on the ongoing remediation, and that's it. And by the way, he's as American as motherhood and apple pie."

"Yeah, well, you'll just have to explain that to the folks at our Homeland Security Interrogation Center in San Jose."

Finally, Olga, in a tone of frustration and disgust, said, "I take back all the nice things I ever said about you. You're just a nasty little man, Mr. Stevenson." She brushed shoulders with him as she walked past.

Stevenson shifted his stance, turning to look at Gavilán, then at Olga, and then at Gavilán again, but Olga had gotten by him. He was slightly disturbed, but he planted himself firmly in front of Gavilán. He turned his head toward Olga and yelled, "S-S-Stop!" but Olga just kept walking.

After Stevenson turned back to look at Gavilán, Gavilán asked, "What is it that you think we are planning to do?"

"Something s-s-s-s-s-s-sinister," Stevenson replied. "I know you're involved in some sort of s-s-s-sinister p-p-p-p-p-pl-pl-scheme."

Gavilán just shook his head and tried to walk past Stevenson, but the young man grabbed Gavilán by the arm, turning both men around so that Gavilán wound up with his back toward Olga. Gavilán jerked his arm out of Stevenson's grip, and the more austere Cuauhtémoc side of his personality appeared. "Keep your hands off me, buddy."

Stevenson stuttered nervously, "I t-t-told you. I'm t-t-taking you in for qui-qui-questioning."

Defiantly, Cuauhtémoc looked Stevenson straight in the eye, raised his right hand, and gave him the one-finger salute. "You've got nothing on me," he said as he turned and started walking away.

"S-S-S-S-Stop," stammered Stevenson as he unbuttoned his suit coat and pulled a service revolver from the armpit holster. He pointed the gun at Gavilán, holding it with two shaky hands, his arms extended. "I s-s-said s-s-s-s-stop!" He cocked the pistol.

Cuauhtémoc Gavilán heard the distinctive sound, paused, but then kept walking. He knew he was gambling, but his instantaneous assessment clearly gave him better odds with Stevenson than with "the agency." He spoke loudly and waved his arms as he walked, "You're working with the wrong crowd, Stevenson. You're not a murderer. Think, man, think! You're not one of them."

"I'm not supposed to think!" the young man shouted nervously. "That's n-n-n-n-not in my job description!"

Oh shit! Gavilán thought to himself. He had an instant of hesitation as he wondered how this throw of the dice would turn out. He knew that all the indoctrination would be hard to overcome for the man with the back of his head in the crosshairs, but he was committed, and there was no turning back. He knew that in an instant he could be dead and only hoped that Olga would know that he loved her. He threw up his hands as a parting gesture and kept walking.

A nervous sweat had begun to appear on Stevenson's forehead. He felt he had just been pushed into the middle of the biggest of all crossroads of his career . . . and of his life. He knew this moral judgment would affect his self-esteem, his being able to live with himself . . . for the rest of his life. Stevenson thought to himself, *Pull the trigger, and just follow the rules . . . but what about being a Christian and loving thy neighbor? What had that man done that he deserved to die?* He licked his lips and started to squeeze the trigger slowly. Then he raised his eyebrows, took a deep breath, and just as slowly pulled back his weapon as he uncocked the hammer . . . and then he whispered to himself, "He's right. I'm not one of them."

Stevenson watched Gavilán walk away as he very slowly lowered his revolver, and he continued for what seemed to be an eternity as Gavilán eventually disappeared from view in the distance.

Gavilán reached the car where Olga was waiting outside on the driver's side. She saw the look on his face and could see he was drained. What he had just been through had left him pale and visibly weak in appearance as though he just had a long bout with the flu. Gavilán took a deep breath and looked at Olga with a solemn face, only to see her gentle smile. She raised her pointing finger to his nose and whispered, "EGBAR."

He smiled gently and nodded. Olga knew just the right thing to say to make him feel more at ease. Olga began to walk around to the other side of the car, and as they were getting into the car, Gavilán's subconscious brain emerged for an instant, placing a thought firmly into his consciousness. *Let's blow this pop stand. Come on, let's go get married.*

As the seat of his pants hit the bucket seat of the car, Gavilán did a double take, asking himself, *What the hell?* He looked at Olga as she shut the door and turned toward him.

She asked, "Are you okay?" and he paused for a few seconds and responded slowly in a low voice, "Let's blow this pop stand."

Out of nowhere, two men in blue suits ran up to Stevenson, grabbed him by his coat's lapel, and tugged and pushed on him, exclaiming, "You let him get away!"

Startled and struggling to maintain his balance, Stevenson shouted, "Who are you?"

The first man hurriedly announced, "We're your DHS safety net. Blakey wasn't going to let you botch this one." The other agent joined in, "We've been tailing you ever since your meeting in his office when you announced your incompetence." Just then a black sedan came screeching around the corner. And as the two men jumped into the vehicle that never came to a complete stop, one of them yelled back at Stevenson, who was left standing in a daze, "Besides, there's been a change in our instructions regarding these two."

Gavilán instinctively looked into the rearview mirror when he heard squealing tires. He then reached for the keys to start the engine as he told Olga, "Buckle up—we're going for a ride!"

At the instant the starter motor disengaged, Gavilán floored the gas pedal, leaving behind two black tire patches and a cloud of smoke and dust. A pair of sharp turns and they were out to Junipero Serra, headed south, with a black DHS sedan in hot pursuit.

They quickly approached the place where Junipero Serra became a divided highway, the Foothill Expressway.

"Now what? Who are they?" Olga was visibly shaken.

Gavilán responded in a low voice, "Cronies of your buddy Stevenson." He glanced at Olga to assess her reaction to the situation that had just befallen them. "We need to shake these guys. What's right on Page Mill [Road]?"

"No! Nothing!" exclaimed Olga. "Not unless you want to go camping at Portola State Park. The road goes on with some hairpin turns near the park, but there are few options other than straight ahead."

Still in a low, calm voice, Gavilán responded, "Okay, I guess it's straight ahead on the world's most beautiful highway—lovely IH 280," as he ran the light at the intersection. Again, he glanced at Olga who was looking back at him with a stern look—head tilted forward, right eyebrow lowered, and left eyebrow raised. Gavilán looked in the rearview and saw the black sedan not far behind. "We need to work our way over to the Bayshore [Freeway]. Suggestions?"

"I think there are a couple of turnoffs up ahead that'll get us there," Olga answered with a hint of a nervous vibrato in her voice.

Gavilán had his right foot all the way to the floor. They continued to weave in and out of lanes of traffic miraculously without his letting up on the gas pedal, but the black sedan continued to advance, closing the gap with every passing mile. "You *are* buckled in, right?" Gavilán grunted as he focused on passing every car in sight.

As she clutched the car seat, Olga abruptly turned her head to the left. Seeing Gavilán chin down, eyes locked on the traffic straight ahead, she uncontrollably shrieked, "Yes!" as the car swerved around a pickup truck. She took a big swallow, regained her composure slightly and continued in a lower tone, "My seat belt is on."

Gavilán kept the gas pedal on the floorboard, but the black sedan slowly, consistently kept getting larger in the rearview. The scenery kept whizzing by, and Gavilán kept maneuvering past the rest of the traffic, which seemed to be moving at a snail's pace. He glanced into the rearview repeatedly, and his adrenaline flow was clearly on the rise.

Olga clutched at her seat with every swerve and recovery that Gavilán skillfully executed. "Something's gotta give soon," he muttered.

Olga turned to look out the rear window, jostled back and forth by Gavilán's passing maneuvers. What was alarming was that not far behind, the black sedan steadily kept closing on them. When Olga turned around to the front, she recognized where they were, took a deep breath, and said in a low, nervous voice, "Gavilán, there's a turnoff a few miles ahead. It's an exit on the left side of the freeway. Take it!"

Gavilán kept weaving in and out of the traffic, darting into any opening he could find. His pursuers were doing the same. Vehicles around them seemed to respond, swerving out of his way, honking as they passed. Gavilán began to look into the rearview more frequently. Their pursuers would soon be upon them. "We've got to lose these guys," he muttered.

Olga refrained from talking in fear of distracting Gavilán from his Formula One driving, what now was clearly a matter of life and death. Olga nervously read aloud the sign that flashed by her, "Construction zone ahead."

Gavilán responded calmly, "I know, but these guys are almost on our tails."

They were in the right lane, and Gavilán knew he had to get back to the left. The slow-down of traffic in the construction zone caused Gavilán to work harder to keep from crashing into the surrounding vehicles as he worked his way to the left. Suddenly, there was a bump from behind. Olga's and Gavilán's heads jerk back slightly, and Olga shrieked upon the mild impact. Gavilán looked in the rearview, and Olga jerked around to look out the rear window, only to see the black sedan speeding forward to bump them again. She turned forward, recognizing they were rapidly approaching the turnoff.

"Gavilán," she yelled frantically, "You have to get in the left lane!" Seemingly out of nowhere, a straightaway appeared, but two large trucks and an eighteen-wheeler were in the left lane. The black sedan was directly behind them. "We've got to take the next exit," Gavilán muttered.

Olga interjected excitedly as she pointed at a sign that was flying by. "The sign said 'Next exit on left!'"

They sped past the two trucks and were approaching the front of the eighteen-wheeler when Gavilán began to honk his horn to alert the driver. They were rapidly approaching the highway exit, but there was construction equipment everywhere and barricades at the exit with a sign that read "Exit Closed." A large gravel truck was on the shoulder just past the exit, and there was gravel all over the road as a front-end loader appeared to be trying to scrape the paved shoulder to gather the gravel. Gavilán knew nothing of this since his field of vision was blocked by the eighteen-wheeler.

Gavilán impatiently looked into his side-view mirror, waiting for the moment he could swerve past the eighteen-wheeler. Suddenly, the mirror exploded. "These guys are playing for keeps!" yelled Gavilán. It was clear that he had to make his move—it was now or never!

Gavilán shouted, "Hold on!" as he leaned to his left, pulling the top of the steering wheel with him and causing the car to swerve in front of the eighteen-wheeler. The big rig immediately sounded its horn with a deafening blast as the car hit the gravel that was spilled in the left lane and extended onto the shoulder. The car crossed in front of the towering cab and began to slide sideways, crashing through several wooden barricades and plowing into a series of orange pylons. Impact with the front-end loader appeared unavoidable. Olga raised and grabbed her knees, assuming a fetal position, tightly closed her eyes, and screamed.

Suddenly, the sound of the eighteen-wheeler's blaring horn was replaced with the sound of squealing tires as Gavilán straightened out the car and sped off the exit ramp into street traffic. As he slowed to the speed of surrounding traffic, Olga raised her head and looked around her in amazement. "I didn't know you were that good a driver."

"I'm not," he responded. Gavilán seemed somewhat stunned as he turned his head to left, peered into the traffic, turned his head to the right, and again peered as though he were looking for something.

Olga let out a sigh of relief and uttered, "I thought for sure we were dead."

Gavilán still appeared stunned as he slowly replied, "Uh . . . I'm not sure we're not."

She reached over and pinched Gavilán's arm. He jerked his right shoulder upward as he yelled, "Ouch! What did you do that for?" His motion caused to car to move slightly into the lane to the left, which drew a honk from the car in that lane. Gavilán immediately corrected his course.

The angry driver gestured at Gavilán as Olga responded coolly, "I guess you're alive."

With a frown on his face, Gavilán asked in a distinctly disturbed tone of voice, "No! What happened back there?"

Olga responded in a very matter-of-fact tone, "You just miraculously got us off the highway, onto the exit ramp, and into street traffic." She rubbed his arm as she finished with a touch of excitement in her voice, "We lost them."

"No, wait! I didn't just pull a miracle out of my ass. What happened back there?" Gavilán was getting agitated as he kept turning his face toward Olga and then back to the traffic ahead. He wanted to see her expression, hoping to see an expression of understanding. "What just happened? Somebody just tried to kill us back there. These guys are playing for keeps! And to top it all off, I have no idea how we wound up on the exit ramp. When I swerved in front of the eighteen-wheeler, we were dead meat!"

A low voice came from the back seat, "Take a left at the next light. I saw a wrinkle in the fabric and I thought we should draw a straight line."

Gavilán slammed on the brakes as Olga swerved around to her left. Their car came to an abrupt stop, and the car behind them came to a screeching halt with horn blaring. Cinz, one of Nivla's drones, continued, "I think you'd better get going if we're going to make that light."

თთთთთთთთთთთთთთთთთთთთთთთთთთთთთთთთთთ

The threesome continued on their journey south. Dr. Welch and Sam left before them, so they were expected to arrive in Los Angeles first. There was ample time for Cinz to share more about himself and his assignment. Gavilán drove, Olga rode in the passenger's seat, and Cinz sat in the middle of the back seat, leaning forward, holding onto the two seats in front of him. "Nivla assigned me the task of protecting you, Olga and Gavilán, when we left your suite on El Camino."

"Oh great . . . an alien chaperone," commented Gavilán under his breath.

Cinz continued, "He was concerned about your safety, and from our recent experience, it appears that his fears were justified."

Olga exclaimed, "You can say that again!"

Cinz tilted his head slightly and repeated, "He was concerned about your safety, and from our recent experience, it appears that his fears were justified."

"No, Cinz, I didn't mean for you to say it again," explained Olga apologetically. "It's just a colloquialism—it's just a saying."

"Ah, yes—one of those Earthling sayings that I keep hearing about. Both Nivla and Suturb are very interested in your quaint and often inconsistent sayings," remarked Cinz.

"Suturb? I'm afraid we haven't had the pleasure of meeting Suturb," noted Gavilán as he glanced to his right to catch a glimpse of Cinz's face out of the corner of his eye before returning his undivided attention to the road.

"No. Unfortunately, he will remain on the ship where he is needed for the rest of our visit," explained Cinz. "He, Nivla, and I are all of the

Kcalb Clan. Because of our size and adaptability to different conditions, we are often assigned tasks of protection. My clan has played an integral part in the struggle against the Muimdac—from our direct involvement in healing the wounds inflicted by the Muimdac to our being engaged in the decision making process at the head of our planetary government. Without our contributions . . . literally, life on our planet would cease to exist. Consequently, members of the Kcalb Clan have been targeted. The Muimdac want to eliminate us so they can advance with less interference."

Olga shared information about Cinz and Reppoc that she had gained during their long conversation the night before. "Did you know, Gavilán, that likewise, Reppoc is essential on certain assignments, but sometimes his clients can tolerate only so much of him."

"Noooo," said Gavilán sarcastically. "I can't imagine why."

"I admit that sometimes," confessed Cinz, "I replace him in such situations and tasks, even though he may be the best suited for the job, simply because he does not demonstrate a significant presence. But in general, we complement each other and work well together."

Olga interrupted, "Gavilán, could you stop at the next filling station because I hear nature calling."

"I heard nothing," remarked Cinz. Olga looked at him with one eyebrow raised. "Oh, I see . . . another of those Earthling sayings."

Gavilán took the next exit and found a convenience store about two blocks beyond the exit. They parked around the back of a convenience store, and everyone emerged from the vehicle to stretch their legs.

"I'll be right back," she said as she stepped inside to get the access key.

Gavilán and Cinz, with his hood over his head, stood outside car. Gavilán nudged Cinz's arm and said, "I guess you saved our lives back there . . . and I apologize for any nasty remarks I may have made. Olga and I are forever indebted to you." Gavilán extended his hand for a handshake as he said, "Thanks."

Cinz took his right hand in his and, with a firm grip, jerked Gavilán toward him so their chests touched, and Cinz was able to pat him on the back with his left hand.

"How long did you say you'd been shadowing us?" Gavilán asked. "No, don't answer that. I don't wanna know!"

Just then, Olga walked up to Gavilán. "Keys, please—my turn to drive. I'll let you get back behind the wheel once we're getting close."

"Deal!" replied Gavilán.

ꖴꖴꖴꖴꖴꖴꖴꖴꖴꖴꖴꖴꖴꖴꖴꖴꖴꖴꖴꖴꖴꖴꖴꖴꖴꖴꖴꖴꖴꖴꖴꖴꖴꖴꖴꖴ

They had officially arrived in the LA metro area, driving through one community after another with nothing separating them but signs at their boundaries. "This next exit is the one we're supposed to take, according to Sam," Olga told Gavilán in a less-than-comfortable tone.

"Well, it's certainly easy access to the highway—easy off and easy on to IH 10," commented Gavilán, trying to look at the positive side of things.

"Are you sure we're in the right place?" asked Olga.

Gavilán shrugged his shoulders, saying in a *don't-blame-me* tone of voice, "I donno. I'm just the driver."

"Surely Sam would have phoned us with an alternative location if he found that his initial choice was inappropriate . . . wouldn't he?" asked Olga as she wrinkled her nose and squinted her eyes.

The motel Sam had identified using his cell phone GPS was indeed convenient but on what seemed to be the seedy side of Los Angeles. Gavilán took the exit, and before they knew it, they were at the motel.

Gavilán went up to the curbside office window to check in, and Olga stayed in the car with Cinz to guard their belongings. The transaction was fast, and before Olga had a chance to call Sam, Gavilán was opening the car door. Gavilán got in the car, turned to Olga with a disturbed look on his face, and said, "He asked if we were renting the room for the night or by the hour." He paused as his look slowly evolved into a snicker. "I asked for a two-room suite, but since he didn't have any, I had to settle for two adjacent rooms, and yes, Cinz can stay with me." His look continued to evolve into a big grin as he watched a relatively attractive woman with heavy makeup and in a short, tight skirt walk by.

Olga was tired and impatient. "Come on, let's get some sleep. I don't know about you two, but I really need some rest after last night."

Cinz responded, "I do not require sleep. My function is to protect you, but if my presence upsets you, I will retire to a less visible location."

"No, no, that's all right," Olga said apologetically. "We already decided you're staying with Gavilán . . . you can watch *him* sleep. I'm just exhausted."

Gavilán moved the car to the parking stall in front of one of the rooms. Everyone got out and grabbed a bag, and they made their way from the car to the building with a long row of identical doors . . . identical except for the room numbers mounted on the doors.

They opened the door to the first room, and they were overtaken by all the mirrors on the walls and ceiling, along with the black box that accepted quarters, mounted on a post at the head of the bed—to make the bed vibrate, of course.

Seeing all the mirrors, Cinz asked innocently, "Is this a meeting room for members of the security cabinet of your country?"

"I don't know. It might be," replied Gavilán with the mischievous grin on his face.

Olga pulled out her cell phone and started looking through her address book. "Where's Sam? He's got some explaining to do . . ." Gavilán shrugged his shoulders slightly, turned slowly, and started to tiptoe away. Olga continued, "And we have the privilege of paying for these accommodations so we can put toilet paper on the toilet seats?"

───

Sam and Dr. Welch went over to talk with Olga. They convinced her that since they would only be there a few hours, their best course of action would be to just get some sleep and move on in the morning. However, the presence of one of Nivla's drones raised questions.

"Well, it's kind of a long story, but the thumbnail sketch is that we ran into Agent Stevenson, and he wanted to take us in for questioning," began Gavilán.

Olga continued, "And we didn't cooperate, so some other agents chased us on the Foothill Expressway. We had to take a certain exit, so we had to cut in front of an eighteen-wheeler, but the exit was blocked . . ." Olga had been accelerating her description, and the pitch of her voice had been rising until this point. She continued in at a slower pace and lower pitch, "And that's when Cinz saved our lives."

They explained in more detail what had happened, and when they had finished, Sam had a question. "So what happened to the agents? Did they try to cut in front of the eighteen-wheeler?"

Both Olga and Gavilán were quiet for about thirty seconds. Then Gavilán took a deep breath and said, "I hope they enjoyed the scenic beauty of the foothills."

Then, out of nowhere, Olga exclaimed, "Wow, Gavilán! You made Steve McQueen's *Bullitt* chase scene look like a bumper car ride at Kiddie Park." Redirecting her conversation to the other members of the party and gesturing at Gavilán, she continued, "I never imagined that he could drive like that!"

The mere mention of the chase caused Gavilán's adrenaline level to rise. He remembered the strange feeling of the blood coursing through his arteries at the end of the chase. It was an uncomfortable déjà vu. In an effort to lighten the mood and not display his discomfort, he followed suit, stating in a very matter-of-fact manner, "Me either, but, well, you see, I've heard a lot of stories about how Americans like to play cowboys and Indians . . . and since I'm not a cowboy . . . well, I just didn't want to have any part of it, thank you."

Olga exhaled a big sigh, followed with a deep breath and a brief whistled chorus of "Do you know the way to San José?"

Gavilán smiled, responding to her unspoken words with, "Actually, I only felt better after I was overcome by the smell of garlic in the air when we passed Gilroy."

It was getting late, but Sam and Dr. Welch still had many questions. At Dr. Welch's request, Olga elaborated on the events that led to their current relationship with the aliens. "Nivla needed to make contact with someone to help him recover the remains of his older brother who died in the 1947 crash near Roswell and is now *still* under observation. Well, he chose me to be his contact, and we thought that his brother's remains were probably in Area 51, Hangar 18. Area 51 is ultrahigh security, and nothing has ever been divulged about an alien spacecraft crash."

Gavilán added sarcastically, "That's because the citizens of the United States don't understand the significance of this event. It would create panic across the nation. Therefore, we need to keep the public calm. We need to hide this from the public—it's for their own good."

Dr. Welch responded, "Son, you're preaching to the choir."

Olga continued, "All documents associated with the 1947 event were classified and, as such, were subject to restricted distribution on the basis of national security. As with any classified document of historical significance, the period that the documents remain classified is twenty-five years. At the end of that period, the Secretary of Defense or any of the heads of the branches of the military has the right to extend the period that the document remains classified. It is now nearly seventy years after the event, and most of the documents related to the event remain classified. Recent interest in the event has caused the formal government position to resurface—it was probably a weather balloon."

Gavilán reacted in an agitated, angry outburst in his native Spanish, "Necesitan ocultarlo porque nos piensan una bola de pendejos, no porque nos quieren proteger." Everyone looked at him with puzzlement and concern.

Olga moved near him, placed her hands on his shoulders affectionately, and proceeded to translate, "They need to hide it because they think we're a bunch of idiots, not because they want to protect us."

Sam then put in his two cents' worth, "No, man . . . it's all about control. Pretend you're the government. You can't tell the public the truth because you're afraid to lose control."

Just then, Cinz interrupted the discussion, "I have received a message from Nivla, and I must leave you now, but I am sure we will be seeing each other soon." He raised his hood and let himself out the door.

Dr. Welch stood from the corner of the bed where he had been sitting and said, "I think we'd better be going as well. We have a long drive ahead of us tomorrow."

ꙮꙮꙮꙮꙮꙮꙮꙮꙮꙮꙮꙮꙮꙮꙮꙮꙮꙮꙮꙮꙮꙮꙮꙮꙮꙮꙮꙮ

Nivla had heard and seen what Olga had to offer. It was time to act—to retrieve the bodies of his brother and other members of the ill-fated crew and return them to Treretum so that their spirits could finally rest. "Tomorrow night, we will enter Hangar 18 in Area 51 to retrieve the remains of Nomis and the others," Nivla announced to his two drones.

In a concerned voice, Reppoc interjected, "But, Nivla, you heard what the Earthlings said—it is unlikely that we will find anything at Hangar 18, and that is why they want to do reconnaissance at Kirtland Air Force Base, a more likely place for hiding the remains of the spacecraft and its personnel."

Nivla explained, "A figure embedded in the placard displayed by one of the doors at Hangar 18 symbolizes three suns—the three suns of our star system. It is a symbol that is not of this Earth, but rather was taken from the control station within the crashed Treretumian spacecraft." There was silence among the aliens. Knowing there was still a question unasked, Nivla added, "I did not want our Earthling friends to get in the way or to get hurt."

The risk was great. There were few wrinkles in the fabric in the vicinity of Hangar 18, but with the aid of Cinz and Reppoc, Nivla was confident he would be successful in restoring the balance of harmony in his family and those of the other crewmembers.

The threesome had experience identifying and sequestering Muimdac transforms from locations on Treretum where they did not belong and only caused disruption. This would not be all that different.

ꙮꙮꙮꙮꙮꙮꙮꙮꙮꙮꙮꙮꙮꙮꙮꙮꙮꙮꙮꙮꙮꙮꙮꙮꙮꙮꙮꙮ

It was nearly two in the morning, and Nivla began briefing his drones on the details of the mission they would be executing shortly before the break of dawn. "Hangar 18 is where Nomis and the others are likely located. It is a highly restricted portion of Area 51, a military complex. Armed military personnel guard the hangar and grounds that surround it, both at the gate of the concertina-wire-topped twelve-foot fence and at the various doors to the hangar. The guards make their rounds routinely, checking on the security of the building perimeter as well as making a sweep of the different areas within the hangar."

Cinz and Reppoc listened attentively and watched Nivla's every gesture.

"We want to avoid contact with the Earthlings, if possible, and take advantage of the anomalies in the space continuum to remove the bodies undetected."

"But that area appears to remain fairly stable," interjected Reppoc.

Cinz immediately continued with the same concern. "Once we are there, will we be relying on an additional instability to roll into the area, as do the high and low pressure areas in the Earth's atmosphere?"

"I'm afraid so," replied Nivla, "unless we can find Nomis and the others and return to the instability portal before it shifts or closes. And remember they are armed. No harm must come to any of the Earthlings."

Cinz and Reppoc turned toward each other exchanging looks of concern.

Just then, Nivla received a communication from Suturb back on the mother ship. He raised his hand to his left ear to activate an earpiece. After listening for a moment, he responded, "Good. Be prepared to get underway as quickly as possible. We will return to the ship to begin the race home . . ." Nivla paused as he turned to look at Cinz and Reppoc, "soon."

Cinz and Reppoc again looked at each other without saying a word.

The moonless night was dark, and the only sound to be heard was that of the chirping crickets. Suddenly, the silence was broken by buzz from the headpieces of communications gear being worn by the armed soldiers standing at the barbed-wire fence. "Johnson and Gonzalez, hit the road. It's your turn to do the rounds," grunted the gruff-looking master sergeant at the main hangar doors.

"Okay, Sarge," and "Yeah, Sarge," responded the two airmen as they started walking to the left side of one of the two huge hangar doors. As they passed a much smaller third door, one airman opened the door and stepped over the threshold into the hangar, while the other continued to do his inspection of the building perimeter.

Inside the hangar, the airman walked the length of the large open space capable of accommodating several large aircraft. He opened a door and entered an area that was finished out as office space. He checked for locked doors to individual offices and quickly opened and closed unlocked doors, scanning with the light from his flashlight for anything that appeared unusual or out of place. He continued down the hallway to a set of double doors with a sign over the doors that read "Forensic Lab."

The impatient airman swung open one of the doors, walked through the portal, and again began checking for locked doors, opening and scanning unlocked lab bays. He proceeded down the hall to an area with a large glass window on the left. Beyond the access door to the lab, the window stretched on for thirty feet, similar to a baby receiving/observation room. But this was not a place where friends and relatives view and make faces at new arrivals. This observation room was a little different. There was an additional long, glass window on the far side of the room. Within the inner room were three tables, on top of which were three long boxes. The Airman passed the door and began to probe with his flashlight beam.

After about a minute, he backed up and jiggled the doorknob, but the lock was secure. He stepped forward and again began to shine his flashlight through the window, lifting his flashlight above his head to inspect the area closest to the window. Next he reached over and flipped a switch between the door and the window, and the lights in the inner room came on. The three boxes were now clearly visible. He glanced through the window, saw nothing, and switched off the light. The airman proceeded down the hallway, and as he walked away, three shadowy figures rose in front of the boxes from behind the inside window. A dim light began to glow within the inner room that, from outside the window, made the backs of the figures appear as silhouettes—one large, one medium, and one small.

From the front, the dim light could be seen to be emanating from the skin that surrounded the eyes of Nivla, Cinz, and Reppoc. The light revealed that the boxes had translucent lids and were attached to a manifold of valves sticking out of piping on the wall by hoses with flexible, braided stainless steel outer sheaths. Within the boxes could be seen the desiccated remains of three creatures.

"Are those our honored dead?" asked Reppoc. There was silence as the three Treretumians gazed into the boxes. The nude remains were almost unrecognizable. It was apparent they had been dissected like laboratory animals. The chest cavities of all three had been cut open, and the skin had been pealed back and pinned to the walls of the boxes. Different internal organs had been removed from the three specimens. An eye from each had also been removed.

"This is my brother Nomis," Nivla mumbled slowly. The others turned toward him as he continued, "I recognize the scar on his arm from a wound that the trainers inflicted during his manhood training."

Cinz recognized that Nivla was emotionally shaken. "Nivla, we must collect the remains and get out of here quickly," he urged as he gave a tug at Nivla's arm. Cinz and Reppoc went into action, moving to the sides of the boxes, and tried to lift the lids with no success.

Nivla regained his composure as though he were coming out of a trance. "The boxes are under a vacuum. Quickly, close the valves at the end of the hoses. There must be additional valves to break the vacuum."

All three Treretumians scrambled to the valve manifold, and almost instantly, the hissing sound of air rushing through several different valves and entering the boxes could be heard. Cinz again tried to lift the lid on the middle box, but this time it opened easily, with the lid rotating ninety degrees on the hinged edge. Within seconds, the other two boxes were opened, and the three Treretumians began hastily folding the skins of their brethren to close the open cavities and prepare the desiccated remains for their trip home.

As the airman continued his rounds inside the hangar, a voice from his communicator rang out, "Gonzalez, motion detectors picked up something in the forensic lab area. Check it out on the double. Backup is on the way." With his weapon grasped firmly with both hands in front of him, the airman turned and began to run back to the forensic lab.

Back in the lab, the three Treretumians were nearing completion of their tasks, inserting the remains in body bags of sorts, which they had brought with them. Suddenly, Nivla raised his head and looked around. He sensed that something was wrong and that they should expect company very soon. He instinctively immediately began to look for the wrinkle in the fabric as he whispered, "Hurry, we must go."

Airman Gonzalez arrived at the outer window and saw movement in the dark lab. He flipped the switch from the hallway, and the entire lab area lit up. There was an immediate locking of eyes between Gonzalez and Nivla's illuminated eyes, while Cinz and Reppoc picked up two of the body bags. The airman was stunned by what he saw, but the noise from the approaching backup personnel made him snap out of it. Gonzalez knew he needed to apprehend the intruders. He fumbled for the key to open the door to the outer lab. He rushed to the window of the inner lab and got a clear view of what was happening, but there was no way out for them, and he knew he had them. As he turned the key to open the door to the inner lab, he heard mumbling from within the inner lab.

Nivla picked up the third body bag as he said directed Cinz and Reppoc, "This way."

Gonzalez opened the door with his weapon pointing ahead of him. Half a dozen additional armed personnel rushed into the outer lab, making a beeline to Gonzalez, standing at the door to the inner lab. Questions came flying: "What happened?"; "Where are the intruders?"; "How many were they?"; and "Where did they go?"

Gonzalez lowered his weapon and muttered, "No one is going to believe what I just witnessed."

CADMIUM POISONING

FACTS

- It is a well-known fact that many of the symptoms and problems associated with Type 2 diabetes disappear upon weight loss. Numerous factors contribute to the return to health. To realize the weight loss, the patient usually changes his/her diet, reducing or eliminating carbohydrates (such as pastas and breads) and fat, reducing overall caloric intake, and increasing exercises. Reducing carbs and calories reduces cadmium intake.

- Zinc does not require sleep. Its function is to protect us. However, its presence or deficiency may not always be obvious, since it, like other heavy metals (e.g., cadmium and lead), primarily resides in the bloodstream during transport to locations where it is needed and is removed from the blood for utilization in bone, muscle, and other tissues.

- The aging process is only marginally related to time. It is more the process of being poisoned . . . to the extent that our vital organs cannot function properly. The Bible cites individuals who lived extremely long lives (e.g., Noah, Lamech, and Methuselah), but their world was far less contaminated than ours.

- Migraine headaches, as you might suspect, are likely related to cadmium poisoning and zinc deficiency, as described in "How to Get Rid of Headaches with Your Diet" (http://www.cybernation.com/livingston/healthstories/meltdown2/headache.html). Different heavy metals are credited for causing headaches in areas of the head. For several (not all) of the types of headaches discussed, zinc deficiency is indicated, and as we know, that is related to cadmium poisoning the majority of the time.

- In addition, the beverages you drink can have a big impact on your headaches: coffee (bad) and water (good). Are you drinking coffee? The caffeine and cadmium contained would be the primary concern, although 20 additional carcinogens (in addition the cadmium) have been identified to be present in trace amounts. And as for water, are you drinking enough cadmium-free (i.e., filtered) water? Insufficient water intake can also lead to headaches.

- Zinc is intimately involved with the storage in the pancreas and regulation of insulin in the bloodstream. Insulin is produced slowly and stored in the beta cells of the islets of Langerhans of the pancreas in groups of six molecules with a zinc ion at the center of each group. These six-packs of insulin molecules remain in the beta cells until an increase in the blood glucose concentration is sensed, at which time the insulin bundles are broken apart, and internal conditions within the beta cells change, casing the infusion of the insulin and the zinc into the bloodstream.

- The use of mercury/silver amalgam in dentistry is bad enough, but it can be even worse if the amalgam comes in contact with a gold crown. The touching of dissimilar metals in the presence of a conductive fluid (i.e., saliva) creates a corrosion cell in which the less noble of the two metals (i.e., the amalgam) slowly dissolves, releasing mercury into the digestive track.

- Selenium is an essential heavy metal for a healthy prostate and is found in high concentrations in foods like garlic. It is directly beneath sulfur in the periodic table, and its chemical symbol is Se. Selenium is involved in enzymatic reactions, like the conversion of glutathione from its oxidized state to its reduced state. It is found in locoweed, and overdosing can lead to other problems. It, like zinc, copper, and other metals, is vital for maintaining health, but only when the dosage is in the proper range. You want to get enough, but too much is toxic.

- With the customary accumulation of cadmium and corresponding depletion of zinc that accompany aging, our immune systems become compromised. We become more susceptible to bacterial infection and less capable of warding off viral attacks. This, together with the direct assault of cadmium and other heavy metals, results in damaged vital internal organs and can eventually lead to cancer and death.

- The number one cause of thyroid problems is cadmium. (The website ithyroid.com has a wealth of information about thyroid issues.) However, iodine deficiency comes in a close second. Both cadmium accumulation and iodine deficiency can induce hypothyroidism (aka Hashimoto's syndrome), slow down the metabolism, and cause weight gain. As with cadmium poisoning, iodine deficiency goes virtually undetected, yet a high percentage of the population (probably over 90%) is currently being adversely impacted. Dr. David Brownstein's website describes an incident where iodine treatments averted surgery for a patient whose primary physician had misdiagnosed a malady. The treatment prescribed by the primary physician was addressing a symptom rather than the underlying cause of the problem.

- Iodine is in the same chemical family as bromine, fluorine, and chlorine, and therefore, it competes with them for reaction sites. Approximately 92% of ingested iodine goes to the thyroid gland, indicating a high selectivity for iodine by the tissues of the thyroid. That is why a common treatment for hyperthyroidism is the administration of an iodine cocktail, containing radioactive iodine-131 with a half-life of just over five days. The doctor's role is to calculate the correct dosage so that the radiation emitted upon disintegration of the iodine atoms kills the right number of cells to achieve the desired result.

- However, as with cadmium and zinc, even though the selectivity for one element is high, introducing overwhelmingly large numbers of atoms of one or more competing elements having similar chemical characteristics can displace it. That is what is happening with iodine. The iodine deficiency problem was recognized decades ago, and that is why iodized salt (sodium chloride spiked with sodium iodide) was promoted. However, the rules of the game have changed. Today, the importance of a low-sodium diet is stressed for controlling high blood pressure, reducing iodine (as iodide) intake for many. Concurrently, more municipal water supplies are adding fluoridation to the chlorination of drinking water, which is standard practice. Increased use of bromides in baked goods, for example, also adds to the antagonistic elements that, when present in high numbers, displace iodine.

Chapter Twenty

The Insurrection

The mission to planet Earth was still in its early stages, but it was already a success in the eyes of many. The Kcalb Clansmen on the Regnellach were a tight-knit group, helping and, whenever possible, protecting each other from what all Kcalb crew members viewed as the capricious mandates of a paranoid and biased mission commander and his elitist Drutsab officers. The consensus was—stemming from his threats of disciplinary actions against all Kcalb Clansmen upon return to Treretum—that Egral Egroeg's punishment pronouncements were generally unfair and biased. It was this comradery among Kcalb Clan crew members that had permitted Nivla and his drones to return to the planet's surface repeatedly, leading to the success of Nivla's personal mission.

With the recovery of the crash victims' bodies behind them, Nivla, Cinz, and Reppoc returned to the spacecraft to make their presence felt among the Regnellach's officers—to keep from being missed. For Nivla it would be a short visit. He assigned his two drones to assist Sucram Suturb with another unsavory but necessary task while he returned to the planet's surface for final discussions with the Earthlings. The drones were instructed that if all went as planned, upon his return to the spacecraft, they would return to the surface before the Regnellach's departure for Treretum, separating Nivla and his drones for many years to come. During his final discussions with Olga and her associates, among other things, he would thank them all for their assistance in mapping out a strategy for combating the Muimdac on Treretum.

For Nivla, the war against the Muimdac was very personal. The loss of his Oleub had led him to become involved with an underground group on Treretum that was helping define the nature and extent of the Muimdac contamination on their planet. They had already identified the means by which the Muimdac were clandestinely spreading their kind across the planet, and a substantial body of evidence pointed at collaboration by the Drutsab Egral with the Muimdac at the expense of the Kcalb Clan. It was in a meeting of this underground group that Nivla first met Suturb. The two were of like mind and spirit.

Reconnaissance into the planning of the current mission to Earth had revealed that Muimdac transforms would be included as crew members. One of those Muimdac transforms was reportedly to be responsible for making all important decisions, and the mission commander, a Drutsab collaborator, would serve primarily as a figurehead. Yenech, the second in command, was thought to be the Muimdac transform who was in charge of the mission for the Muimdac.

In his final conversation with Cinz and Reppoc before returning to the Earth's surface, Nivla left strict instructions that under no circumstances was Yenech to be cut or his skin injured in any manner that would cause bleeding. He also reminded them that their involvement was a critical part of gaining control of one of their planet's most sophisticated aircraft—something that was essential for their planet's survival.

॒॒॒॒॒॒॒॒॒॒॒॒॒॒॒॒॒॒॒॒॒॒॒॒॒॒॒॒॒॒॒॒

It was nearly time for Suturb's weekly report to Egroeg. But this was to be an early-morning briefing and different from other briefings in many ways. Cinz and Reppoc accompanied Suturb as the trio walked down the dimly lit, curved hallway with what was clear to be great deliberation. The curvature of the hallways was more pronounced in the upper decks where Egroeg's and his officers' quarters were located because of the diminished diameter of the aircraft. Fortunately for Reppoc, he had the inside track so that his short legs didn't have to cover as much ground.

They arrived at Egroeg's suite. Cinz and Reppoc took their posts on either side of the door. Suturb looked to his left and then to his right, making eye contact with the two drones that stood with their backs to the wall, looking in his direction. Suturb raised his left hand to look at his Earth chronometer. The white digital display stood out against the black screen. It read, "03:15 MAR 15."

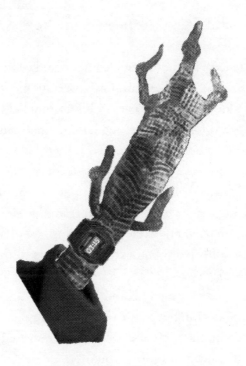

"It is time," mumbled Suturb. He raised his head, looked at the door, took a deep breath, and extended his right arm. A large hand with long, bony fingers and bulging knuckles emerged from the loose sleeve of his robelike uniform. He slowly clinched his fist into a massive sledge. Suturb looked capable of knocking down any door with a single blow of the heel of his fist, but as though he had changed his mind, he slowly rotated his fist and knocked. It was a slow and deliberate knock. Three solid impacts and then a long pause. Reppoc turned toward Suturb, but Suturb extended his arm with the palm of his massive hand toward Reppoc's face. They paused for a moment, and then Suturb knocked again, a bit harder this time.

"Who dares to disturb me at this hour?" could be heard coming from within the chamber.

Again, Suturb looked to his left and then to his right, making eye contact with his two companions. "It is Sucram Suturb. I came to report some important findings about the Earthlings."

"Can this not wait until morning?" asked the muffled voice.

Suturb responded, "Sir, these findings have to do with something that could jeopardize the mission."

His tone softened a bit, but the reluctance could be heard in Egroeg's voice as he said, "Very well, Sucram. Give me a moment."

Suturb again looked into the eyes of his accomplices. "Wait for me here, but be prepared for the worst," he said in a nervous voice.

The two drones stood as sentinels with their backs to the wall on either side of the doorway. Cinz remained steadfast, standing tall with his feet spread slightly—solid as a rock. Reppoc, on the other hand, was fidgety, shifting his weight back and forth from one side to the other.

"Sucram, you may enter," came from within the officer's chamber.

Suturb touched his palm and extended fingers to the sensor panel on the door, and in an instant, the door seemed to evaporate. Suturb entered, and the door reformed behind him.

The lighting was dim, but Suturb could easily make out the shapes and locations of the numerous cubes that were arranged differently from the last time he had been in Egroeg's quarters.

Egroeg was dressed in a white, loose-fitting, toga-style robe; he walked slowly from the back of the room toward his favorite chair, the canary-yellow chaise longue. "Sit," he said as he arrived at the chaise longue, pointing at the one of the stacks of cubes in front of him. The cubes were covered with a multicolored cloth that extended from the top cube to the floor. It was draped over the cubes in a way that it resembled a volcano. At the top, it was mostly red, the red of a molten spray from an exploding volcano, against a black backdrop. The cloth covered the seat portion of the stacked cubes, making it appear like a throne of lava, overflowing down to the floor. Suturb walked over to the cube chair, tugged at the cloth gently, and slowly lowered himself into the chair.

Suturb sat erect, squinting due to the poor lighting but looking around him at the many reminders of Treretum. Egroeg slowly wandered around the chaise longue to the backside of the cube chair where Suturb sat. He placed his hands on the top cube that served as the back of the chair and asked sleepily, "Now, what was so urgent that it could not wait? And jeopardize the mission? How could any Earthling jeopardize our mission?"

"Sir," Suturb responded as he stood quickly, turning to face Egroeg, "they are aware of our presence."

"Absurd! Why, that's impossible!" exclaimed Egroeg in total disbelief as he began to retrace his path to the backside of the chaise longue. Turning abruptly to directly face Suturb, he continued emphatically, "Sucram, they don't have the intelligence, much less the technology, to detect our presence."

"Sir, it was one of the landing parties," responded Suturb briskly. "They chose to let themselves be seen."

"What? Who led the party? Who is responsible?" demanded Egroeg in anger.

"Nivla, I am ashamed to say . . . my fellow Kcalb Clansman," Suturb responded as he moved to the side of the chaise longue, knelt, and bowed his head. "Please, sir, do not judge all Kcalbs for the actions of a few."

"I knew it. I knew that he would betray our mission for the sake of finding the remains of his brother. I felt it from the moment you told me of his participation in the expedition." He stepped over to where Suturb knelt, placed his hand on his shoulder, and said, "Sucram, thank you for recognizing you duty and coming to me."

Suturb raised his head and rose gracefully to his feet, towering before Egroeg. "That is why I am here. I knew that you would want to be informed as soon as possible, regardless of the hour."

"Praise Avohaj that there are still loyal Treretumians like you that value the good of the many over the self-interests of a few." Egroeg turned, saying as he slowly walked away from Suturb, "I know that it must hurt you to turn in a member of your own clan." Turning his head toward Suturb, he continued, "But your loyalty will not go unrewarded. As for Nivla . . . there are grave consequences for his actions, and he will be dealt with accordingly."

The choreographed scene of cat and mouse continued. "Thank you, sir," responded Suturb as he slowly turned to walk the opposite side of the chaise longue. The two Treretumians with strikingly different physical features met at the end of the chaise longue, standing before each other, face-to-face.

"I had mentioned to you that I felt surrounded by tyranny," Egroeg said. "And I am sure that Nivla did not act alone. That is all the more reason I praise Avohaj that you are by my side." He turned slowly, giving his back to Suturb, and continued. "All I have to do is close my eyes, and I see them. All around me they stand as I walk down the corridor. Reaching out to snatch a little piece of my life, glancing blows when their extended arms can reach me."

Egroeg continued describing his paranoid delusion as Suturb's hand emerged from the sleeve of his uniform as it had in the corridor, but this time, it held an ornately decorated ceremonial dagger. The blade curved back and forth in a serpentine fashion, and two outwardly pointing spikes protruded from the ends of the handle. He lunged toward Egroeg and sank the long blade into his back with a single, forceful thrust. Silently, Egroeg arched his spine, throwing his head and narrow shoulders back. He slowly turned his head toward Suturb, uttered in a pained and surprised voice, "And you, Suturb?" With the same forceful deliberation as before, Suturb extracted the blade from his victim. The light began to dim in Egroeg's eyes. A pea-green stain appeared on the robe where the dagger had been.

Egroeg slowly raised his right hand as his knees began to buckle. The sleeve of his robe slid back to his elbow, exposing the object he held. Suturb recognized the object. A combination of fear and desperation appeared on his face as he lurched for the object, but not before Egroeg set off the alarm that he clinched in his fist.

In an attempt to snatch the alarm, Suturb grazed the back of Egroeg's hand, sending the object flying forward. Suturb knew that now, any attempt to silence the alarm would be futile. He stopped, stood erect with his bloodstained dagger at his side, still in a clinched fist, and watched Egroeg's body go limp and fall forward.

The noise of the alarm was deafening, but the pounding on the door could be heard above the alarm. The door to the suite slid open, and Cinz and Reppoc rushed in, only to grab Suturb by the arms, pulling him out of Egroeg's suite and into the corridor. In an instant, a dozen or more of Egroeg's officers emerged from their quarters and ran down the corridor toward Egroeg's suite with their modern weapons in hand. As the disheveled, out-of-uniform officers converged upon Suturb and company, Cinz raised his left wrist to his mouth and calmly uttered a single word: "Now."

Out of thin air it seemed, swarms of Kcalb warriors and their drones appeared, dressed in ornate ceremonial robes and equipped with curved-blade ceremonial daggers similar to that of Suturb. Their actions were swift and effective. A few rays were fired, but within seconds, the brief struggle was over. All of the officers that had come to rescue, instead had fallen victim. They fell to the floor almost in unison, and the corresponding daggers in the hands of Kcalb warriors dripped with the pea-green blood of the dead.

Suturb raised his wrist to his mouth and said solemnly, in a low voice, "Nivla, it is done." He lowered his hand to make an adjustment on his communicator. The warriors began to pick up remains of the dead for transport to the expulsion chamber. He again raised his wrist to his mouth. "Treretumians, this is Suturb. Look at those around you. I did not have an opportunity to speak with all of you, but there are enough among you with all the information about what just happened. You all have a decision to make. Egroeg and the officers of this vessel are dead, and each of you must now decide where your loyalty lies—with our mother planet, Treretum, or with those responsible for the treachery and tyranny that has befallen us."

As he was finishing the sentence, one of the Kcalb Clansmen rushed up to Suturb, caught his breath, placed his hand on Suturb's shoulder, and said, "Yenech."

"What?" asked Suturb in a somewhat startled voice. "What about Yenech?"

"He was not among them." The second in command of the mission was still alive somewhere within the spacecraft.

Rumors had run rampant for years that Yenech, a member of the Drutsab Egral Security Cabinet, was not of their world. His behavior had always been "unusual," and it was not uncommon for those around him to have "accidents."

"Find him! And quickly!" Suturb exclaimed. "The head of the serpent remains." All knew that the real officer in control was not Egroeg but instead Yenech. His capture was vital to minimize the possibility of conflict within the rest of the crew.

Everyone in the corridor scurried, and soon the corridor was deserted except for Suturb, who stood silently, looking down at his dagger . . . reflecting on what he had just done.

ꗠꗠꗠꗠꗠꗠꗠꗠꗠꗠꗠꗠꗠꗠꗠꗠꗠꗠꗠꗠꗠꗠꗠꗠꗠꗠꗠꗠꗠꗠꗠꗠ

In the control center, several Treretumians of various clans monitored the ship's instrumentation and control panels. Each had distinct distinguishing features that identified the clan of origin. Suturb stood among them, directing the various search teams that were combing the vessel for Yenech. A large segmented screen with the layout of each of the levels of the spacecraft was displayed. On the screen, small moving dots that represented the search teams could be seen moving on all levels.

Suturb muttered to himself, "The focus of the search has to be the potential escape routes from the spacecraft."

Yttocs, the chief controller on duty, standing next to Suturb, heard the comment and asked, "What is the urgency with capturing Yenech?"

"We have reason to believe that Yenech and possibly several others on this vessel are Muimdac transforms. His interests are very different from those of Treretumians. And now that he has been discovered, he and his henchmen will try to escape." Suturb paused and then continued slowly, "Or he may do something to infect the rest of the crew to regain control."

Suturb adjusted the communicator on his wrist so that only the heads of the search parties would receive the message. He raised it to his mouth and directed, "Inspect all escape pods and launch chambers. If you encounter any suspected Muimdac, *do not* cut or wound them. And above all, avoid contact with their blood."

The search parties put their methodical sweeps of all levels on hold and headed directly to all the launch chambers. The door to the launch chamber on level 7 failed to open properly, and a request for a security override was sent to the control center. Neves, the head of the search party, received a message from Suturb that the override was in place but that he must proceed with great caution.

Neves touched his palm and extended fingers to the sensor panel on the door, and the door evaporated, exposing five individuals boarding an escape pod. Yenech was among them. All five were noticeably startled and turned their heads toward the doorway in unison.

"Stop! You are detained and relieved of your duties. You must come with us for interrogation," shouted Neves from the doorway.

Yenech said calmly, "Dlefsmur, you must go." One of the larger individuals, standing at the back of the escape pod, turned and began to walk toward the search party. He gazed upward as he raised a clinched fist to his chest. He then raised his hands to the sides of his head as he walked. His face changed radically to that of someone in anguish, as though he were in great pain from a terrible sound he was trying to escape by covering his ears.

Neves and his party instinctively moved back, and Neves slowly reached for the door closure panel. Dlefsmur leaned forward, bending at the waist, and suddenly, his head came off in his hands. A blinding light and an atomized spray came pouring from the neck to which Dlefsmur's head had been attached. With lightning-fast reflexes, Neves pressed the closure panel, and the door appeared instantly.

Neves, acting instinctively, shouted, "Everyone remain calm and stay where you are!" He pressed a corner of the closure panel, and a translucent observation portal about the size of his head appeared at eye level in the door. He looked inside and observed Dlefsmur's body continuing to go forward until it bumped up against the door. He raised his communicator to his mouth and exclaimed frantically, "Suturb, seal off this quadrant on the seventh level and open the exit hatch to the launch chamber." Suddenly, Dlefsmur's hand slammed up against the closure panel, clutching for something to grab onto. Neves's tone became still more frantic as he yelled, "Quickly! *Now!*"

In the control center, Suturb simply looked at Yttocs and nodded. Yttocs turned to the override panel and made several keystrokes on a keyboard filled with cryptic markings. He then leaned to his left and pressed the seventh of ten bright orange-colored buttons.

Several members of Neves's party looked up and around when they first heard the hiss indicating that a separate life support system was taking over on the sealed-off portion of the seventh level. Neves continued to watch through the observation portal as the hatch "evaporated," and everyone and everything that was not secured was sucked into the vacuum of space. In the ejected debris, five small detonations could be discerned, with a spray of a million tiny luminescent fragments emanating from each. Neves raised his communicator and uttered a single word: "Flush." Through the portal, what appeared to be a purple fluid was discharged from nozzles that sprayed all surfaces within the launch chamber. The fluid was also sucked into the void of space, and a few seconds later, the hatch reappeared in the exit portal. This was the first step in the decontamination process.

Suturb's concerned, almost-frantic voice could be heard over Neves's communicator. "Neves, is everything under control?"

Neves responded, "Yes, but it is as you suspected . . . Muimdac. We are initiating full decontamination of the entire quadrant with a double-decon of the launch chamber."

രു

Suturb stood next to Yttocs in the control center, relieved that the events on the seventh deck would not jeopardized the safety of the rest of the crew or their spacecraft.

Yttocs commented, "We are fortunate that the Muimdac were detected in a launch chamber. It made their containment and expulsion relatively easy thanks to Neves and his team. Now we can take a deep breath and relax while we wait for Nivla."

"Not so fast!" exclaimed Suturb. "You have to prepare for a high-speed return to Treretum. It will be taxing on our engines, and you have to be prepared for the unexpected." Suturb paused and appeared pensive, thinking about how he also should be prepared for the unexpected. "Yttocs, can you detect if there has been any activity in any of the other launch chambers?"

"Of course, Suturb, but with all the searches that were just conducted, all will show activity," replied Yttocs.

"All right, Yttocs. Let's put our heads together. How can we know with certainty that Muimdac transforms were not trying to escape using multiple launch chambers? When the Muimdac were detected on deck seven, others may have been alerted and abandoned their escape attempts."

Yttocs responded with stunned surprise, "Suturb, you're right."

"As the Earthlings say," declared Suturb, "We're not out of the woods yet."

CADMIUM POISONING

FACTS

- Cadmium is silent and goes unnoticed until it has reached a critical concentration in vital organs. Then, unless something drastically different from the status quo is done, additional ingestion will lead to disease (e.g., diabetes, kidney failure, cancer) and death. Changes such as adjustments to the diet to minimize cadmium intake to an absolute minimum and supplementation of zinc and other minerals and vitamins will be essential for survival and recovery from cadmium poisoning.

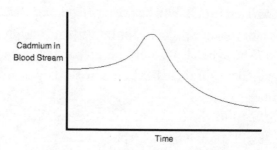

- Flush, flush, flush! Mobilization of cadmium is not sufficient. Like the Muimdac, cadmium must be expelled from the body to ensure it doesn't cause problems elsewhere. For example, an increase in the blood cadmium concentration can cause lesions of the sciatic nerve. But stay the course; the sciatica will subside as the cadmium is excreted from the body. However, you can do something to alleviate the problem sooner by taking vitamin E (gamma tocopherol), which soothes and lubricates nerves.

- Fruits that grow on trees are among the lowest cadmium-containing foods, and they keep you regular. And feces contain higher cadmium concentrations than urine. Regular bowel movements represent the most effective means of expelling the toxic metal from our bodies. Shoot for a minimum of five pieces of fruit per day.

- In addition to getting the digestive track going, a challenge for most who are suffering from cadmium poisoning is getting the cadmium out of the cells and into the bloodstream for subsequent expulsion from the body. Many diabetics, for example, suffer from impaired circulation. Niacin (vitamin B_3) is a natural vasodilator that aids in increasing the diameters of our capillaries by as much as 100%. This is beneficial in that it improves the efficiency of the circulatory system, not only for removing accumulated toxins (including heavy metals like cadmium), but also for supplying nutrients and minerals to the cells of the extremities, thereby reducing the likelihood of diabetics developing complications that could lead to amputation. Note that one of those minerals in the blood supply is zinc—an element required in the healing process. Impaired circulation means restricted flow of zinc and other materials that are essential for cell maintenance and repair, along with retained toxins. Niacin is needed to flush—on the cellular level.

- Another aspect of flushing cadmium from the body is to maintain a high metabolism rate. Exercise is an absolute must . . . it opens blood vessels, facilitating the transport of oxygen and nutrients to the cells while enhancing removal of toxins. However, a little *intense* exercise goes a long way. Reports of as little as a few minutes of intense exercise (e.g., pushups—as many as you can do in two minutes) a couple of times per week will not only increase your heart rate for those short period of exercise, but it will also increase your metabolism rate for the rest of the week, which burns fat, even when you are not working out.

- An aspirin a day is a good thing to consider, not only because it reportedly reduces heart attacks, but also because it is a vasodilator, and dilation of blood vessels, during exercise or otherwise, reduces the accumulation of plaque (and, therefore, the likelihood of a heart attack) and enhances transport of cadmium so that it can be removed from the body.

- Things are not always as they appear.

  o Myth: As stated previously, dogs shouldn't eat high-protein foods because the kidneys are the first to go, and they start passing protein.

Fact: Accumulation of cadmium in the kidneys causes them to malfunction, with the passing of protein being one of the symptoms of cadmium poisoning.

  o Myth: Kidney disease and a host of other diseases are complications associated with diabetes.

Fact: While there are diseases that result from diabetes, complications that are attributed to diabetes are more often than not symptoms of diseases that are developing concurrently due to cadmium poisoning, the same cause of the Type 2 diabetes. (Zinc is required for the biosynthesis of insulin.)

  o Myth: People should avoid drinking or eating things that are acidic because it causes disorders like acidosis of the blood, and acidic conditions promote cancer.

Fact: Acidosis of the blood is an indication that the kidneys are not clearing sufficient acid from the bloodstream, a malfunction that is most likely due to the accumulation of cadmium. On a small, localized scale, acidic conditions inhibit the accumulation of heavy metals like cadmium, keeping them mobile for subsequent sequestration and expulsion from the body.

  o Myth: The gout is a result of eating foods that are too rich, like pate, made of goose liver.

Fact: It is now known that gout results from high uric acid concentrations in the blood and precipitation of crystals that cause pain, primarily in the joints of the feet and ankles—again because the kidneys are not functioning properly—a symptom of cadmium poisoning. Cherry juice is supposed to suppress crystal formation, but again, drinking cherry juice is treating a symptom, not the underlying cause. And while goose liver or other organ meats may be involved in the problem, it is more likely due to their high cadmium concentration rather than the fat they contain. Eskimos thrive on a diet of whale blubber with none of the symptoms of cadmium poisoning that are commonplace elsewhere; but then, Eskimos don't use phosphate fertilizers or otherwise have a diet that is high in cadmium.

- Cinnamon (canela) and ginger are reportedly beneficial because they help bind heavy metals. Cinnamon is said to prevent diabetes. But caveat emptor (buyer beware), because that cinnamon or ginger you put in your body may already be loaded with cadmium, and beginning on a regimen of, for example, several cups of cinnamon tea each day can be counterproductive, resulting in the release of the cadmium contained in the cinnamon as the organic chelating agent to which the cadmium was originally bound is digested.

Chapter Twenty-One

The Uphill Battles

Olga, Gavilán, Dr. Welch, and Sam arrived in Albuquerque the night before the scheduled balloon flight to Kirtland Air Force Base, and they had coordinated to stay at a motel of Gavilán's choosing. Orville had been contacted during the day on the drive in, and he was expecting a call some time in the late morning after they had checked out of their rooms. As customary, Olga and Gavilán shared a suite. Everyone was famished after the long drive, and they decided to indulge in a late night/early morning meal at a place that advertised as being Albuquerque's only all-night Mexican restaurant. It was an opportunity to unwind. After a relaxing meal, everyone returned to the motel to freshen up because there were still more details to pin down regarding the next day's balloon ride/photo shoot.

Because they anticipated additional discussions with Dr. Welch and Sam, Olga and Gavilán moved the tables from their individual rooms into the commons area and positioned them on either side of the small table in the room, creating what appeared to be a single, long table surface.

Just then Dr. Welch and Sam arrived, and before they had had a chance to sit down, there was another knock at the door. Gavilán peeked through the eyepiece mounted in the middle of the door and then opened the door wide open. "Greetings to our unexpected guests.

Please come in," he said as he bowed, extending his arm into the room as a gesture of welcome.

"Thank you" in semiunison emanated from the three robed Treretumians as they entered room. Nivla, Cinz, and Reppoc entered and removed their hoods as they greeted everyone.

Olga entered the room with a pitcher of water and glasses on a tray. She set the tray on the table and asked everyone to take a seat. She then directed herself at the aliens, "I'm glad you're here. We decided to meet before embarking on another airborne reconnaissance adventure. And—"

Nivla interrupted her, saying, "That won't be necessary." Puzzled looks came over all of the Earthlings' faces. Nivla continued, "The remains of our fallen comrades are already in our possession, retrieved from Hangar 18."

Expressing the sentiments of all, Olga mumbled, "I don't understand," in a confused tone of voice. She went on, "We examined all the footage, and we found nothing. How could you have known?"

"When you showed us the scans of the hangar doors," Nivla said, "I noticed a three-sun symbol embedded in one of the placards mounted next to one of the doors. The inspiration for that placard had to have originated from the crashed Treretumian spacecraft. I said nothing because I did not want to involve any of you in what was a potentially dangerous mission." Nivla motioned at Cinz and Reppoc as he continued, "My capable drones and I were able to successfully complete our mission. We were detected, but don't expect to hear about it in a news broadcast—that would only affirm our existence."

As usual, Cinz and Reppoc just sat quietly.

〰〰〰〰〰〰〰〰〰〰〰〰〰〰〰〰〰〰〰〰〰〰〰〰〰

They sat at a table like an abbreviated intergalactic version of the Last Supper. "Before I leave, I must thank you for your help in recovering the remains of Nomis," declared Nivla. "For this, my brother Rodoet and I shall be forever in your debt. My mission would have been much more difficult had it not been for your assistance.

"But more than that," he continued, "Treretum is in your debt for the revelations that you have provided and the beginning strategy that we will attempt to follow to regain our planet from the Muimdac invaders.

"There is no way that I can ever repay you for your assistance with our ongoing battle with the Muimdac. It is a matter of survival for Treretumians. But in a small way, I will try to express our gratitude by sharing some information with you that we uploaded from a peculiar, five-sided building in your nation's capital. It is of no consequence to Treretum, but it may personally impact you or your children."

Nivla stood up and began to gaze at a white wall almost as though he were going into a trance. The brown covering that everyone had assumed was the surface of his eye began to retract in a fashion similar to that of ancient reptiles, revealing a source of light behind it. Nivla mumbled in a low voice, "This document may be of interest to you," as he raised his head and stared at the wall.

An image of a document marked "Top Secret" appeared on the wall, projected by the light emanating from Nivla's eyes. The document was an executive summary from a report submitted to the President by the Secretary of Defense. The next thing Olga was viewing on the left half of the screen, much to her disbelief, was the agenda on the program passed out at the beginning of the Houston conference. On the right were the names of the attending scientists and engineers who were leaders in their fields related to the various conference topics, along with handwritten notes containing the terms "friend" and "foe—liquidate."

The text went on to describe in great detail the objectives of Operation Houston Control, including the global conditions that were anticipated to set the operation into motion. Following the onset of massive global unrest and starvation, it was anticipated the focus of the masses would eventually turn to American assets around the world. In a series of preemptive strikes, the United States military, supplied by the industrial might of this country's war machine, would launch simultaneous attacks from strategically positioned satellites on most of the capitals of the nations of the planet. The propaganda machine would follow with announcements, using all available means of communication, stating the United States was stepping in to save the people of each of the countries from tyrannical governments.

Immediately thereafter, all orbiting communication satellites would be destroyed, effectively cutting off all contact with the outside world and isolating the population of each country in individual states of turmoil. The goal was to liquidate approximately three-fourths of the population and seize assets, focusing on natural resources that could be exploited by the United States. That would get the planet back to its more manageable, pre–World War II population. Internal instability and civil war were sought because that would reduce the United States' unsavory task of ensuring that at least three-fourths of the population was eliminated.

These actions were viewed as necessary and a favor to the masses. By eliminating three-fourths of the mouths that required feeding, the available food resources would be sufficient for many additional years, and the turmoil and disease that was anticipated would greatly reduce the birthrate. And certainly, if the disease did not appear naturally, the clandestine United States Department of Biological Warfare Research would be able to assist. Furthermore, recovering from the mass death and destruction would keep people around the world busy and preoccupied with worthwhile endeavors such as survival rather than posing a threat to the United States and its assets. These were measures that were necessary to protect the interests of the United States around the world in a time of global crisis.

Olga read the text in horror and disbelief. "This goes against all that I hold sacred, against all that is human, against all that is holy in heaven and on earth."

Gavilán, also stunned, simply uttered, "It makes the Holocaust look like child's play."

Sam was speechless, while Dr. Welch shook his head as he mumbled, "I can't believe this," several times.

To put Dr. Welch's doubt to rest, Nivla added, "By the way, picking up on a previous conversation that we had, it is no coincidence that in addition to the Space Vehicles Directorate, the Directed Energy Directorate of the Air Force is also housed at Kirtland Air Force Base in Albuquerque. This is the home of the Air Force's high-energy 'attack laser,' an aircraft that had a nose job and other alterations to equip it for laser attacks from the air. Equip a few reverse-engineered 'alien aircraft' with the high-energy attack lasers capabilities, and we could say that it was all an alien attack on planet Earth." He then mumbled under his breath, "Thank you, Orson, for setting the accepted standard."

Nivla had shocked his audience, but there was more they had to know, so he continued, "I will share something else with you that, again, will be of little consequence in my lifetime to the Treretum that I know and love, but it may set the stage for a different type of encounter in the millennia ahead. The primary goal of the current mission to your planet was to see what progress had made over the centuries—to assess your readiness for interaction with Treretumians."

Olga responded sarcastically to the new topic by interjecting, "Oh, that's cool. You sought collaborators—other souls on the same journey through time, right?" The lack of sincerity in what she had just said was evident to all.

"It was not exactly like that. We planted seeds on Earth to see you progress, to see you conquer your environment. We planted seeds that would allow you to extend your life expectancy to several centuries. But it is clear that the information was not understood, and your progress has been much slower than expected . . . and that, perhaps, is your salvation. Your environment is out of control, and in fact, segments of your society are responsible for the continued and worsening contamination of the planet's surface at the expense of the masses. The contaminants spread through the food chain and accumulate in your bodies." Nivla paused. It was clear that what he was describing was very difficult for him, and what he was about to divulge was more difficult still.

"You see, the Treretumians are carnivorous, and our appetite for flesh made us cannibals in the ancient times. As we progressed, we took control of our environment, and our life span increased accordingly. This resulted in a major stress on our food supply. On neighboring planets, we established favorable environments that would support healthy, flesh-bearing species, with minimal accumulation of contaminants— feed colonies. But our numbers grew, and our appetites were insatiable."

Nivla paused once again then continued, "When the Muimdac invaded Treretum, shipments from the feed colonies came to a stop. Our cannibalistic side resurfaced and became very active, perceived by many to be out of necessity. Not until the apparent victory over the Muimdac did the shipments from the feed colonies resume. Life on Treretum appeared to return to normal, but our population growth rate seemed to explode, and the popularity of cannibalism increased because the feed colonies could not keep up with the demand for flesh. It was not until many centuries later that an unthinkable discovery was made. It was actually less of a discovery and more of a revelation, an attempt to find a solution that would mean survival for two species."

"Nivla, this lesson on Treretumian history is very interesting, but where is all of this going, and what does it have to with us?" Sam queried impatiently.

"Patience, Sam." Nivla turned toward Olga and Gavilán in a gesture of gratitude for their patience and unwavering support. He continued, "The Muimdac are masters at adapting to new environments, but the apparent victory over the Muimdac was not a victory at all. The Muimdac were insidiously infecting the Treretumian population. They took control of individuals by fighting their battles within the bodies of their enemies. They conquered one organ at a time, one Treretumian at a time. They took control of the individuals responsible for the operation of cleansing stations and the associated replacement filters of toxic metals that every Treretumian is obliged to maintain to forego a premature death by environmental contaminant poisoning.

"Unknowingly, Treretumians were being inoculated with Muimdac that would ultimately overtake the internal organs of their victims. Today, most of the members of the Drutsab Egral are actually Muimdac transforms—that is, Muimdac that have taken the form of the Treretumians whose bodies they invaded. The coup was especially effective because of the demonstration at the Drutsab Egral Security Cabinet where a Muimdac transform was decapitated and had his right arm severed from his body. What was not recognized prior to that demonstration was that the natural response of the Muimdac to a cut in the skin of the transform is to emit spores from the wounds until the skin reforms over the wound.

"The demonstration resulted in the inoculation of every member of the Drutsab Egral Security Cabinet with Muimdac spores and the rapid assent to power of the Muimdac through the influence of the cabinet members. The true Treretumians are deceived by their leaders and are decreasing in numbers. Because the Muimdac are not cannibalistic, they will not consider feeding on Muimdac transforms. They feed the Treretumians to each other and feed on them, as well—consequently, the true Treretumians population continues to dwindle. The food situation is critical." Nivla took his long slender fingers and touched his right cheek. It was as though he was struggling with what he was about to say. Finally, Nivla turned to look directly at Sam and uttered in a low voice, "Sam, our mission to Earth was to assess the suitability of this planet as a feed colony."

Sam, Olga, and Gavilán looked at each other in silence, their eyes opened wide while Dr. Welch pushed back from the table and peered at Nivla and company. In response, Cinz and Reppoc also pushed away from the table, in case they need to take control of the developing situation.

Sam stuttered nervously, "I-I-I really didn't mean to be so impatient, Nivla, a-a-and you have my un-n-n-n-divided at-t-t-tention."

Then Gavilán mumbled slowly in a low tone, "Years ago, my grandfather told me that *the teachers* had come to this planet to teach us and protect us. What he didn't know was that it was protection with strings attached, protection with ulterior motives. Huh, some protection."

Nivla showed concern in his face over Gavilán's comment, but he continued, "At some point in the future, certainly after I am no longer alive, a mission from Treretum will be launched to again assess the situation on Earth. The interaction between our descendants," Nivla explained, "will depend on the paths of history taken by our two planets and the influences that we can have on those paths. Your battles here on Earth will be first—to conquer your environment. But before you can do that, you must conquer greed. The greed of few at the expense of all has been the downfall of your society."

Sam, Olga, Gavilán, and Dr. Welch exchanged glances, at first in disbelief. But the expressions on their faces changed as it became clear to each of them that what Nivla said was true.

He continued, "Your next challenge then will be to keep from destroying each other, and to do this, you will need to regain control and establish a benevolent government that will be able to deal rationally with the challenges of an expanding population. This planet that you occupy is your box. You must think outside the box." Nivla again lowered his voice and slowed his speech. He looked downward as he said, "You have difficult times ahead." He paused. No one said a word, and the silence was deafening.

Nivla raised his head and again spoke with renewed energy, "With the actions of our crew on this mission, the beginning of a change in direction may have been initiated for Treretum. The Egral officers of my spacecraft have been eliminated, and the situation may be considered to be mutiny back on Treretum. At this point in our history, many Treretumians are aware of the continued presence of the Muimdac and their continuing activities through the Drutsab Egral to promote the ever-expanding grip that the Muimdac have on our planet. The growing Muimdac transform population of Treretum needs to find additional sources of food even more desperately than true Treretumians. They realize that the current supplies of flesh, including the true Treretumian population, will eventually be exhausted, and they will need additional sources of flesh to feed an insatiable hunger."

Sam gulped loudly as he swallowed and gasped for air. "Relax, son," whispered Dr. Welch as he reached behind Sam with his right arm. He squeezed Sam's upper arms with his two hands in a fatherly way as he continued his whisper, "Nothing is going to happen in your lifetime or the next." Sam nodded his head.

Nivla again spoke with a trace of hope in his voice, "The fact that the Drutsab sent mostly true Treretumians rather than Muimdac transforms on this mission may be our salvation. Our taking control of the spacecraft from an incompetent Drutsab Egral and his officers may be viewed as a Treretumian squabble and not draw as much attention as it would have, had it been a mutiny against a team of mission officers made up of solely Muimdac transforms." Again Nivla paused. "At this moment, my fate and that of my crew are uncertain. If our spacecraft is not blown out of the Treretumian atmosphere by

Muimdac transform-controlled anti-invasion defense rays at reentry, we may stand a chance of surviving the incident. Our mission is clear. The Muimdac must truly be expelled from Treretum, but the struggle will be a difficult one—as much of an uphill battle for my planet as the one you have before you."

Olga took Gavilán's hand. They looked at each other solemnly. They realized the rest of their lives would be spent trying to save the planet, save humanity, save their sanity, and save their descendants from being the filet mignon on the dinner plate of an alien life-form.

Dr. Welch leaned forward and spoke, almost defiantly, "But how are we going to get anyone to believe anything that we say? No one will ever believe that we had this conversation. If I even mention this to one of my colleagues, my credibility will be destroyed, even if I am a bigwig at the CDC. And what's worse is that we will be dealing with an oppressive government that has concealed the existence of life on another planet—your race—for nearly seventy years. And the public"— he let out a low, sarcastic chuckle—"they think that the government is their great protector." Dr. Welch began to appear agitated.

Then, to everyone's surprise, Sam stood from his seat and declared, without a trace of a stutter, "You can't just up and leave without helping to set things straight."

Nivla calmly raised one finger in front of his nose. "Your answer awaits you in your office. On the top shelf of the bookshelf against the east wall of your office, you will find an *etnafele*, a small spherical container the size of a man's fist, made of one of the hardest materials known and designed to preserve the environment within." Nivla paused and turned slightly to look directly at Sam, saying, "Oh, by the way, Sam . . . cute dog . . . very perceptive."

Sam scratched his head as he responded sluggishly, "Thanks."

Nivla continued, "Do not use a blade or saw to attempt to open the *etnafele*. You will fail. Do not try to open it with a heat-emitting flame of a cutting torch. You will fail."

"What is it made of?" inquired Gavilán and Olga simultaneously.

"It is made of common elements found on your planet, but you do not fully understand their interaction," responded Nivla. "A sample of this material, including the recipe for making it, was left behind on a previous Treretumian visit to your planet. But that seed, as many other seeds left behind, failed to germinate. It is not until now, with the accidental discovery of graphene, that your species is beginning to understand the potential of common materials that have surrounded you since the beginning of your existence."

"How will we open the *etnafele*, and what does it contain?" asked Dr. Welch in a low, calm voice.

Nivla responded, "You will need to construct an electrosonic torch that will simultaneously focus both electromagnetic and high-intensity sound waves of specific frequencies onto an area of a fraction of a square millimeter. The details of its construction and the specific wave frequencies and intensities needed to open the *etnafele* are awaiting Sam in an e-mail from Star Traveler. I apologize, Dr. Welch, but at the time, I was only aware of Sam's involvement, and I did not have your e-mail address." Random glances were exchanged until the silence was broken by what appeared to be a Treretumian chuckle.

All eyes were on Nivla. He continued, "The *etnafele* contains a map of the locations where seeds were planted by previous Treretumian expeditions, along with descriptions and desired outcomes in your development."

Dr. Welch responded, "From what you've described, it sounds as though there will be many things that will help advance our technology."

Almost cutting into the end of Dr. Welch's sentence, Nivla leaned his head back slightly, interjecting, "Beyond your imagination." He paused, but everyone looked at him, expecting him to say more. Nivla continued, "You will have tools to help conquer your environment, and this, in turn, will help you conquer disease stemming from environmental contamination, reversing what appears to be a rising wave of pain and suffering among the populace of your planet. The intent is to share the information with all Earthlings."

In a low, sarcastic tone, Olga's voice was heard. "That may be a challenge if it gets into the hands of our beloved governmental officials . . . you know . . . the ones that are intent on protecting us."

"And in our global environment of distrust, aggression, and terrorism," added Sam, directing his comment at Nivla, "it will be a *real* challenge to disseminate the information without it being altered, twisted, and distorted to suit the interests of powerful individuals and interest groups even if we try to share it with everyone, as you intend."

"Son," said a fatherly but authoritative Dr. Welch, "we may just need to get a little creative. And we will certainly need the help of present company . . . and I mean everyone." Everyone mumbled in agreement.

Nivla again took center stage. "In retrospect, several things become clear about Treretumian society, and perhaps your society is not in the same place as was Treretum, but my sharing what I am about to tell you may help your society to keep from making the same mistakes, now and in the future. Three sets of societal conditions have led Treretum to its current state, and you must guard against the same. These are conditions that it appears your society may already be experiencing."

Olga and Gavilán looked at each other in puzzlement. Nivla continued, "The first is misguided and overprotective leadership, coupled with the greed of a few individuals in high places. At the time of the invasion by the Muimdac, most of the leaders of the planet were dedicated to the safety and happiness of all Treretumians. They were, as you would say, the shepherds of the flock, and virtually every shepherd believed that he or she was a member of a sacred group charged with overseeing the well-being of all living things Treretumian, including maintaining peace and tranquility on the planet. In principle, this type of benevolent oversight should work well, but in practice, a handful of Drutsab shepherds let their focus shift to the accumulation of personal wealth without regard for the hardship and suffering inflicted on other Treretumians and their families. They took the carrot that was dangled in front of their collective nose and betrayed the trust of the entire planet."

Olga, Gavilán, Sam, and Dr. Welch exchanged glances in total amazement. None could believe what was coming from Nivla's small, pale, wrinkled lips as the time of his departure approached.

"All of this is intriguing, but, Nivla, you are speaking in riddles," Olga uttered impatiently.

Nivla gently tilted his head to the left and then straightened it. He ignored Olga and continued, "The second societal condition is complacency and skepticism of the masses, including blind and unquestioning confidence in organizations and individuals. On Treretum, over the millennia, the Drutsab Egral had protected the inhabitants of the planet, and the population had come to rely on having someone or some group of individuals vigilantly overseeing and directing all matters on the planet to serve the best interests of the entire population. But all that changed with the invasion. Today, the supreme council on Treretumian Environment and Agriculture, appointed by the elder members of the Drutsab Egral, is responsible for ensuring a safe living environment and food supply for all Treretumians. When exposed to the truth about the Muimdac presence on the planet and the dwindling uncontaminated food supply, some Treretumians fail to show concern because they assume that the TEA has things under control. Others reject the truth because they believe that, first of all, the TEA would never let this happen, and secondly, even if it were true, the TEA would alert the public of the situation."

Sam interjected, "Sounds like our FDA."

"Yes, well . . ." continued Nivla, "and the third societal condition that you must guard against is mass ignorance and the associated vulnerability. There is power in knowledge, and without it, the masses are vulnerable to being exploited. Again, in the case of Treretumians, most are still unaware of a Muimdac presence on the planet, and this has led to their exploitation, no . . . our exploitation, carrying out missions expressly designed to benefit the Muimdac. The result is that native Treretumians now serve as the primary food stock for the invading Muimdac forces. Unchecked, the existence of these conditions will surely lead to the extinction of my race."

All were silent, somewhat stunned at what they had heard.

Nivla sensed the desired impact had been made. Changing topics slightly, he continued as he stood to his feet, "Upon my departure, you will have the tools to keep your own planet from suffering the same fate. However, in the grand scheme of things, all that we see and do is of little consequence."

"Of little consequence?" reacted Sam and Dr. Welch in unison. Olga and Gavilán also appeared puzzled, but they remained quiet.

Nivla responded, "Yes. I must share with you something that I have already shared with Olga and Gavilán but in a different context. I was referring to everything that we do, everything that we experience, from the perspective of our current universal cycle. The universe that we know is in a damped periodic cycle that inevitably . . . everything that came to be during this cycle—every planet, every solar system, and every galaxy, every bit of unexpended energy, and every life-form, large and small, that originated and evolved in the less hostile reaches of the vast universe—will be annihilated. Our expanding universe is slowing down and will come to a virtual stop. It will then begin to contract. It will eventually fall in on itself, culminating in all the mass and energy of the universe occupying a very small space, triggering the beginning of the next cycle."

Olga turned to Gavilán and mumbled in puzzlement, "The next cycle?"

Nivla continued, "The next cycle will begin as did the cycle of our time—with an Explosion of Conception. Not so much a single explosion but more a period of time during which everything is exploding, colliding, disintegrating, and reforming—free flow between energy and matter. An epoch of unimaginable cataclysmic proportion, involving all matter and energy that exists."

Again, there was silence, until Nivla once again spoke. "During my brief tenure of existence as a Treretumian, I am thankful, honored, and privileged to have shared a tiny spec of time and space during this universal cycle with creatures like you that value life, not just of your species, not just on your planet, but all life—creatures of honor and integrity. If we only view things in terms of the universal cycle, we can only conclude that our existence is of little consequence. That is why we must realize that what gives our lives and the lives of any life-form meaning is the impact that we make during the span of a lifetime. Though my lifetime is twenty times that of an Earthling of this millennium, the impact that you have made on me is very great, and it will likely change the course of life on Treretum."

Olga, Gavilán, Dr. Welch, and Sam exchanged glances. Everyone rose from the table.

Then Olga spoke, "Nivla, we have been fortunate to have known you, and the information that you have shared will hopefully change the destiny of our planet as well. It seems that my whole life I have been gazing at the stars, wondering. I never really knew my place in the universe—my reason for living . . . but now I do." Olga's eyes began to tear up, and in a slightly shaky voice, she continued, "You truly amaze me. Thank you."

Gavilán chimed in, "Your ambitious goals for saving your race and saving your planet strangely strike a chord in my heart. It reminds me of a Mexican song, movie, and book, all of the same name. All I can say is '¡Jalisco, no te rajes!' The song is a love song to the entire Mexican state of Jalisco, and the literal translation may not make sense, but the slang interpretation is one of encouragement—don't be scared, don't back down, don't chicken out, keep on going in spite of adversity. Amigo [friend], if there is anything, and I mean *anything* we can do to help you . . . if it is humanly possible, we will do it."

Nivla walked over to Olga. His massive presence dwarfed her petite frame. He held out his hand, closed as thought he had something to give her, but he kept his hand closed as he continued, "As I said when we first arrived, very soon I will be leaving, but Cinz and Reppoc will remain to help protect you. I am certain that you will need their assistance. Keep this amulet on you—around your neck, on a charm bracelet, or on a key ring—and we will always be able to find you."

Olga looked at Cinz and Reppoc in confusion as Nivla took her hand and placed the amulet in her palm. Olga's mouth fell open. It was a gold airplane, just like the one Gavilán wore around his neck. Olga looked up at Nivla's face and then quickly turned around to show Gavilán. The instant he recognized the figure, he pulled the Mayan airplane amulet his grandfather had given him out from under his shirt. The two were virtually identical.

Dr. Welch continued with the goodbyes, "I have not had the privilege of sharing as much time with you and your associates as my friends, certainly not as much as I would have liked, but I assure you that the time you have shared has been impactful"—Dr. Welch looked around at his companions and completed his thought as he raised his eyebrows and again looked into Nivla's chestnut eyes—"on all of us. The information you have shared will certainly result in great change, and the future of this planet will change for the better due to our interaction."

Nivla responded, "Yes, I hope so."

Sam was virtually speechless. He walked over to Nivla, reached out, and took the hand of the alien to shake it as he said in a mild, sincere voice, "Thank you."

ꗃꗃꗃꗃꗃꗃꗃꗃꗃꗃꗃꗃꗃꗃꗃꗃꗃꗃꗃꗃꗃꗃꗃꗃꗃꗃꗃꗃꗃꗃꗃ

It had been another eventful day, the kind that changes the rest of your life. Sam and Dr. Welch were already on their way back to Atlanta with a mission: finding and opening the *etnafele* without destroying its contents. The success of their mission would catapult mankind into a new era of technological advancement, enlightenment, and understanding.

Gavilán opened the door to their two-bedroom suite, letting Olga lead the way. They were returning from Orville's warehouse where they had explained the reasons for the change in plans and cancellation of the balloon ride. Olga flicked on the light in the common area illuminating a small sofa, a sitting chair, a small kitchenette, and the prominent row of three tables and chairs they had assembled previously. They dropped their things on the tables, kicked off their shoes, and proceeded to seek out the comfort of the sofa (Olga) and sitting chair (Gavilán). They both sat, somewhat stunned, for a moment.

Olga had been bombarded with information that rocked the foundations of her beliefs, changing her perspective on many levels. She needed a sounding board, and as always, Cuauhtémoc Gavilán was her choice. "What do you make of all this?"

"Amazing . . . all of it!" he responded. "I guess we have our work cut out for us."

"I'll say," she quickly agreed. "But nobody's going to believe us, and after seeing the documents Nivla showed us, who do you trust?"

"I don't know . . . and there's no magic bullet to get us out of this either," replied Gavilán, sounding somewhat disillusioned. "But I think I owe our f-f-f-friend Mr. Stevenson a visit. Clearly, he's not one of them. If he were, I would have already been laid out on a marble slab."

"I think you're right. We need to first identify friends and foes," responded Olga with a display of renewed energy and enthusiasm. A strategy was about to begin to evolve. Olga continued, "Several obstacles have to be overcome. Everyone—every man, woman, and child on the planet—needs to know what's going on."

Gavilán added, "Yeah, except as the saying goes, you can lead a horse to water, but you can't make him drink." Gavilán noticed that Olga was starting to squint—a sure sign the discussion was getting too serious.

Olga retorted with a scowl on her face, "But if the horse's caretaker keeps hiding the water from him, he may die of thirst without much of a choice."

"Yeah . . . horses," Gavilán responded. "My grandfather told me of a distant cousin in Texas—not too bright, but he was the only son of a widow who lived out in the country but not too far from the outskirts of town. His mother gave him a list and their weekly grocery allowance and asked him to walk into town for the groceries." He then lifted his right hand, palm up, about chest high, and said as he slowly shook his head, "They didn't have a horse."

Olga had to pause, "unsquinted" her eyes, and take a deep breath. She then tilted her head slightly and looked at Gavilán in puzzlement. But the horse connection kept her from saying anything.

Gavilán continued, "She made sure that he had his backpack and that the list was short, because she didn't want her son out in the hot Texas sun for too long, especially not carrying heavy groceries. Well, according to my grandfather, my cousin crossed paths with a man leading an old horse. The man stopped him and asked, 'Hey, kid, wanna buy a horse?' My cousin stopped, pulled out and looked at the money in his pocket, and said, 'Naw, I have to go into town for groceries.' The man was a swindler who sensed that my cousin wasn't too bright and said, 'Son, I'll sell you my magic horse for the money in your hand.'"

By this time, Olga smelled a rat. She knew she was being set up. She began to squint again as she queried, "And then?"

"So my cousin asked, 'What's magic about him?'" Gavilán continued. "The man responded, 'You know how most horses get hot when they run? Well, this one cools off and how much depends on how fast he's running.' My cousin couldn't contain himself. He knew that his mother had been saving money to buy a horse, and he wanted to please her. He agreed to the deal, handed over the money, climbed onto the horse, and started for home. Atop the horse he felt a slight breeze, and he thought to himself, *Gee, I can feel him cooling off already.*"

Olga sat up on the edge of her chair and interrupted, "Gavilán—" but Gavilán raised his hand, palm out, in front of his chest as he continued, "So he swatted the old horse on the backside to make him go a little faster. The horse broke into a trot. Most people would have realized that this was really stressing the old guy."

Olga pushed herself back into the chair and just listened.

"My cousin thought to himself, *Gee, I guess that man was right—I can really feel him cooling off now.* With the house in sight, my cousin slaps the horse's backside to get him to go into a full gallop. The horse complies, but his tongue is hanging out his mouth, and my cousin's mother sees him from the kitchen window. She runs out of the house toward her son, but just as they are about to meet, the horse drops dead from heat exhaustion. His mother is obviously very upset and yells, 'What happened?' My cousin scratched his head as he looked at the poor dead animal before him and said, '*Duh* . . . gee, Maw, I guess he musta froze to death!'"

With a big smile on her face, Olga shook her head, exclaiming, "Loco!" [Crazy!] as she stretched to punch him in the arm. "That's one of the things I love about you—your bizarre sense of humor." Olga went over to Gavilán and landed a gentle punch to his upper left arm. "Come on, let's get these tables back where they belong."

Gavilán glanced at his wristwatch, and his weary eyes became wearier. "It's after one o'clock," he muttered. They had been talking all evening about the events of their great adventure. Gavilán was exhausted, not so much from physical exertion but rather from the mental and emotional stress they had experienced. Gavilán was ready for some much-needed sleep.

Olga too was exhausted, but she still had to get his opinion on one more. "And what do you make of all this business about the 'damped periodic cycle, inevitable annihilation of all life, and the next big bang initiating a new cycle'?"

Gavilán took a deep breath, let out a sigh, and began to describe what he perceived. "Well, to me it seems plausible, but there are many questions that come to mind. How long does each cycle take—twenty billion, forty billion, a hundred billion years? And what about the mass/energy loss per cycle, or are they fairly uniform? How many cycles will there be with the mass/energy of our universe—a thousand, a million, a trillion? And what about the final curtain? How does it all end? With the annihilation of the last two atoms in the universe—a relative whimper? But even if it is only slightly damped, no matter how many years per cycles and how many cycles, you're talking about a finite duration of time. No matter how large the number, it is finite. What happened before the first big bang, and what happens after the final whimper? In other words, what about the real beginning?" Gavilán paused, shook his head slowly, continuing, "What about infinity?"

"I know," Olga responded in a low, descending tone—one that expressed awe. "Back when I was a little kid, we always thought in terms of the universe being infinite, and therefore, the mass of the universe would have to be infinite. A couple of years ago, for grins, I did a Google search on the total mass of the universe." Olga continued parenthetically, "You know, Google knows all." Gavilán just nodded in affirmation as Olga continued, "Well, you know what I mean—Google knows all, at least as a starting point for doing your own personal research. I looked up a bunch of the cited references to see how they had come up with their estimates, and then I did calculations of my own. And it looks like the total mass is somewhere between ten to the fiftieth and ten to the sixtieth kilograms. Granted, there's quite a bit of slop in the calculations—it's a pretty broad range, but whatever the number is, it's a pretty damn big number . . ." At that point, Olga tilted her head to the right, squinted her eyes, and raised the pitch of her voice as she continued, shook her head slowly, saying "and it's not infinite."

Gavilán was amazed at the energy Olga still displayed. He struggled to pull himself out of the easy chair, looked at Olga, and said, "I'm wasted. I have to get some sleep. I'll take that one," he said as he gestured at the door to the next room with an extended arm and his shoes in hand. "You take this one."

"I have to think a little more," Olga replied as she curled up on the sofa.

Gavilán staggered away as he muttered, "See you in a few hours."

Gavilán entered the room, closing the door behind him. He went to the air conditioning unit by the closed drapes, turned it on, and sat on the edge of the large bed for a few seconds, looking down toward his knees, contemplating whether he had the energy to get ready for bed and slip under the covers. He shook his head as a dog would to get his ears dry after being given a bath. He then leaned back and raised his feet onto the bed—he was out like a light.

In dream, Gavilán kept going over everything that had transpired since he and Olga had agreed to rendezvous in Houston. Bits and pieces swirled around in his head in a big jumble as though he were in the middle of the tornado that had swept Toto and Dorothy to another world in the *Wizard of Oz*. He could see flashes of the faces of all the living creatures he had encountered during this, his most amazing adventure. But the single strong and consistent image that persisted was that of Olga. Then images in his dream changed suddenly, and he felt the bare shin of his right leg rub against Olga's leg, and he instinctively mumbled, "Oh, I'm sorry." It was Olga . . . he could relax. His dream finally left him alone so that he could get some rest.

A sliver of the morning sun flowed into the room from the edge of the drapes that had not been drawn completely closed. The beam of light seemed to caress Gavilán's face to awaken him. He slowly opened his eyes, raised his right arm to rub his right eye with his hand. He looked at his shirtsleeve and realized he must have opted to not prepare for bed and slip under the covers. Instinctively, he slowly turned his head to the right. To his surprise, he saw Olga lying a respectable distance from him, propped up on her left elbow, looking at him as he came back to life.

Olga smiled gently, saying, "You must have had *some* nightmare. I heard you from the other room, mumbling as you tossed and turned."

Gavilán took a breath and began to respond, but Olga placed the first finger of her right hand on his lips to keep him from speaking. "It's all right," she said. "Everything's going to be all right. EGBAR, remember?"

Her presence made him feel at peace. He slowly blinked his eyes and said in a near-whisper, "Yeah."

CADMIUM POISONING

FACTS

- Never eat carrots that haven't had the outer skin removed. Approximately one-third of the cadmium is in the outer skin. Soak the carrots in cadmium-free water for 24 hours, and you just removed half of the remaining (one-third of the original) cadmium. By removing a total of two-thirds of the cadmium, that makes them marginally acceptable as part of a low-cadmium diet. The bad news is that soaking them in water also removes much of the flavor and possibly reduces their nutritive value. Consider supplementing with Vitamin A and/or beta carotene.

- Don't overeat, except maybe for non-fat, phosphate-free, sugar-free, HFCS-free, plain yogurt for the probiotics.

- The death toll of WWII was over 72 million, which accounted for approximately 3.7% of the world population of 1.9 billion. Since then, the population of planet earth has nearly quadrupled to over 7.1 billion.

And just when you thought you were starting to get the picture, you get additional information that shows the situation is more complex than you had anticipated. You know you're being poisoned with cadmium, and you think zinc is the answer: take a therapeutic dosage of zinc to displace cadmium; take vitamins and minerals to chelate cadmium and to compensate for the high dosage of zinc, respectively; and flush the cadmium from your body by taking niacin and eating lots of fruit and drinking lots of low-cadmium (not from concentrate unless *you* add the filtered water) fruit juice (e.g., orange). Then you are in an accident, and they administer steroids or cordicotorpin to control swelling and inflammation.

Oops! Beware of possible development of Cushing's disease (Cushing's syndrome), a disease that sometimes results from steroid overdoses. The cordicotorpin that is normally released by the pituitary gland within the brain readily adsorbs zinc and becomes more effective and longer lasting in the stimulation of the adrenal glands (by the kidneys) in the production and release of anti-inflammatory steroids like cortisone. The result is a potential steroid overdose—and Cushing's disease. Steroids should always be respected and administered with caution. Always let medical professionals who have access to your veins and arteries know that you are taking supplements, and specifically zinc, and don't assume they'll understand the significance because they probably won't. If this is a concern, consider taping a notice onto your insurance card since hospitals are unlikely to do anything without knowing they will be paid. That is the first thing they will look for in your wallet or purse if you are injured, taken to a hospital, and unable to interact with attendants. Alternatively, consider wearing a medical alert bracelet.

ꝏꝏꝏꝏꝏꝏꝏꝏꝏꝏꝏꝏꝏꝏꝏꝏꝏꝏꝏꝏꝏꝏꝏꝏꝏꝏꝏ

Epilogue

He stood on the observation deck, staring into the dark void of space. Nivla, on his return voyage to his beloved Treretum, found himself in the role of the leader of mutineers, a role he had not sought but accepted without hesitation. In this capacity, he, his comrade in arms and friend, Suturb, and his two faithful drones, Cinz and Reppoc, had been ultimately responsible for the safety of all members of the crew. And now, with the bond that had been formed with a select few Earthlings, he somehow felt responsible for their future as well. He regretted the loss of life that had occurred and ultimately felt responsible for the death of Egroeg and his clique of elitist officers. They were not Muimdac but Treretumians entrenched in the Muimdac system that eventually would have led to the death of all native Treretumians.

Because of the distance between Earth and Treretum, the distress signals Yenech had surely sent would take over eight and one-half years to reach home. At maximum cruising speed, their spacecraft would reach 0.9 times the speed of light, so they would arrive home a brief year after the signal. Much could happen on Treretum during that span of time. Nivla was apprehensive about the nature of the welcoming committee that would be awaiting them. He was also acutely aware that from his perspective and that of everyone aboard the Regnellach, the 8.6-light-year return trip would take less time than it would appear to stationary observers on either Earth or Treretum. Although they would seem to lose time, traveling near the speed of light, he and his crew would have to make good use of the years they would spend aboard their spacecraft. They had to prepare for every contingency. Nivla knew that the fate of his race depended upon their ability to cope with their dubious reception on Treretum. Nivla also knew he would miss Cinz and Reppoc in the years to come.

In the doors of the CDC bright and early just before 7:00 a.m., evading questions from his early-bird peers regarding how he had spent his vacation, Dr. Billy Ruben Welch returned to work as scheduled, ready to tackle the first item of business: locating Nivla's *etnafele*. He had discussed things with Sam, and they had agreed they would go in at their normal times to keep from raising additional questions among the CDC staff, and Sam was an eight-to-five sort of guy. After setting down his briefcase and cranking up his CDC laptop, he made his way into the bullpen to Sam's cubicle.

He looked on the top shelf of the bookshelf in Sam's cubicle, and there it was. He took the *etnafele* in his hand and viewed it in amazement, knowing the contents of the small sphere would dramatically change the world he knew. Just then, Sean, Sam's boss who was strolling by with a cup of coffee in hand, saw Dr. Welch and stopped to say hello.

"Whacha got there?" he asked.

A startled Billy Ruben turned as he lowered the *etnafele* near his waist, replying, "Oh, nothing . . . I have a touch of arthritis, and my doctor suggested that I exercise my hand with a squeeze ball. Do you know when Sam will be getting in?"

Sean replied, "Oh, probably around eight. Anything I can help you with?"

"No, no thanks, Sean," answered Dr. Welch coolly. "I have a long-term project that's just gearing up, and I may need his help on it, so if you see him before I do, could you ask him to drop by my office?"

"Sure. You got it."

"Thanks, Sean," said Dr. Welch as he patted Sean's upper left arm and squeezed out into the aisle between the rows of cubicles.

Once in his office, he placed he *etnafele* in the top-right drawer of his desk and locked it. He contemplated the next step he and Sam would take. A few phone calls to friends at the Georgia Tech engineering department were in order. They would be able to help with the equipment that would be needed to open the *etnafele*. In his get-things-done style, he mentally mapped out how he would approach his engineering friends and began looking up phone numbers on his computer. Suddenly, he stopped, unlocked the top-right drawer of his desk, opened the drawer and stared at the sphere that it contained, and wondered what destiny held in store for the rest of his life.

"I accept your letter of resignation, Mr. Stevenson," said Blakey, sitting behind his desk.

"And here are my service revolver and badge, sir," Stevenson said as he stretched forward to surrender his holstered firearm and badge.

Blakey took the gun and badge and placed them in the drawer of his desk. "Now that you've turned in your service revolver, I can tell you that if you hadn't resigned, I personally was going to make sure you were booted out of the DHS and never had another government job as long as you live. You're a sa-sa-sa-sorry son of a bitch, and a pu-pu-pu-poor excuse for a DHS agent."

Stevenson stood there calmly and replied, "You really should do something about that stutter, sir. It'll probably hinder your advancement in the DHS. You might try lowering your stress level—I did . . . and my stutter is gone."

He turned and walked out the door to Blakey's office, feeling good about himself, uplifted, and free. Stevenson didn't know what he would do next, but that didn't seem to bother him. He felt a sense of euphoria by the time he got to the front door of the building. He paused and whispered to himself, "I'm not one of them," as a big smile developed on his face. He stepped out the door and didn't look back.

Sam sat on the back porch with his dachshund in his lap. "Coop," he said, followed by a deep breath, "what does all this mean? What's going to happen now?" Cooper turned his head and looked up at master's face and proceeded to comfort him the best way he could. Cooper began to lick Sam's right hand repeatedly. "I missed you too, boy," Sam said. He turned his eyes to the heavens and gazed into the starlit night sky as he continued to stroke his trusty friend. He went on, "Nivla, we've been oblivious to the toxins in our environment since the beginning of our time on Earth, and because of that, every man, woman, and child—*everyone* on the face of my planet—is destined to unknowingly self-inflict tremendous abuse. As soon as a baby emerges from the womb, the poisoning process begins. How can we undo the harm? How can we undo decades of abuse?"

Again, Cooper looked up, and the two gazed into each other's eyes for a few seconds. Sam continued, "Or does any of this matter? Aww, heck, I don't know . . . . And what have I been doing to you? I know now that I should have paid more attention to what I feed you. I'm sorry, little trooper." A tear rolled down his cheek and landed on Cooper's back. "I promise I'll do better now that I know more about what's going on." Sam paused as he thought about the all the tales Nivla had shared, but the one that had evoked the most visceral reaction from him was the one regarding Earth becoming a feed colony. He looked at Cooper and said, "And you know, I would never think of eating you." Suddenly Cooper's ears went up and his head jerked back. Sam noticed Cooper's reaction, so he snatched him up and clutched him to his chest as he continued in a higher-pitched baby talk, "But that's not because you're full of cadmium . . . it's because your my buddy, and I wuv you."

Olga and Gavilán walked in the park near the JPL at dusk, still stunned from what they had experienced. They strolled leisurely, Gavilán's arm draped around her shoulder and Olga's arm around his waist. It was clear that this, for them, was just the beginning in many ways . . . but it was the beginning of a future they would be facing and sharing together.

As they walked, Gavilán slowed to a halt, turning toward Olga. Olga looked up at his face with a mixture of confusion and concern. "What's the matter?" she said gently. Gavilán took her by the shoulders, leaned forward, and kissed her. It caught Olga by surprise, but it was welcomed. She wrapped her arms around him, and he responded in kind as Olga went up on here toes. It was a long, tender kiss. Both closed their eyes, and they were in another world . . . alone together. His left hand went up to Olga's head, under her hair, to cradle the back of her head. When either moved, ever so slightly, the other responded with the complementary motion. They were in sync. Much was said, although no words were spoken. For both of them, it was the perfect kiss, and neither wanted it to end, but both knew when Gavilán slowly began to raise his head that it was time to resume their walk. The separation of their lips was slow and sensual, with a small area on the right side of Olga's top lip sticking slightly to Gavilán's. They both opened their eyes at the instant when their lips finally parted, and there they stood, arms around each other, looking into each other's eyes. From out of nowhere, they both heard faint music. It was Tchaikovsky's "Love Theme" from *Romeo and Juliet*.

When they realized it was emanating from Olga's purse, Olga scrambled to get to her cell phone. With her usual flair, she reached into her purse and flipped open her cell phone. She had just received a text message from Star Traveler. As she retrieved the message and focused on the screen of her cell phone, Olga said, "It's a message from Nivla. 'Yenech and four others escaped. More to follow.' What do you think that means?"

Just then, Gavilán looked up and pointed at what appeared to be a small meteor shower, but this one was different. "Look!" he exclaimed, pointing into the sky. "I've seen a few meteor showers in my day, but this one seems to have a luminescent glow."

Almost as a reflex, Olga explained, "That's usually caused by a high concentration of very fine particles that descend with the larger objects. The thing is"—she pointed to the sky—"these fines that would usually burn up upon entering the atmosphere are somehow surviving the intense heat. They glow like crazy, and it looks like they may actually survive the descent all the way to the earth's surface."

CADMIUM POISONING

FACTS

- The problems associated with the "small" quantities of cadmium that accumulated in your body over the years don't end with a bowel movement. Since this is the primary disposal pathway for cadmium, wastewater treatment plants are collection centers for cadmium. And since sewage sludge, which is rich in cadmium, is an accepted fertilizer for organic vegetables and fruits, the cadmium that caused problems in one person's body is recycled and made available for ingestion by another. While recycling is generally a good practice that reduces our adverse impact on our environment, recycling is not necessarily good for your internal environment.

- To clarify the issue of sewage sludge usage in organic farming, we need to examine the difference between "organic produce" and "certified organic" produce. Sewage sludge is not allowed in the growing of *certified* organic crops, but it is permitted for use in growing noncertified organic crops. In addition, to my chagrin, 40 synthetic pesticides *are allowed* to be used in growing certified organic crops. Farmers say that it's okay since they spray the soil before the crop grows and that the crop is never exposed to the pesticide. However, since the pesticide is in the soil, it may not be *on* the crop and still be *in* the crop. Furthermore, a crop can be advertised as 100% organic, but if it is not *certified* organic, that means that 30% of the substances used by the farmer can be of a non-organic nature. The "100%" refers to 70% of the substances used in crop production. So you could buy something labeled "100% organic," and it may have been grown using sewage sludge.

- There is no such thing as a "small" dose of cadmium—it all adds up. Cadmium poisoning is cumulative.

- After knowing about the situation associated with cadmium in the food supply, some people will say "I only eat oysters once a year and shrimp once every few months." Is the immediate gratification from tainted food worth the risk of future long-term pain and suffering? Unless you've seen someone you love suffer or you have personally felt the pain, you may think yes. After you have cancer, it's a little late to change your mind.

- It is a fact of life and a cause of suffering and death: cadmium is in our food supply. Cadmium accumulates primarily in the pancreas, liver, lungs, kidneys, and bones, so any ingestion or inhalation of cadmium has potential cumulative adverse effects. It is present in relatively high concentrations in, for example, many grains (e.g., wheat and rice), vegetables, organ meats and associated meat products, shellfish, mushrooms, chocolate, and coffee. The carcinogenic heavy metal does not belong in our bodies, and it often causes severe autoimmune system reactions that are given other names, depending on what outward symptoms. When threshold concentrations are reached, it causes critical organs to malfunction, and typically, it eventually leads to cancer.

- Informing the public of the problem, removing cadmium from phosphate fertilizers (currently contaminated with cadmium) to be used for food crops, decontaminating the cadmium-laden soils of our farmlands, and requiring that the FDA to perform its function of protecting public health would be the initial steps in tackling this issue. There will be substantial economic impacts, and therefore, there will be opposition to doing what is best for human health and the environment. This is why government intervention is needed. The road will be long and tenuous, and the inevitable results of improved public health and lower cancer rates will not be achievable in a few short years. As with lead and mercury, legislation is needed to limit exposure, and your continued pressure on responsible parties in government is vital for successful enactment of laws to protect all of us from cadmium poisoning.

- In the meantime, each of us must take responsibility for his/her own health, doing what is necessary to counter the impacts of cadmium exposure as much as possible. For example, taking phosphate-free zinc supplements (only with meals) would mitigate the assimilation of ingested cadmium. The recommended daily allowance (RDA) for zinc is 15 mg, a quantity that may have been appropriate for a typical human before the widespread use of phosphate fertilizers; however, our environment has changed, and this RDA is woefully inadequate for humans in today's environment. Because the public generally accepts RDAs to be the dosages they should take, the FDA is neglecting its responsibilities by not taking a changing environment and individual conditions (e.g., weight, pregnancy) into account. The pregnant woman who religiously takes her prenatal vitamins containing 15 mg of zinc daily is likely to experience zinc deficiency by the end of her pregnancy due to the zinc requirements of the fetus that will likely be met before her own. Recall that the placenta has a zinc concentration about 1,000 times that of the rest of the mother's body tissues to protect the baby, drawing the zinc from other parts of the body. Also recall that the biological half-life of zinc in the human body is about 78 days, a fraction of the time needed for development of a full-term baby, resulting in the diversion of nutrients and essential trace metals to the developing fetus and away from its mother.

- In short, be informed. Do whatever is necessary to protect yourself and your loved ones, and do something to affect change in our society to end the needless and almost universal suffering, both physical and financial, for those exhibiting the signs of cadmium poisoning (e.g., diabetes, breast cancer, kidney failure) and their families.

- We are treating the symptoms of many diseases like diabetes, kidney failure, and the associated cancers . . . not the underlying cause(s).

- Recognizing underlying causes of illness can be a challenge, but for most of the medical community, public health officials, and the public in general, cadmium appears to be off the radar screen.

- Spread the word. *Everyone* needs to know.

POINTS OF CONTACT IN THE FEDERAL GOVERNMENT

Office of the President and Vice President The White House 1600 Pennsylvania Avenue Washington, DC 20500 (202) 465-1414 www.whitehouse.gov	USDA Forest Service 1400 Independence Avenue, SW Washington, DC 20250-0002 (202) 205-8333 www.fs.fed.us
U.S. Senate (Senator's Name) Senate Office Building Washington, DC 20510 (202) 224-3121 www.senate.gov	Department of the Interior Interior Building, Room 6151 1849 C Street, NW Washington, DC 20240 (202) 208-3100 www.doi.gov
U.S. House of Representatives (Representative's Name) House Office Building Washington, DC 20515 (202) 224-3121 www.house.gov	U.S. Fish and Wildlife Service Interior Building, Room 3156 1849 C Street, NW Washington, DC 20240 (202) 208-4416 www.fws.gov
Environmental Protection Agency Ariel Rios Building 1200 Pennsylvania Avenue, NW/1011A Washington, DC 20460 (202) 272-0167 www.epa.gov	Department of Energy James Forrestal Building 1000 Independence Avenue, SW Washington, DC 20585 www.doe.gov
Centers for Disease Control and Prevention For regional offices, see https://wwwn.cdc.gov/dcs/	Food and Drug Administration For regional offices, see http://www.fda.gov/AboutFDA/ContactFDA/ucm2005604.htm

Additional Points of Contact	
Greenpeace 702 H Street, NW, Suite 300 Washington, DC 20001 (800) 326-0959 www.greenpeace.org	The Environmental Working Group San Francisco, California (510) 444-0973, ext. 302 www.ewg.org
Food & Water Watch 1616 P Street NW Washington, DC 20036 (202) 683-2500 info@fwwatch.org	NRDC Headquarters 40 West 20th Street 11th floor New York, NY 10011 For regional offices, see https://www.nrdc.org/contact-us

Appendix A

SUGGESTED STRATEGY FOR
RECOVERING FROM CADMIUM POISONING

- Eliminate further insults to the body—as much as possible, eliminate all identifiable sources of cadmium from the air you breathe, the food you eat, and the beverages you drink—as much as possible, eliminate cadmium from your life.

- Stop smoking, legal or otherwise.
    - o Cigarettes
    - o Cigars
    - o Pipes
    - o Marijuana
    - o Secondhand smoke (It's your responsibility to protect yourself and the ones you love—you can always leave.)
    - o Smoky bars
    - o Smoke-filled parties, meetings, and concerts
    - o Smoking sections in restaurants and airports

- Avoid foods that are high in cadmium.
    - o Sugar—more than half of he U.S. sugar production comes from sugar beets

o Bread—especially white bread (because the cadmium resides in the white inner portion of the grain, and the zinc is concentrated on the brown outer portion)

o Flour tortillas (tortillas de harina)—very high due to addition of wheat gluten

o All pastas made of wheat—typically made with Durham wheat, which is higher in cadmium than other strains

o All wheat products—especially those not made from whole wheat (substitute oat flour or corn flour for wheat flour [most of the cadmium absorbed by oats stays in the roots of the plants])

o All rice products—especially those made of white rice (Rice flour is not a suitable substitute for wheat flour, from the perspective of cadmium intake.)

o All shellfish, including shrimp and oysters—they are bottom dwellers and typically contain 1,000 time the concentration of cadmium compared to beef, pork, fish, or chicken

o Organ meats (e.g., liver) and sausages that typically contain organ meats

o Beets—used to phytoremediate soils that are contaminated with cadmium

o Mushrooms—they grow low to the ground and are commonly grown with commercial fertilizers, cow or horse manure, or sewage sludge so they can be categorized as "organic"

o Lunch (i.e., deli) meats (usually loaded with phosphates, and therefore, cadmium—*Do not* ingest anything with phosphates.)

o Cheese (Although dairy products, in general, are considered to be low in cadmium, it takes a lot of milk to make a little cheese, and the concentration factor catapults cheese out of the "low-cadmium dairy" category. If you eat cheese, eat it in small doses. It has been identified as a food that causes internal inflammation on numerous Internet sites—a dubious honor typically reserved for foods with high cadmium concentrations.)

o   Peanuts and peanut butter (which likely also contains high-fructose corn syrup)

- Avoid beverages that are high in cadmium.
    - o   Coffee (contains some beneficial compounds—along with trace amounts of over twenty known carcinogens)
    - o   Chocolate (contains some beneficial compounds, but also contains both cadmium and lead)
    - o   All soft drinks (In addition to having a low pH and promoting tooth decay, they are laden with cadmium—from the water used, from the processing equipment, and from the additives like phosphoric acid [aka hydrogen *phosphate*, typically obtained by reacting sulfuric acid with phosphate rock— cadmium usually goes with the phosphate.])
    - o   Green tea
    - o   Tap water (not because treatment was inadequate and the quality of water in the purveyor's distribution system does not meet standards but because water is recontaminated when it enters the plumbing system of your home—cadmium leaching from galvanized or PVC piping)

- Reestablish the dominance of zinc in your bodily functions by shifting the equilibrium away from cadmium.
    - o   Take phosphate-free zinc supplements (The RDA of 15 mg/day is woefully inadequate; a therapeutic dosage might be around 200 mg/day—*always with a meal.*)
    - o   Eat zinc-rich foods (that are also low in cadmium—e.g., peas)

- Eat foods that will benefit your body.
    - o   Clean, fresh fruits from trees—low in cadmium, provide roughage, and keep you "regular" (the primary means of eliminating cadmium from the body is through the bowel)

o Vegetables—focus on foods that are not in direct contact with the soils—ones that grow on tall stalks or long vines (e.g., beans and legumes, peas, green beans, squash, corn, and broccoli [rich in vitamin C and it's green, and therefore, contains magnesium in chlorophyll])

o Tree nuts (e.g., cashews, pecans, walnuts, almonds), avocados, and berries for essential oils and antioxidants (avoid peanuts since they are not tree nuts— they grow in the ground [not real nuts])

- Take supplements that will assist in chelating the cadmium and make up for nutrients that were eliminated from your diet.

  o Vitamin A—not only good for the eyes but also chelates cadmium

  o Vitamin B complex—B vitamins usually work best together)

  o Vitamin B_1—thiamine (in addition to vitamin B complex) chelates cadmium

  o Vitamin B_3—niacin opens the capillaries, enhancing delivery of zinc and removal of cadmium on the cellular level

  o Vitamin B_6—precursor to hemoglobin and combats anemia, one of the symptoms of cadmium poisoning

  o Vitamin B_{12}—contains cobalt, helps prevent cadmium accumulation in the kidneys, and is essential for brain function

  o Vitamin C—an essential component of a healthy immune system, and it chelates cadmium

  o Vitamin D_3—essential for healthy bones and assimilation of calcium, which is essential for repairs of sites where cadmium has been removed from the bones

  o Vitamin E—lubricates and sooths nerves, enhancing healing of lesions (e.g., on the sciatic nerve) caused by high concentrations of cadmium in the blood.

  o Magnesium—essential element for bone and nerve health and necessary supplement to offset the reduction in chlorophyll intake associated with removal of lettuce and spinach from the diet (A deficiency in magnesium is sometimes accompanied by anxiety and tightness in the chest.)

o Copper—essential element in connective tissue and reportedly important in maintaining hair color (Supplementation is likely needed for those doing long-term zinc supplementation, since it is preferentially removed by metallothioneins [even more so than cadmium], which are proteins synthesized and released into the bloodstream in response to the increased zinc concentrations.)

o Selenium—sister metal of sulfur and essential for a healthy prostate.

- *Flush! Flush! Flush!* Take niacin (vitamin B₃) to open your capillaries (by as much as 100% of their normal diameter). Cadmium is an element that cannot be broken down or detoxified. It is essential that it be removed from the body as quickly as possible, or it may be liberated from one location only to cause harm in another. This will also facilitate access to many of the beneficial elements and compounds, such as zinc, vitamins B, and vitamin C.

- Drink purified water (typically filtered)—and lots of it—to help flush cadmium from your body and to stay regular, while helping to maintain a youthful appearance.) Water should be filtered with activated carbon or by reverse osmosis, distilled, demineralized via ion exchange, or treated by some other means to eliminate cadmium.

- Drink orange juice (with no phosphate additives) but not orange juice from concentrate unless you are the one adding the filtered (cadmium-free) water. Or better yet, eat oranges—that way you also get the fiber. I try to eat at least five pieces of fruit per day.

NOTE: If you are diabetic and cannot currently tolerate the high sugar content, just drink lots of filtered water until after your pancreas begins to respond to changes in blood glucose concentrations.

- Don't overeat. Because the amount of cadmium we ingest is the product of the concentration of the cadmium in our food and the volume of food we ingest, eating twice as much of something that has half the concentration of cadmium does nothing to reduce the level of cadmium intake. If you *have to* overeat, eat *phosphate-free*, sugar-free, HFCS-free, nonfat or low-fat, plain yogurt, which will help the biota in your intestines (probiotics). Make your own nonfat or low-fat fruit yogurt by adding fruit (e.g., blueberries, cranberries—fresh or freeze dried) and a little honey. Honey has been shown to reduce the immediate adverse body response (as indicated by changes in blood chemistry) following cadmium exposure more effectively than vitamin C or zinc. Also, honey is rich in zinc and niacin.

- To ensure that other minerals removed from the body are not depleted, especially those that, like zinc, compete with cadmium, consider taking additional supplements (e.g., copper, magnesium, calcium). Eat a banana a day for potassium, and consider eating banana slices that include the peal, which is the part of the banana with the highest potassium content.

SO WHAT ELSE IS A GIRL (OR BOY) TO DO?

- Take responsibility of your health, make the necessary changes in you diet, and take control of your life.

- Spread the word, but be prepared to be thought a crackpot.
    - o   Tell the people you love
    - o   Tell your friends
    - o   Tell those who demonstrate cadmium poisoning

    o   Tell those who don't demonstrate cadmium poisoning (*everyone* needs to know)

- Inspect the products you purchase, read the list of ingredients, and know what you are putting into your body.

- Put on the pressure (at home, at stores, at restaurants, on doctors, on pharmacists, on school officials, on legislators, on health officials) to inform the public and do something (e.g., push for laws to require removal of cadmium from phosphate fertilizers) to minimize public exposure.

- Optimize—once you have the regimen/routine down, consider optimizing the timing on your supplementation. Assess the potential interactions between different supplements, especially those that can form cations and anions. For example, zinc ions interact strongly with sulfides (and, probably selenium in its reduced form). Time your supplementation so that you don't take zinc when you're eating a lot of garlic (selenium) or onions or eggs (sulfur). This could reduce the availability of the zinc, selenium, and sulfur before they have a chance to enter the bloodstream. That is not to say that you should skip supplementation but rather that the timing can be adjusted to maximize the associated benefits.

Appendix B

COMMENTS MADE AND ASSOCIATED QUESTIONS
ASKED DURING VARIOUS ONLINE SUMMITS

The following are comments, responses, questions and corresponding answers, all from various online health-related "summits" involving guest speakers/interviewees. Names have been deleted from the comments "to protect the innocent." All speakers will be referred to as Dr. X.

COMMENT #1

CADMIUM, CADMIUM, CADMIUM!!!!!!! The reason that today's airmen are showing a four-fold increase in celiac markers in their blood compared to Airmen from sixty years ago is the chronic exposure to cadmium in the food supply due to the use of phosphate fertilizers. Massive use of fertilizers was not commonplace back then. Cadmium concentrations in the soils where fertilizers are applied and our food is grown have been documented to be increasing with each season of fertilizer application. Cadmium accumulates in the human body (average biological half-life of 30 years), and it competes with zinc (biological half-life of 78 days), impacting the immune system and countless other systems in the body in which zinc plays a vital role. (Cadmium is located directly below zinc in the periodic table.) Cadmium is especially high in wheat gluten, but it is also in coffee, chocolate, mushrooms, beets, lettuce, shellfish of all types, organ meats, etc. It accumulates primarily in the pancreas, kidneys, liver, lungs, and bones, and long term exposure results in zinc deficiency. Celiac disease is a manifestation of cadmium poisoning, and yes, a restricted diet will help. Zinc supplementation (free of phosphate fillers) and other vitamins and minerals that will help mobilize and chelate cadmium help tremendously. I am my own guinea pig, and with today's environment, the RDA for zinc is woefully inadequate. Stay away from cadmium and THINK ZINC!!!!

Summit Coordinator and Moderator (C&M) response:

You have done your homework Mr. Riojas-congratulations. Very useful information. I agree with all that you say except for the statement "Celiac Disease is a manifestation of cadmium poisoning." I personally would modify that statement by saying 'Cadmium poisoning may be "the straw that broke the camel's back" in loss of oral tolerance and pushed the body's ability to cope beyond its threshold, thus initiating or fueling the development of celiac disease. An important difference. All celiac disease is not caused by cadmium poisoning, but all cadmium poisoned genetically-sensitive people may be vulnerable to developing celiac disease.

Response to C&M response:

Thanks for the comment, and sorry for the delayed response. I would agree with you that there is more to celiac disease (CD) than just cadmium poisoning, but I feel strongly that cadmium is what pushes *many* (if not most) people who suffer from CD over the edge. Cadmium, a carcinogenic heavy metal, has been linked to countless diseases. And thanks for saying that I'd done my homework. Actually, I watched almost everyone in my family from my parents' generation suffer from various illnesses (e.g., diabetes, kidney failure, osteoporosis) only to develop cancer (e.g., pancreatic cancer, kidney cancer, stomach cancer, breast cancer) and die. Both my parents died in their mid-sixties, and all the cancers are linked to cadmium. For years I thought I would share their fate, thinking that the issue was genetic and beyond my control. Everyone developed multiple conditions that were signs of cadmium poisoning, but the medical community doesn't have cadmium on their radar screen, and I didn't know anything back then. Zinc is key in getting our bodies (including our immune systems) to function properly, and most of us are suffering from zinc deficiency. It has made a huge difference in my life! However, there is one thing I failed to mention in my original comment: NEVER TAKE ZINC ON AN EMPTY STOMACH! I have a friend whose daughter suffers from CD. I convinced him to have her start taking zinc, and she is doing much better. It's a long road to "recovery," and it's sooooo true that "you are what you eat."

Q #1a: Should we not eat as much foods with cadmium, or just take zinc supplements?

A #1a: Both! Stay away from high-cadmium foods (e.g., wheat, rice, chocolate, coffee, shellfish, and generally things that grow low to the ground), and focus on low-cadmium foods (e.g., fruits and nuts that grow on trees, corn, broccoli, peas, green beans, and things that grow far from the ground or are connected to the ground by long vines). Also, consider additional supplements (phosphate free!) that help chelate cadmium (e.g., vitamin A, vitamin C, vitamin B_1) and minerals that you may need as a result of your dietary changes and zinc supplementation (e.g., magnesium due to reduced chlorophyll intake, copper since it also competes with zinc and cadmium). Also, consider niacin (vitamin B_3) to open your capillaries to help flush out the cadmium and let in the zinc, vitamin B_{12} that helps block cadmium accumulation in the kidneys . . . and the list goes on. My entire diet has changed, focusing on how I can minimize my cadmium exposure and promote its removal from my body. Now when I go to the grocery store, I continue to be amazed at all the poison on the shelves.

Q #1b: Do you recommend measuring cadmium, via hair test analysis or RBC analysis? Certainly I think that in general, many people are zinc deficient.

A #1b: Sorry for the delay in responding! Knowing what the concentrations are in your body would be nice, but it is difficult to determine, first and foremost, because most labs are not used to doing cadmium analyses, and they generally do not look for low enough concentrations (looking for parts per billion rather than parts per million). So, first of all, find a lab that is used to doing this and knows what they are doing! Secondly, the hair or blood or urine sample that is analyzed is only a general indicator, and it may not give you an accurate read on how much and where the cadmium in your body is located. I think that a better indicator would be based on a combination of (1) how you feel, (2) how old you are, and (3) knowing what your diet has been like all your life. For people who have grown up on a typical "American diet," signs of cadmium poisoning start to appear at around age 50. For Mexican Americans in my hometown, it is typically about 40. Note that there is a big difference between a maintenance zinc dosage (RDA) and a therapeutic zinc dosage, which would be MUCH higher.

Q #1c: I find all this very interesting; all the different perspectives on the cause and ways to fix this. Our son sees a Homeopathy practicioner who says Gaps is not needed and that he can reverse this damage via Homeopathy. I've also read this. I'm still considering doing Gaps in addition to the Homeopathy, but then that raises the question to me as to why are people reacting to gluten. Perhaps it's not the wheat/gluten itself, but something that has changed; environmental/chemical, something causing guy dysbosis, etc. . . .

A #1c: I think you hit the nail on the head. I first made the connection when a good friend was telling me about her sensitivity to gluten, and how she was changing her diet. The diet that she described is very similar to mine, but my focus is on minimizing ingestion of cadmium. As it turns out, the product from wheat processing that contains the highest cadmium concentration is WHEAT GLUTEN! Wheat gluten is added to many food products, so when you eat something with added wheat gluten, you are getting a higher dosage than you would otherwise. Take flour tortillas, for example. Some tend to dry out and get brittle, and generally, people like the ones that stay soft and pliable. The two main ingredients that are added to keep them soft and pliable are wheat gluten and lard. People love their breakfast tacos on flour tortillas in my hometown.

COMMENT #2

Thank you, Dr. X! You stressed how important glutathione is, and I agree 110%. Glutathione, the master antioxidant, is like hemoglobin in that it goes back and forth between the oxidized and reduced states. One of the causes of low levels of glutathione is CADMIUM, a carcinogenic heavy metal that enters our food chain as a contaminant in phosphate fertilizers that are spread on the fields where our food is grown (including sewage sludge used in organic farming). While oxidants temporarily inactivate glutathione, cadmium is chelated by two glutathione molecules that escort it out of the body via the biliary system and intestinal tract. Therefore, cadmium permanently eliminates glutathione from the body. Unfortunately, cadmium is generally found in relatively high concentrations in foods that grow in or near the ground—INCLUDING GREEN LEAFY VEGETABLES. Foods that grow on long vines, tall stalks, and on trees are generally low in cadmium. I know that we need folate, but until we clean up our act (and our fields), the green leafy veggies may be doing more harm than good. Cadmium typically has a 30-year half-life in our bodies, compared to 78 days for zinc. It is in the same column in the periodic table as zinc, and competes with zinc in our bodies. It accumulates primarily in the liver, kidneys, lungs, pancreas, and bones, and to a lesser extent in the thyroid, prostate and other vital organs. It typically goes unnoticed because it doesn't cause problems until it reaches organ-specific threshold concentrations. As it accumulates beyond those concentrations, it causes the organs to cease functioning properly, and eventually leads to cancer. Zinc, on the other hand is essential for a healthy immune system, essential for proper brain function, essential for healing, and is found in every strand of DNA in our bodies. The accumulation of cadmium (i.e., cadmium poisoning) results in the pushing out of zinc from our bodies (i.e., zinc deficiency). The bottom line: beware of those green smoothies!!!

Q #2a: I liked your post, so what do you suggest for someone who has just been diagnosed with the A1298c mutation heterozygous and also has a high level of cadmium 0.001?

A #2a: I can tell you all about cadmium, but first, I found the following quote regarding A1298C mutation on Dr. X's website: "My current stance on the heterozygous MTHFR A1298C mutation is that it is very common and does not seem to pose too much concern unless there are other methylation or cytochrome mutations present. Obviously, if one leads a lifestyle which is unhealthy (smoking, high stress, toxic exposures) and consumes an unhealthy diet (refined carbs, processed meats, saturated fats), then having a heterozygous A1298C mutation may contribute to cardiovascular disease, depression, fibromyalgia and others." My guess is that the mutation is common because it is caused by cadmium. Anyway, in a nutshell, I would suggest that you do the following: (1) avoid cadmium in every way possible—it is in the food you eat, the water and other beverages you drink, and the air you breathe (i.e., avoid all forms of wheat and rice [breads, pastas, wheat cereals, etc.], mushrooms, beets, lettuce, spinach, organ meats, shrimp, oysters, and all shellfish, chocolate, coffee, sugar, soft drinks, unfiltered water [RO and activated carbon filters are good], and stay away from cigarette smoke); (2) take zinc to compete with cadmium and replace the zinc that has been pushed out by cadmium over the years—the 15 mg/day RDA is ridiculously low—ten (or more) times that is more reasonable, as long as you don't get close to the 800 mg/day toxic threshold (per U of Iowa Dept of Nutrition); (3) take vitamins and minerals to compensate for things you are removing from your diet (e.g., a magnesium supplement to compensate for the reduced magnesium in chlorophyll); (4) take vitamins and minerals that chelate cadmium (e.g., vitamins A, B_1, C); (5) FLUSH cadmium out of your system by opening up your capillaries (with vitamin B_3—niacin) and eating at least five pieces of fruit (from trees) per day (cadmium is mostly removed from the body through bowel movements); (6) for long-term zinc supplementation, evaluate your copper intake and supplement with copper (higher zinc intake will generate metallothioneins that will chelate copper, cadmium, and zinc, in that preferential order); (7) take vitamin E, because with the mobilization of cadmium, you may experience sciatic nerve pain, and vitamin E sooths and lubricates nerves to keep lesions from developing; (8) take vitamin D_3 to help with assimilation of calcium, because cadmium poisoning causes loss of bone mass; (9) take vitamin B_{12}, which inhibits accumulation of cadmium in the kidneys; 10) take Vitamin B_6 because cadmium usually induces anemia, and vitamin B_6 is important in the generation of hemoglobin; and (11) read all labels on food you buy at the grocery store, and never buy anything with phosphates (the same goes for your pet foods). Multiple vitamins may contain all this stuff and more, but they are in woefully low quantities. And after doing a little homework on iodine, you may want to make sure you're not iodine deficient, because in addition to being involved in all the thyroid hormone issues, it is key in the vital role that apoptosis (scheduled cell death) plays in keeping us healthy. I think that if you take care of the cadmium, your body will take care of the rest, including the A1298C mutation.

Response: Thank you so much for your in-depth reply, I appreciate it.

Reply: I should have mentioned a couple of more things: ALWAYS TAKE ZINC WITH A MEAL, AND MAKE SURE YOUR ZINC IS FREE OF PHOSPHATE FILLERS. Also, spread the word. People need to know about the cadmium issue. Take care.

Response: Definitely spreading the word about Cadmium, thank you, I'm surprised my functional medicine doctor, never suggested anything though, apart from pointing out it was high!

Q #2b: Besides the Summit info, your cadmium poisoning does make sense, lots of sense. I just took all of your great info on a piece of paper. Please, which would be the best test for heavy metal contamination and if I will do IV chelation you think that may help? I struggle to stay functional these days. After many years of symptoms, seeing 7 different doctors that diagnosed me with Hashimoto's and Grave's I found out last November that I have Celiac. Now I am off grains, dairy and wheat, also having lots of food allergies due to the leaky gut. I have to limit my fruit intake and I am super sensitive to any supplement that I take. Which type of Zn should I consider? Please, I really appreciate your help. Thank you and have a lovely summer!

A #2b: First of all, let me say that the initials after my name are PhD, not MD, and I'm sorry to hear that you are having difficulties. Let me try to answer your questions:

(Q1) Which would be the best test for heavy metal contamination? (A1) Hair, nail, blood, and urine samples are often analyzed to assess heavy metals in the body. Because heavy metals tend to go into the tissues of specific organs, they don't stay in the blood or urine for very long, and those analyses would only tell you about your most recent exposure. Hair and nail samples are usually analyzed for longer-term exposure. However, all results are subject to interpretation, and none of these analyses can accurately indicate the total body burden, because the heavy metals started accumulating with the first solid food we eat as infants . . . If you just want to know if heavy metals are present—I'd go with hair and nails.

(Q2) If I do IV chelation you think that may help? (A2) I have heard of an IV chelation treatment where the patient credits it for saving his life, but I have also heard of concerns regarding possible adverse effects on the kidneys. Although some chelating agents are better at removing a particular heavy metal than others, chelating agents, in general, are not usually specific to one metal. Since the metal or metals we want to remove may have characteristics similar to those that we require to stay alive (e.g., cadmium versus zinc and copper), it can be a little tricky keeping things in balance during the treatment. It sounds as though you feel you are running out of options; therefore, I recommend that you talk to someone who has had success in treating patients with IV chelation. It is definitely an option that should be considered. Also, talk to their patients, if possible. Ultimately, when considering putting a chelating agent in your body, choose the right doctor. Close monitoring by competent, experienced personnel is a must.

(Q3) Which type of Zn should I consider? (A3) Zinc is available as gluconate and picolinate. The most common form of zinc sold is zinc gluconate. It is a lot cheaper than the picolinate, which is said to have a slightly higher absorption efficiency. I take zinc gluconate, Mason brand, in 100 mg tablets. Whatever you do, ALWAYS TAKE ZINC WITH A MEAL, AND MAKE SURE YOUR ZINC IS FREE OF PHOSPHATE FILLERS. I get my zinc from drugstore.com, but any zinc gluconate that you may find at Walgreen's, CVS, Walmart, etc. should be fine, as long as it is phosphate-free. I hope this helps, and best of luck!

Response: What excellent advice thank you!! I'm just about to start a course of Zeolite (pure powder) to commence heavy metal detoxification, any comments or recommendations? Thank you again, your information is a critical adjunct to this session in particular.

Reply: My only suggestion is to make sure you know what you're putting in your body. Zeolites are often used in water treating, for example, to remove unwanted contaminants (e.g., heavy metals). It is important to know that the zeolite you will be using isn't already loaded with the same heavy metals you are trying to remove. The same thing goes for any natural chelating agent (e.g., cinnamon, cilantro) that may have been grown in cadmium-rich soils. If the zeolite or chelating agent is already loaded with heavy metals, changes in the conditions that surround them (e.g., acidic environment of the stomach) can cause the heavy metals to be released inside your body (counterproductive!!!). Good luck with your detox program!

Response: Wow! Thank you again, there is, as always, so much more to consider. I will definitely do more research!

COMMENT #3

Thank you Dr. X for touching on so many different interrelated issues. One key message that you shared was the need for balance. But what causes the imbalances to develop? I would like to suggest that one pervasive contributor to many hormonal imbalances is our chronic exposure to CADMIUM, a carcinogenic heavy metal that is in our food supply. It is a contaminant in the phosphate fertilizers used in agriculture. Once it is in our bodies and it reaches organ-specific threshold concentrations, the organs cease to function properly. In the pancreas, for example, the beta cells of the Islets of Langerhans cease to release insulin into the bloodstream in response to changes in glucose levels (Type 2 diabetes). You mentioned Type 3 diabetes (Alzheimer's disease). The brain is one of the largest reservoirs of zinc in the body, but the brains of Alzheimer's patients tend to be zinc deficient. Cadmium and zinc have similar chemical characteristics, and they compete with each other within our bodies. Cadmium tends to concentrate primarily in the liver, pancreas, kidneys, lungs, and bones, but it also accumulates to a lesser degree in the thyroid, prostate, and other vital organs. Because of its long biological half-life (30 years compared to 78 days for zinc), it pushes zinc out of the body, and the body responds by robbing the brain of zinc. Initial symptoms of occasional memory loss could lead to Alzheimer's disease. You mentioned testosterone imbalance. Testosterone chelates cadmium for removal from the body, as does glutathione. The daily dosing of cadmium results in the depletion of these two compound that are vital for our health. Furthermore, cadmium has been linked to prostate cancer, pancreatic cancer, liver cancer, kidney cancer, lung cancer, etc., etc., etc.—talk about an added stress on the body! Cadmium is found in high concentrations in high-carb foods made from wheat and rice, but it is also present in coffee, chocolate, mushrooms, and, of course, SUGAR. Approximately 56% of the sugar production in the US comes from sugar beets. Beets, in general, are so efficient at absorbing cadmium from their surroundings, that they are used in the phytoremediation of cadmium-contaminated soils. I could go on . . . . I think we are singing the same song, but have different perspectives. I see the imbalances that you spoke of as being induced by cadmium poisoning. I realize that cadmium is not the only toxic heavy metal in our environment, it just happens to have the greatest impact because it is associated with phosphates, and phosphates are everywhere—just check the labels of the products you buy at the grocery store. Again, thank you Dr. X. Interesting discussion!

COMMENT #4

Thank you Dr. X for spending some time on the importance of zinc. You mentioned pyrrole disorder as being responsible for zinc deficiency, but here in the US, chronic exposure to cadmium is likely the primary reason for zinc deficiency. Cadmium is a contaminant in the phosphate fertilizers used to grow the food we put on the table. (I probably sound like a broken record.) Cadmium and zinc are in the same column of the periodic table and, therefore, have similar chemical characteristics and compete within our bodies. The difference is that zinc is required for a healthy immune system, healing, proper brain function, proper thyroid function, and is involved in hundreds of enzymatic reactions; while cadmium, on the other hand, is a carcinogenic heavy metal that accumulates until it builds up to organ-specific threshold concentrations, above which it interferes with the function of those organs (e.g., production and release of insulin). Cadmium concentrates primarily in the pancreas, liver, kidneys, lungs, and bones, and to a lesser extent in the thyroid, prostate, and other vital organs. With its 30-year biological half-life, compared to the 78-day biological half-life of zinc, it slowly but surely pushes zinc out of the body, causing zinc deficiency and a compromised immune system. The results are devastating, and include maladies like Type 2 diabetes, kidney and liver disease, gout, Alzheimer's disease, adverse impacts on blood pressure, plaque formation in the circulatory system, and of course, cancer of the pancreas, liver, kidneys, and lungs. I try to minimize my cadmium intake while supplementing with zinc and other vitamins and minerals, all of which in one way or another are involved in protecting against assimilation of cadmium or chelating and removing cadmium from the body. IN GENERAL, I eat things that grow on trees or long vines or stalks and stay away from things that grow on or in the ground. So we are in agreement about staying away from peanuts and peanut butter, but for different reasons. And as for sunflower butter, unfortunately, sunflower seeds are high in cadmium, so I'll pass on that one too.

COMMENT #5

Thank you, Dr. X, for a very interesting, informative, and entertaining talk. I have three questions, though. First, are there any concerns regarding heavy metals in desiccated thyroid? I remember in the old days diabetics feared that if they were put on porcine insulin, they would never get off it, and that was probably due to cadmium, which was likely the original cause of their problem. My second question is related to the underlying cause(s) of the imbalances that you discussed and are treating. Since cadmium also accumulates in the thyroid and drives out zinc in the process, could cadmium be part of the cause of the imbalances? Cadmium is a carcinogenic heavy metal that is a contaminant in the phosphate fertilizers used to grow the crops we ingest, and it competes with zinc in our bodies. Third question: Could zinc supplementation assist in treating an underlying cause of the hormonal imbalances you discussed? (Several of the other speakers stressed how important zinc is for the thyroid, the immune system, etc.)

COMMENT #6

Thank you, Dr. X, for an informative discussion on prostate cancer prevention. Your comments on gamma versus "dl" synthetic alpha tocopherol was an eye opener for me! As I recall, you only mentioned cadmium in passing one time as a potential cause of prostate cancer. I suggest that this topic deserves much more attention, since, in my opinion, chronic exposure to cadmium is a leading cause of prostate cancer. Your comment that the presence of "Gleason 6s" was an indication that the body was "cancering" was interesting, because I have long contended that the spread of cancer in the body was usually an indication that cadmium has accumulated in various organs in the body and is initiating cancer in several locations at the same time. Cadmium, a carcinogenic heavy metal, endocrine disruptor, and estrogen emulator, is ubiquitous in our food supply. It is a contaminant in the phosphate fertilizers used to grow most crops that we eat. In the periodic table, cadmium and mercury are directly below zinc, so they have similar chemical characteristics. Zinc is essential for a healthy immune system, essential for healing, essential for proper brain function, and it is found in every cell of our bodies. Cadmium, on the other hand, is one of only three heavy metals (up to atomic number 92) that is not used by the body. The other two are lead and mercury. Because cadmium has a biological half-life of 30 years, compared to the 78-day half-life of zinc, it slowly drives out the zinc and accumulates primarily in the pancreas, kidneys, liver, lungs, and bones, but also to a lesser degree in the thyroid, prostate, adrenals, and other vital organs. For people with a typical American diet, the accumulation of cadmium goes without notice until around age 50, when it begins to interfere with the function of specific organs (e.g., pancreas—type 2 diabetes). Soon thereafter, cancer appears. For Hispanics, and more specifically Mexican Americans, this begins about 10 years sooner, not due to genetic factors, but rather due to cultural and dietary customs. The focus in my diet is to eat low-cadmium foods, and stay as far away from high-cadmium foods (e.g., sugar, wheat products, rice products, mushrooms, beets, shellfish [e.g., shrimp and oysters], all products containing organ meats, soft drinks, chocolate, coffee, lettuce and spinach, and all processed foods and supplements containing phosphates [e.g., bacon, evaporated milk, cereals, puddings, and soft drinks—phosphoric acid is hydrogen phosphate]). You have to look at the labels on all products on the grocery store shelves. My general rule of thumb is that if it grows in the ground or on the ground, it is likely high in cadmium, while if it grows on a tree, long vine, or tall stalk, it is likely low in cadmium. With regard to supplements, zinc is key. The 15-mg RDA is woefully inadequate. The U of Iowa Department of Nutrition states that 800 mg of zinc per day is toxic. I have been taking 200 mg/day for the last ten years. Elevated dosages of zinc result in the synthesis of more metallothioneins, proteins that preferentially bind to copper, cadmium, and zinc, enhancing the removal of all three metals from the body. (Yes, I am also taking copper supplements.) I sincerely hope that you will look into cadmium poisoning, because it likely plays a much greater role in the development of prostate cancer (and MANY other cancers) than is generally acknowledged. Again, thank you for an informative talk, and I will make an immediate adjustment with respect to my tocopherol supplement.

COMMENT #7

Dr. X, I loved your presentation. It was VERY informative. You mentioned heavy metals were a problem, but what can you tell us about cadmium, specifically? It is a carcinogenic heavy metal that accumulates primarily in the pancreas, kidneys, liver, lungs, and bones, but also in the thyroid, prostate, and other vital organs to a lesser degree. It causes the beta cells in the pancreas to stop responding to changes in glucose in the bloodstream (Type 2 diabetes), and it has an average biological half-life of 30 years. On the periodic table, it is located directly beneath zinc, so it competes with zinc, which has only a 78-day biological half-life. That is why zinc deficiencies are more common among older people. Zinc is essential for healing, a healthy immune system, brain function. It is involved in 300 enzymatic reactions and if found in every strand of DNA in our bodies. Zinc deficiency generally means compromised immune system. Cadmium is a contaminant in the phosphate fertilizers that are used to grow the crops we eat. Some crops accumulate cadmium more efficiently than others. Some of those that accumulate cadmium more efficiently include wheat, rice, mushrooms, and beets. In general, if it grows on the ground or in the ground, it is likely high in cadmium, while if it grows on a tree, tall stalk, or long vine, it is probably low in cadmium. BTW, 56% of the US sugar production comes from sugar beets, and beets are used to phytoremediate cadmium-contaminated soils, so most products that contain sugar are contaminated with cadmium. Similarly, most products that contain phosphates are likely to contain cadmium. Check the labels of the products on your grocery store shelves. You will find phosphate additives in cereals, puddings, evaporated milk, deli meats, bacon . . . and soft drinks (phosphoric acid is hydrogen phosphate). Cadmium is also found in chocolate, coffee, shellfish (e.g., shrimp and oysters), and organ meats (e.g., liver, sausages containing organ meats). In wheat and rice, the cadmium concentrates inside the grain, while zinc concentrates on the outside. Simultaneous ingestion of zinc and cadmium reduces the assimilation of the cadmium. That is why whole wheat bread and brown rice are better for you than white bread and white rice. Cadmium is a silent killer that is off the radar screen of the medical profession, while we are all experiencing chronic exposure to cadmium. It has been linked to countless diseases (e.g., diabetes, kidney failure, and cancers of the breast, stomach, kidneys, pancreas, lungs, liver, to name a few), and zinc is key to counter the deleterious impact of cadmium. The current RDA for zinc is 15 mg, woefully inadequate to compete with the amount of cadmium in a typical American diet. Supplements of 30, 50, and 100 of zinc gluconate, for example, can be found in drug stores and on the Internet. However, make certain that they don't contain phosphate fillers, or you may be "shooting yourself in the foot" due to the cadmium that would accompany the phosphate. Our food supply is complex, and we all need to research the possible impacts of known contaminants and potential supplements. Again, thank you, Dr. X for sharing your insights into the many nutrient/vitamin-related topics you covered in your presentation.

COMMENT #8

Thank you, Dr. X, for a VERY interesting discussion on many factors that can affect the pancreas and cases of diabetes that result from factors that are difficult to identify. You mentioned that your patients were individuals who were "eating perfectly," indicating that their diets were "perfect" and beyond suspicion as possible causes of their diabetes. However, I am curious how you define a perfect diet. I used to think I had a good diet with lots of lettuce, spinach, mushrooms, seafood that occasionally included shrimp, whole grain bread, etc., but I later learned that these foods are high in cadmium. And I wonder if some of the people that you have as patients, the ones with the perfect diets, may actually have diets with relatively high cadmium content. Cadmium is a carcinogenic heavy metal that is involved in numerous autoimmune diseases, including osteoporosis and multiple sclerosis. Cadmium and mercury are directly beneath zinc in the periodic table, so that they have similar chemical characteristics. Also, cadmium accumulates primarily in the pancreas, kidneys, liver, lungs, and bones, and to a lesser degree in vital organs such as the thyroid and prostate. Since zinc is in every strand of DNA in the body, and cadmium is competing with it, is it possible the some of the autoimmune response in the pancreas is due to cadmium being incorporated in the pancreatic tissues? Cadmium also has some of the other characteristics that you mentioned in your presentation. It is an endocrine disruptor. It is generally found in high concentrations in products containing gluten. It has been linked to the incidence of both hypothyroidism and diabetes. It is present in relatively high concentrations in wheat and rice. It induces oxidative stress and changes in the 24-hour pattern of the pituitary circadian clock. Should cadmium poisoning be added to the list of factors that may be responsible for the symptoms in those hard-to-diagnose diabetes cases? Again, thank you for a very informative discussion.

COMMENT #9

Thank you, Dr. X, for your informative presentation/discussion. I would like to add a couple of comments on what, by my tally, were Myths 3, 5, and 7. Myth #3: Type 2 diabetes is caused by eating too much sugar and being overweight. Certainly, high sugar consumption and being overweight do not help, but something that is being overlooked here is the cadmium that accompanies the sugar. Cadmium is a carcinogenic, heavy-metal contaminant in phosphate fertilizers that are used to grow crops that we consume. It concentrates primarily in the pancreas, liver, lungs, kidneys, and bones, and to a lesser degree in the thyroid, prostate, and other vital organs. In the pancreas, it causes the beta cells to stop responding to changes in blood glucose levels. It also contributes to insulin resistance. In the US, 56% of the sugar production comes from sugar beets. However, beets are very efficient at removing cadmium from soil, so much so that they are used to phytoremediate soils that are contaminated with cadmium. Hence, high sugar intake is directly related to high cadmium intake. Myth#5: Once you are on insulin, you're on insulin forever. This is likely a carryover from the old days when insulin for treating human diabetes was extracted from porcine pancreas. Just as cadmium accumulates in the human pancreas, it accumulates in the pancreas of pigs. No special measures were taken to remove cadmium in the processing of insulin, so that with every injection of insulin, the patient was also receiving a dose of cadmium, making it virtually impossible for the pancreas to recover from cadmium poisoning. Myth #7: Diabetes will go away if you just get off sugar and start exercising. Certainly, eliminating sugar from the diet will reduce cadmium consumption, and exercise will help to mobilize and expel cadmium from the body. However, sugar is not the only source of cadmium. A few of the high-cadmium foods and beverages that I have eliminated from my diet include the following: wheat and wheat products, rice and rice products, sugar, chocolate, coffee, mushrooms, beets and most root vegetables, soft drinks, processed foods containing phosphates, lettuce, and spinach. My general rule of thumb is the following: If it grows in the ground or on the ground, it is likely to be high in cadmium; while if it grows on a tree, tall stalk, or long vine, it is likely to be low in cadmium. The other key in addressing cadmium in our diets is zinc supplementation. Cadmium is directly beneath zinc in the periodic table. The two metals, therefore, have similar chemical characteristics and compete with each other within our bodies. Cadmium assimilation is reduced when zinc is present; however, its biological half-life is about 78 days, compared to 30 YEARS for cadmium. The current RDA of 15 mg/day is woefully inadequate. Zinc supplements of 30, 50, and 100 mg are available in drug stores and on the Internet. Just make sure that they contain no phosphate additives. Long-term, the changes in diet and zinc supplementation may call for additional adjustments, such as magnesium and/or copper supplementation, or growing your own vegetables in a cadmium-free environment. I hope this helps put things in perspective, and again, thank you for an excellent discussion on diabetes myths.

COMMENT #10

Dr. X, much of your presentation is on the psychology of diabetes treatment. Without buy-in from the patient, it doesn't matter what you tell them they need to do, it's not going to happen. Also, you hit a couple of nails on the head regarding cultural issues. I am Hispanic, and I can tell you that most Hispanics in south Texas love their breakfast tacos on those delicious flour tortillas. And especially in Corpus Christi, who can resist shrimp and oyster platters, when the seafood is delicious, abundant, and affordable? The main reason diabetes and cancer run in families is not the genetics, it's the eating habits and the choices we make in our diets. We usually eat the same kinds of foods that we grew up with. When you get your patients to drop things from their diets, one item at a time, consider getting them to drop flour tortillas and shellfish, and here is why: Both are loaded with cadmium, a carcinogenic, heavy-metal contaminant in the phosphate fertilizers used in crop production. Cadmium tends to accumulate in the pancreas, liver, kidneys, lungs, and bones, and to a lesser extent in the thyroid, prostate, and other vital organs. It causes the beta cells of the pancreas to stop responding to changes in glucose levels in the blood, and it increases insulin resistance in muscle and fat tissues. Wheat and rice are efficient at absorbing cadmium out of the soil, so wheat flour contains cadmium. However, because we all like the tortillas that stay soft and pliable, the flour used to make them is typically spiked with lard and wheat gluten. Of all wheat products, wheat gluten has the highest cadmium concentration. As for the shellfish, shellfish from the Gulf of Mexico have cadmium concentrations that are about 1,000 times the concentration in a cut of beef or pork or a piece of chicken (excluding organ meats). This is about 10 times that of shellfish in the Pacific or Atlantic Oceans. Runoff from the fields in the bread basket of our country plus countless discharges from sewage treatment plants flow into the Mississippi River, which flushes into the Gulf of Mexico. The general flow of water in the Gulf along the coast is from east to west, so that the cadmium-laden water is directed toward your location. A single quarter-pound meal containing shrimp or oysters has about the same amount of cadmium as three years' of meals, each containing a quarter-pound of steak, pork chops, or chicken. An additional suggestion: consider increasing patients' zinc intake with phosphate-free supplements. Cadmium is directly below zinc in the periodic table, so it competes with zinc within the body, and the current RDA is woefully inadequate. The problem is that zinc has a biological half-life of about 78 days, compared to 30 YEARS for cadmium. For people with a typical American diet, symptoms of cadmium poisoning (which includes Type 2 diabetes, kidney failure, etc.) start to show up at around age 50. For Hispanics, it's more like age 40. This is just a small part of the cadmium/zinc story, but I thought you might want to know, and that your patients might benefit. Keep up the GREAT work.

COMMENT #11

Thank you, Dr. X, for your presentation on Hashimoto's and hypothyroidism. I think your discussion is very relevant for individuals suffering from diabetes, in particular your comments on various diagnostic tests and toxins such as fluoride. I especially appreciate your digging down past symptoms to get at the "Root Causes" of apparent thyroid problems. I similarly try to identify underlying causes of exhibited symptoms. You identified the following five root causes of Hashimoto's disease: food sensitivities, nutrient depletions, impaired ability to handle stress, impaired ability to detoxify, and infections (inside/outside gut). Thinking on a still more fundamental level, I think that three elements (cadmium, zinc, and iodine) are the root causes of your root causes— specifically: cadmium poisoning, zinc deficiency, and iodine deficiency. Cadmium is a carcinogenic, heavy-metal contaminant in phosphate fertilizers. It is in our food supply, and when ingested, it accumulates primarily in the pancreas, liver, kidneys, lungs, and bones, and to a lesser degree in the thyroid, prostate, adrenal glands, and other vital organs. Cadmium typically accumulates until it reaches an organ-specific threshold concentration, at which time it interferes with the function of the organ. Later it causes cancer. Cadmium induces insulin resistance in muscle and adipose tissues and makes the beta cells of the pancreas unresponsive to changes in glucose concentrations in the blood (Type 2 diabetes). The human body uses every element in the periodic table up to element 92, except for three metals: lead, cadmium, and mercury. Many autoimmune diseases are actually the body's attempt to rid itself of these toxic metals. Osteoporosis and multiple sclerosis, for example, have been linked to cadmium. The following are a few examples of how cadmium, zinc, and iodine are related to the five root causes you cited.

FOOD SENSITIVITIES

Cadmium binds strongly to wheat gluten. It is the wheat product with the highest concentration of cadmium. Other high-cadmium foods are commonly associated with food allergies.

NUTRIENT DEPLETIONS

Because of the relative magnitudes of the half-lives of cadmium and zinc (30 years compared to 78 days), chronic exposure to cadmium in our diets drives out zinc, resulting in zinc deficiency. Halides compete within our bodies, so that increased fluoride, bromide, chloride exposure results in reduced iodine assimilation. It is estimated that over 90% of the population is iodine deficient, and iodine is essential for proper thyroid function.

IMPAIRED ABILITY TO HANDLE STRESS

Cadmium affects adrenal gland function and cortisol production. Zinc deficiency induces oxidative stress.

IMPAIRED ABILITY TO DETOXIFY

Cadmium inhibits liver function and can eventually cause liver cancer.

INFECTIONS (inside/outside gut)

Zinc is an essential part of a healthy immune system. Cadmium poisoning, accompanied by zinc deficiency, results in a compromised immune system and increased susceptibility to infections.

Again, thank you for sharing your insights into the complex subject of Hashimoto's disease and hypothyroidism.

COMMENT #12

Thank you Dr. X for an interesting discussion on the interrelationships among various hormones. I particularly found your comments on "estrogen pollution" interesting. You indicated that the rise in estrogen levels in young girls today is due to things like meats (and especially the fatty tissues) from Concentrated Animal Feeding Operations (CAFOs), where cows are injected with six different hormones, and eating too much sugar. I would like to elaborate on the sugar issue and suggest that the problem is much more widespread. Sugar production from beets accounts for approximately 56% of the sugar consumed in the US. Beets are very efficient at absorbing cadmium, a carcinogenic heavy metal, out of the soil. Unfortunately, cadmium is a contaminant in the phosphate fertilizers used in crop production, so that it is ubiquitous in our food supply. Cadmium accumulates primarily in the pancreas, kidneys, liver, lungs, and bones, and to a lesser extent in the thyroid, prostate, adrenal glands, and other vital organs. Cadmium is an endocrine disruptor and estrogen emulator, so that the source of something that acts like estrogen is coming from much more than just sugar. High concentrations can be found, for example, in all wheat and rice products, mushrooms, chocolate, coffee, soft drinks, shellfish, deli meats and sausages containing organ meats, and processed foods containing phosphate additives (e.g., puddings, cheese, bacon, evaporated milk—you HAVE to read the ingredients listed on the labels). In general, things that grows in or on the ground is high in cadmium, while things that grow on trees, tall stalks, and long vines are low in cadmium. One of the big messages from your discussion was that we all need to minimize stress in our lives. Because of the cadmium contamination of our food supply, I suggest that there are AT LEAST two additional things that we should all consider, and they are (1) adjust our diets to minimize cadmium consumption, and (2) augment our zinc intake with a phosphate-free zinc supplement. Cadmium is located directly beneath zinc in the periodic table, so the two metals have similar chemical characteristics, and they compete with each other within our bodies. However, cadmium has a 30-year biological half-life, while that of zinc is only approximately 78 days. Cadmium is not used by the body, while zinc is involved in over 300 enzymatic reactions, it is essential for proper brain function, it is essential for healing, it is essential for a healthy immune system, and it is found in every strand of DNA in our bodies. Living in an environment where our food supply is laden with cadmium, we move closer and closer to zinc deficiency condition unless we take strong measures to avoid it. Additional supplementation may be called for (e.g., magnesium), depending on what items are eliminated from the diet. I hope that this comment provides a glimpse of the extent of the problem. Again, thank you for sharing your experiences and perspectives. It is greatly appreciated.

COMMENT #13

Thanks, Dr. X, for a VERY interesting discussion on the adrenals and related hormones. One thing I would like to ask about that was not covered in your discussion is the impact of heavy metals. Specifically, cadmium, a carcinogenic heavy-metal contaminant in phosphate fertilizers, is in our food supply. It accumulates primarily in the pancreas, kidneys, liver, lungs, and bones, and to a lesser extent in the thyroid, prostate, adrenal glands, and other vital organs. Cadmium is an endocrine disruptor, and it has an impact on adrenal function and cortisol production. At the end of your discussion, you mentioned coffee and chocolate. Both are high in cadmium. There are many other foods and beverages that are high in cadmium. I checked on the Internet, and found a food list from your book, Adrenal Reset Diet. Other foods that I would stay away from include shrimp, oysters, mushrooms, and beets, strictly based on their cadmium content. Shellfish, for example, contain 100 or 1,000 times the cadmium concentration compared to beef, pork, or chicken (excluding organ meats), depending on whether the shellfish come from the Pacific/Atlantic Oceans or the Gulf of Mexico, respectively. Similarly, beets are VERY efficient at extracting cadmium from the soil, so much so that they are used to phytoremediate cadmium-contaminated soils. I loved your presentation, but personally, I would have to make a few adjustments to the list of foods presented in your book. Again, many thanks.

COMMENT #14

Thank you, Dr. X, for a great discussion on hormones, body types, the importance of bile to the liver and gallbladder, applying acupressure to organs and glands, diet, and so much more. I am a firm believer that cadmium, a heavy-metal contaminant contained in the phosphate fertilizers used in crop production, is a major contributor to many if not most of the ailments plaguing today's society. Cadmium is an endocrine disruptor and estrogen emulator. It accumulates primarily in the pancreas, liver, kidneys, lungs, and bones, and to a lesser degree in the thyroid, prostate, adrenals, and other vital organs. It directly affects insulin production (impairs pancreatic beta cell function) and contributes to insulin resistance throughout the body. I have theorized that the disease that develops first (e.g., diabetes versus kidney failure) depends on where the cadmium accumulates fastest. Your discussion on body types reinforces my suspicion. Oftentimes people have characteristics of more than one of the body types you discussed, probably because cadmium has reached critical concentrations in more than one of the vital organs that influence those body types. I think that a discussion of heavy metals, particularly cadmium and zinc, would have been appropriate. Since cadmium is located directly beneath zinc in the periodic table, they have similar chemical characteristics, and they compete with each other within our bodies. However, because cadmium has a 30-year biological half-life, compared to 78 days for zinc, it slowly accumulates, pushing zinc out of the body and leading to zinc deficiency. Zinc is essential for a healthy immune system, essential for healing, essential for proper brain function, involved in over 300 enzymatic reactions, and contained in every strand of DNA in the body. The concentration of zinc in the placenta is about 1,000 times the concentration in any other tissue in a woman's body. Many women's body types change after a pregnancy, and I would speculate that is due to the accumulation of cadmium and depletion of zinc in certain vital organs. At the end of your presentation, you stated that diabetes is not a disease—it is a symptom—and we need to find the root cause. In today's environment, I contend that cadmium is that root cause! Again, thank you for an excellent discussion. It is greatly appreciated.

COMMENT #15

Thank you, Dr. X, for an interesting and informative discussion that, I am sure, will guide people in the right direction with regard to their diets. However, I think that perhaps we need to dig a little deeper in the search for the root cause of type 2 diabetes. You stated that the causes were (1) sugar, and (2) insufficient fiber. What is it in sugar that makes it so toxic? In the US, 56% of the sugar production comes from sugar beets, and beets in general are loaded with cadmium. Cadmium is a carcinogenic heavy metal that accumulates primarily in the pancreas, liver, kidneys, lungs, and bones, and to a lesser extent in the thyroid, prostate, adrenals, and other vital organs. It occurs naturally in phosphate deposits that are mined and used as fertilizers in crop production. So, cadmium is in our food supply, with some crops having higher cadmium concentrations than others. Beets are so efficient at absorbing cadmium from the soil that they are used in the phytoremediation of cadmium-contaminated soils. High cadmium foods and beverages include wheat and rice products, chocolate, coffee, soft drinks, mushrooms, any product containing organ meats (e.g., sausages and frankfurters), shellfish (e.g., shrimp and oysters), beets, lettuce, spinach and MANY processed foods. So, I agree with you when you said that obesity was not the cause of diabetes, and that processed foods were a big part of the problem. Thin people can suffer from cadmium poisoning too. We all need to look at the labels of the products on our grocery store shelves. If you see "phosphate," it is likely contaminated with cadmium. They are adding phosphates to many foods these days (e.g., bacon, deli meats, cereals, evaporated milk, pudding, and even vitamin supplements). The key is to go "LOW CADMIUM," and eliminating sugar from our diets will help tremendously (a GREAT FIRST STEP), but so will eliminating wheat, organ meats, shellfish, and processed foods containing phosphate additives. Again, thank you for an excellent presentation.

Q #15a: Arturo, Joseph Pizzomo, ND is coming out with a book next year on the topic of heavy metals, pesticides, herbicides, etc. correlating with type 2 diabetes. It's titled *The Detox Cure*.

Curious as to where I can learn more about what you're sharing here. Also, if I eat organic beets, would that lessen the cadmium exposure?

A #15a: Hi there. I started doing Internet research on this topic about 10 years ago, since I was experiencing severe bone pain at that time. I saw my bone pain starting to go away after about two weeks by changing my diet and taking zinc supplements (phosphate free). I kept reading and added other supplements to compensate for things that I had eliminated from my diet (e.g., magnesium), to help chelate and remove cadmium from my body (e.g., vitamins A, B_1, C), and to help open blood vessels to flush the toxins out (vitamin B_3—niacin). Eventually, I realized that all my relatives and several friends had died of cadmium poisoning. They all exhibited multiple symptoms of cadmium poisoning, most with diabetes, and all with the final symptom—some sort of cancer. All the cancers were linked to cadmium. I don't know of any single document that explains things, but I try to give a thumbnail sketch of the problem. As for organic beets, "organic" doesn't guarantee anything with regard to heavy metals. Sewage sludge is an accepted and widely used fertilizer in organic farming. You may not have all the pesticides and herbicides, but you could still get a dose of heavy metals. I hope this helps.

Q #15b: I hadn't thought about organic foods being contaminated with heavy metals [sigh...]

I recently listened to a 3-hour lecture by Nicholas Gonzalez, M.D. in 2010 on YouTube, Titled "Dr. Nicholas Gonzalez – What Should I Eat?" (Part 1 and Part 2). In it he discusses the history of the treatment he used to treat and prevent chronic health conditions including cancer using individualized diet, supplements, enzymes, and detoxification.

When he was interviewed by Dr. Mercola in 2011—(do a search on Dr. Mercola: Kelley Treatment: The Cancer Treatment So Successful—Traditional Doctors SHUT It Down") —he talked about the protocol he and his staff used to detox from heavy metals every 6 months, using sodium alginate (a brown seaweed extract), also that he personally used coffee enemas daily (which were used by conventional medicine through the 1960s and described in the Merck Manual through the 1970s). He shares a funny story about a doctor stating at a meeting that coffee enemas were "unnatural." He responded that living in a toxic world was unnatural too.

Based on what I've learned over the last year, I now believe we all need to pay more attention to what we're consuming while at the same time finding ways to regularly detox.

Thank you for sharing your story, and that of your friends and family. I wish you continued good health.

A #15b: Thanks for your kind wishes and best wishes to you and yours. A parting thought: Is it better (1) having to detox every 6 months, or (2) changing your diet to minimize heavy metal (and cadmium, specifically) consumption? I chose the latter. Take care.

Q #15c: Arturo, to clarify, like you, Dr. Gonzalez and his staff also did everything they could to remove POPs [persistent organic pollutants] and heavy metals from their diet. For example, Dr. Gonzalez didn't eat chocolate, which is considered a health food, I assume because he know it's often contaminated with varying levels of cadmium and lead.

Interestingly, the foods I have an inflammatory reaction to are coffee and chocolate, so I've had to remove both from my diet. I've been gluten free for five years, and last year removed all grains from my diet. I now believe glyphosate is damaging our health.

I have more questions.

You wrote: "I started doing Internet research on this topic about 10 years ago, since I was experiencing severe bone pain at that time. I saw my bone pain starting to go away after about two weeks by changing my diet and taking zinc supplements (phosphate free). I kept reading and added other supplements to compensate for things that I had eliminated from my diet (e.g., magnesium), to help chelate and remove cadmium from my body (e.g., vitamins A, B_1, C), and to help open blood vessels to flush the toxins out (vitamin B3—niacin)."

Q: How specifically did you change your diet? (What did you stop eating? What did you start eating?)

Q: Do you take other supplements in addition to zinc supplements (phosphate free), magnesium, vitamins A, B_1, B_3 (niacin), and C?

Your experience is of great interest to me.

A big question these last 15 months, since I was re-diagnosed with type 2 diabetes, following my initial diagnosis 10 years earlier, is WHY do I still have fasting and 2-hour posgt meal blood glucose levels in the pre-diabetes range—(though my A1c of 5.4% is in the non-diabetic range) —if I'm eating all the right foods, have eliminated the foods that cause inflammation in my body, am walking daily, and am additionally taking high quality, whole food supplements?

It's got to be due to POPs (persistant organic pollutants) and heavy metals, so that's becoming my new focus. My understanding is that heavy metals are contained by the body in our fat cells, so when I begin losing weight again, it will be important to move them out of the body quickly.

Something interesting has happened to me in the last couple of weeks. My blood glucose levels dropped an average of 20 mg/dL. Why?

At first I thought it was because of the Alpha Lipoic Acid I'd been taking 200 mg in the morning, but recently added an additional evening dose of 200 mg in the evening for a total of 400 mg daily.

This improvement continued for two weeks, then stopped, so I began asking what had changed?

I was still taking the ALA but I realized I'd run out of my whole foods, B-complex that included probiotics and enzymes that I had begun taking for the first time a month earlier.

So I stopped taking the whole foods B-complex I've been taking for the last year, and restarted the new B-complex. Blood glucose levels dropped again to their previous low levels. (I haven't had blood glucose levels in the '80s since I was initially diagnosed with diabetes 11 or 12 years ago; I don't and have never taken diabetes medications or insulin.)

In addition to all 8 B vitamins, the new B-complex contains lipase, protease, aspergillopepsin, beta-glucanase, bromelain, phytase, lactase, papain, peptidase, pectinase, xylanase, hemicellulase, [lactobacillus bulgaricus, lactobacillus plantarum] (500 million CFU), saccharomyces ceraviciae; organic apple (fruit), beet (root), broccoli (stalk and flower), carrot (root), spinach (leaf), tomato (fruit), strawberry (fruit), tart cherry (fruit), blackberry (fruit), green bell pepper (fruit), brussels sprout (leaf), blueberry (fruit), ginger (root), garlic (bulb), green onion (bulb), raspberry (fruit), parsley (leaf), cauliflower (flower and stem), red cabbage (leaf), kale (leaf), cucumber (gourd), celery (stalk), asparagus (flower and stem) [All are listed as organic] Don't know which ingredient caused the change: the enzymes? the probiotics? the whole food co-factors? a combination with or without the ALA? I eat many of these foods, a few every day.

Are some of these ingredients binding with POPs or heavy metals? Are some of the food sourced co-factors providing something I've been missing nutritionally?

I eat an organic, whole foods diet, primarily fresh vegetables, frozen berries, butter from grass-fed cows, extra virgin olive oil, a variety of vinegars, unrefined, virgin coconut oil, eggs and meat from free-range chickens, beef from grass fed steers, leafy greens, avocado, olives, nuts, black and green tea, red wine, and fresh lemon juice with stevia and water. No sugar, no grains, no omega-6 vegetable oils, limited dairy.

I have no answers yet. My plan is to continue taking with my regular supplements the ALA and B-complex for a week or two, then the ALA without the B-complex for a week or two, then the B-complex without the ALA for a week or two to see how my blood glucose numbers trend.

I also take a whole foods multi-vitamin and mineral supplement (which includes 2,000 IU vitamin D3 as well as 100% of the RDA for iodine, zinc, selenium, copper, manganese, chromium (GTF), and molybdenum), cod liver oil, B-complex (listed above), vitamin C, fish oil, curcumin phytosome, magnesium citrate, alpha lipoic acid (listed above), and CoQ10.

Apologies for the lengthy, detailed post. It's a bit much, I know. I'm very interested in understanding how specifically you healed your body. I greatly appreciate the time you've taken to share what you've learned and to warn us.

I facilitate a local diabetes group for those interested in using diet, supplements, and walking to restore their health.

A #15c: Hi there,

I would be interested in knowing what you think of my approach, and if you and/or members of your group decide to follow this approach, I would be very interested in knowing what it's impact is. Going through your message I have the following comments:

1) Coffee and chocolate are both high in cadmium. Chocolate is also high in lead.

2) Wheat gluten has the highest cadmium content of any wheat product, so going gluten-free is a major step forward.

3) Glyphosate is a carcinogen, and it was originally developed as a boiler scale remover. Therefore, it should come as no surprise that in the human body, it mobilizes cadmium. Unfortunately, that mobilized cadmium winds up getting stuck in the kidneys, resulting in kidney failure. That is why thousands of agricultural workers in Latin America are dying if kidney failure each year! Glyphosate is now being used, not only to control unwanted weeds, but also to dry crops prior to harvest (i.e., used as a desiccant).

4) I changed my diet by eliminating everything that I could identify as having a high cadmium content. As I stated in my original comment to Dr. X, "High cadmium foods and beverages include wheat and rice products, chocolate, coffee, soft drinks, mushrooms, any product containing organ meats (e.g., sausages and frankfurters), shellfish (e.g., shrimp and

oysters), beets, lettuce, spinach and MANY processed foods . . . If you see 'phosphate,' it is likely contaminated with cadmium. They are adding phosphates to many foods these days (e.g., bacon, deli meats, cereals, evaporated milk, pudding, and even vitamin supplements). The key is to go 'LOW CADMIUM,' and eliminating sugar from our diets will help tremendously (a GREAT FIRST STEP), but so will eliminating wheat, organ meats, shellfish, and processed foods containing phosphate additives." Also, my general rule-of-thumb is that if it grows on the ground or in the ground, it is likely high in cadmium, while if it grows on a tree, tall stalk, or long vine, it is likely low in cadmium. I now eat more things like beans, broccoli, avocados, corn, eggs, various kinds of squash, cashews and pecans (no peanuts), and I choose low cadmium alternatives (e.g., I make pancakes using oat and/or corn flour, eat quinoa or corn pasta, choose corn tortillas over flour tortillas) whenever possible.

5) Yes, I take other phosphate-free supplements, and they are all related to my efforts to remove cadmium from my body. My list of includes numerous Vitamins (A, B Complex, B_1, B_3, B_6, B_{12}, C, D_3, E), zinc, magnesium, copper, selenium, and iodine. Some of these chelate cadmium and aid in its removal (e.g., vitamins A, B_1, C), some replace things I no longer get enough of in my diet (e.g., magnesium [found in chlorophyll]), some help flush toxins (including cadmium) from our bodies (e.g., vitamin B_3—niacin), and some to replenish other elements that are being removed due to supplements being taken (e.g., copper). Taking greater quantities of zinc stimulates the synthesis of proteins called "metallothioneins." These proteins chelate heavy metals in the following preferential order: copper, cadmium, zinc. Therefore, long-term zinc supplementation also removes copper from the body.

6) You may still be diagnosed as "diabetic" because you may not be reducing cadmium consumption sufficiently (i.e., your diet and supplements may not be as good as you think), and you may not be flushing it from your system very fast. I used to eat lots of

green salads, with lots of lettuce, spinach, and mushrooms (all high in cadmium). The zinc supplement that I began with had phosphate fillers. You have to stay clear of high-cadmium foods and beverages, and examine labels carefully to make sure the products you ingest do not contain phosphate additives. These additives can be accompanied by small amounts of cadmium, and because cadmium has a 30-year biological half-life, a little goes a long way. As I mentioned previously, I take 200 mg of zinc per day to push some of the cadmium out. The 15 mg/day RDA for zinc is totally inadequate. Niacin helps flush it out, but most of the cadmium leaving the body is through the digestive tract. That's why I drink lots of water and try to eat five pieces of fruit every day. BTW, just because something is labeled "organic" does not mean it is low in heavy metals, since sewage sludge is an accepted organic fertilizer (loaded with cadmium).

7) Cadmium competes with zinc, and zinc is in every cell in your body, so cadmium eventually goes everywhere, not just adipose tissue. However, it accumulates primarily in the liver, pancreas, lungs, bones, and kidneys, and to a lesser extent in the thyroid, prostate, adrenal glands, and other vital organs.

8) Beets, sometimes included in supplements, pet foods, etc., are very efficient at extracting cadmium from the ground, so much so that they are used in the phytoremediation of cadmium-contaminated soils. Also, 56% of the US sugar production is from sugar beets, so that sugar is loaded with cadmium.

9) Whenever you know you will have increased cadmium exposure in a meal, take extra zinc. The rate of cadmium assimilation decreases when high concentrations of zinc are present. That is why whole wheat bread is better for you than bread made of bleached flour, and brown rice is better for you than white rice. The cadmium is concentrated within the grains, while zinc is concentrated in the brown, outside portion.

10) For many nutrients (e.g., zinc, iodine), the RDA is an inaccurate indicator of our daily requirements. Things change in our

environment, and our requirements change accordingly. For example, cadmium in the bones of modern-day humans is 50 times higher than in the skeletal remains of ancient Native Americans. And the greatest part of that increase is since the end of WWII, which coincides with the widespread use of phosphate fertilizers. Cadmium is in our food chain, and zinc has major competition occurring within our bodies. Similarly, the RDA for iodine was set to address the widespread incidence of goiter in the Great Lakes area where soil iodine concentrations are low. However, today iodine competes with other halides, which include chlorine, fluorine, and bromine. These competitors are in much higher concentrations in our diets today, causing over 95% of the US public to be iodine deficient.

Well, that's it for now. I am looking forward to hearing from you again.
Q #15d: Arturo, I've copied and pasted our conversation into a file to share with our diabetes group's members. I introduced them to the problem of POPs (Persistent Organic Pollutants) and heavy metals a month ago. This will further reinforce and add to what we've already learned.

My concern is not just diabetes, cancer is a concern too. Since I last wrote you, I did some research online and learned that its the digestive enzymes in the new B-complex supplement I'm taking that is coming very close to normalizing my blood glucose levels, something I didn't think possible when I began this journey 15 months ago.

But I'm not going to stop there. Next step is to get the POPs and heavy metals out of my body. I'm in my mid-50's now, so this will be my focus for the next couple of years. Following that, I'll continue to limit foods that contain POPs, cadmium, and other heavy metals.

I eat organic, whole foods only, an important first step. And I've already eliminated most of the foods you've listed from my diet. Checked my supplements tonight. None have phosphate listed. Will add a zinc supplement now.

I've also noted your email address, and would very much like to revisit our conversation from time to time. You've done an amazing amount of research, and more importantly, you've put into practice what you've learned.

When Joseph Pizzorno's book, *The Toxic Cure*, comes out next January, I'll begin educating the larger diabetes community about this problem. I do understand now that organic foods can be contaminated with heavy metals too - (perhaps it's time to start a garden). Thank you.

For me, story is powerful. It saddens me to learn that by eating foods contaminated with heavy metals, farm workers are dying, not just us. What you've written is potentially life changing. I wish you continued good health Arturo.

A #15d: Again, thank you for your kind wishes, and I wish you the best, as well. I am fairly certain that the zinc will help in many areas, including building a strong immune system that will ward off cancer. Vitamin C and iodine are also very important in that regard. Final thought: Remember that it's not just what supplements you are taking, but also the quantities. If things are out of kilter, the RDAs are not applicable, and in many cases, RDAs don't apply because of changes in our environment. I consider my zinc dosage to be a "therapeutic" dosage rather than a "maintenance" dosage. Best of luck, and keep me posted.

COMMENT #16

Thank you, Dr. X, especially for the discussion on heavy metals and the link between heavy metal poisoning and schizophrenia, bipolar disorder, and other mental health issues. Your discussion of lead, mercury, and arsenic was informative, as was your treatment of chelating agents used to remove them from the body. I think, however, that including a detailed discussion on the cadmium, its toxicity, its occurrence in our environment, and its relationship to diabetes and mental health would have been appropriate. Cadmium is a carcinogenic, heavy-metal contaminant in phosphate fertilizers used in crop production, and therefore, it is in our food chain. It is off the radar screens of the FDA and the medical profession, probably because it is generally found in "low" concentrations in the food products we eat.

However, it has a biological half-live of 30 years, compared to that of zinc, which is approximately 78 days, so that I still have cadmium in my body from the first chocolate Easter egg I ate as a toddler, and I am more than two cadmium half-lives old. I compare it to zinc because on the periodic table, it appears directly beneath zinc and directly above mercury. These metals have similar chemical characteristics, and therefore, they compete with each other within our bodies. The difference is that zinc is essential for a healthy immune system, essential for healing, essential for proper brain function, involved in 300 enzymatic reactions, and present in ever strand of DNA in the body, while cadmium and mercury (and lead) have no business in our bodies. They simply accumulate, disrupt organ functions, and cause disease. In the case of cadmium, it accumulates primarily in the pancreas, kidneys, liver, lungs, and bones, and to a lesser degree in the thyroid, prostate, adrenals, and other vital organs. It accumulates without being noticed until it reaches organ-specific, function-disrupting concentrations (e.g., accumulation in the beta cells of the pancreas and Type 2 diabetes). Cadmium contributes to violent behavior and many mental illnesses.

In my opinion, the cadmium problem is at least as important, if not more important than the lead and mercury problems combined, because everyone is being exposed, unknowingly, and the amount of cadmium that is introduced and then recirculated in our environment has been on the rise since about the time of World War II. It is no coincidence that the rates of diabetes and various forms of cancer have increased to pandemic proportions since that time. You mentioned that diet was very important in treating heavy-metal induced mental illness. Avoiding high-cadmium foods and beverages (e.g., sugar, chocolate, mushrooms, shellfish [e.g., shrimp and oysters], beets, coffee, soft drinks, products made from organ meats, wheat products, rice products, and processed foods containing phosphates [e.g., bacon and most deli meats, puddings, evaporated milk]) has become essential for maintaining health. As with lead and mercury, cadmium does not stay in the bloodstream for very long, and when asked to analyze a blood sample for cadmium, inexperienced labs will test for concentrations in the parts per million range, when concentrations in the parts per billion could be indicative of cadmium poisoning issues. I particularly liked your closing statement that each of us needs to take responsibility for and control of his/her own health! Again, thank you for emphasizing the harmful role that heavy metals play in our environment and our health.

Printed in the United States
By Bookmasters